PETERSON'S

W9-BMA-122

THE INSIDER'S GUIDE TO
Medical Schools

**Current Students Tell You What
Their Medical School is Really Like**

*Edited by Ivan Oransky, M.D.; Eric J. Poulsen, M.D.;
Darshak M. Sanghavi, M.D.; and Jay K. Varma, M.D.*

PETERSON'S
Princeton, New Jersey

About Peterson's

Peterson's is the country's largest educational information/communications company, providing the academic, consumer, and professional communities with books, software, and online services in support of lifelong education access and career choice. Well-known references include Peterson's annual guides to private schools, summer programs, colleges and universities, graduate and professional programs, financial aid, international study, adult learning, and career guidance. Peterson's Web site at petersons.com is the only comprehensive—and most heavily traveled—education resource on the Internet. The site carries all of Peterson's fully searchable major databases and includes financial aid sources, test-prep help, job postings, direct inquiry and application features, and specially created Virtual Campuses for every accredited academic institution and summer program in the U.S. and Canada that offers in-depth narratives, announcements, and multimedia features.

Visit Peterson's Education Center on the Internet (World Wide Web) at www.petersons.com

Editorial inquiries concerning this book should be addressed to the editor at: Peterson's, P.O. Box 2123, Princeton, New Jersey 08543-2123.

Library of Congress Cataloging-in-Publication Data

Peterson's the insider's guide to medical schools, 1999 : medical students tell you what you really want to know / Jay K. Varma ... [et al.].
     p.   cm.
  Includes index.
  ISBN 0-7689-0203-7 (paperback)
  1. Medical colleges—North America Directories. I. Varma, Jay K., 1971– . II. Title: Insider's guide to medical schools, 1999.
  [DNLM: 1. Schools, Medical—United States Directory. 2. School Admission Criteria—United States.
W 19 P485 1999] R743.P48 1999
610'.71'173—DC21
DNLM/DLC
for Library of Congress   99-23444
                                                   CIP

Printed in Canada

10   9   8   7   6   5   4   3   2   1

CONTENTS

ABOUT
University Wire

What Are U-Wire Student-To-Student Guides?

University Wire (U-WIRE) is a free wire service for college newspapers that connects all college media to each other and to the world. Membership consists of more than 450 campus newspapers.

U-WIRE shares Peterson's respect for information to provide students with the tools they need to make solid choices about their education and their future. Peterson's student-to-student guides mark a dramatic innovation in communicating the thoughts and voices of students to other students. In recognition of this parallel approach to providing information, U-WIRE has agreed to lend its name to Peterson's student-to-student guides.

How Was the Insider's Guide to Medical Schools Compiled?

There is nothing wrong with official information. If gathered and published by a reliable publisher, it will touch all of the important bases and be dependable and accurate, worthy to form the base for a decision. However, if you ask students what their schools are like, what they say will not be at all similar to the official guidebooks and usually it will be a lot more interesting.

Four physicians and recent medical school graduates, all former editors of *Pulse* (the medical student section of the *Journal of the American Medical Association*), decided to make use of their national network of medical school student-writer contacts to put together a new kind of college guide, one that really tells you what it is like at a particular medical school. As far as we know, this is the first systematically organized guide to medical schools written by students for students.

Our goal was to cover all the accredited allopathic medical colleges in the fifty United States and the District of Columbia and as many of the accredited osteopathic colleges as we were able to. We have profiles of 122 accredited colleges of allopathic medicine in the United States and D.C. and sixteen accredited schools of osteopathic medicine. We did not extend our scope to Puerto Rican schools or to schools outside of the United States. We were not able to secure articles from students at two osteopathic colleges: West Virginia School of Osteopathic Medicine and University of Health Sciences College in Kansas City. Profiles for the medical colleges at the University of Cincinnati, University of Hawaii, University of Indiana, University of Massachusetts, and University of Texas at Galveston were composed by a professional writer from publicly available information. The remaining 129 profiles were written either by current upperclass students or recent graduates of the institution described. Names of these authors and their articles appear beginning on page 330.

The authors were asked to describe, as only a student could, their school's overall image, admissions and financial aid characteristics, preclinical and clinical curriculum, school-based social life, living arrangements, locale, and student body, and provide a brief bottom-line summation. Length of the sections, emphasis, style, and focus were then left to each writer to shape. Articles vary from school to school in these details as well as the overall tone and reflect both the nature of the college and the individual writing the piece. The data immediately following the head of each profile, which represent the number of applications, size of the entering class, numbers and percentages of women and men students, Web site address, and information/admissions contact name, address, and telephone number, were gathered during spring and summer 1998 through Peterson's Annual Survey of Graduate Institutions, supplemented by data from Peterson's annual survey of accredited medical colleges. This data comes from the institutions.

Except for the above-cited data, the information within each profile represents the opinions and views of each author and not necessarily those of Peterson's. In most cases, officials of the institution did not review or approve the content of the article that describes their institution. Peterson's did not verify and cannot vouch for the accuracy of information contained within these profiles.

WHAT TO
Look for in a Medical School

by Jay K. Varma, M.D.

Medical education continues to fascinate researchers, clinicians, and the popular press—how physicians are trained, many believe, directly impacts how they care for patients. Since the standardization of medical curriculums in the early twentieth century, there have been numerous attempts to update medical education to meet public health goals and the evolving images of the physician in society. Educators in the 1960s expanded basic science training, hoping to create physicians who were also scientists. The 1980s brought great praise for Harvard's New Pathway program, which sought to train physicians to be better clinicians, both more humanistic and more analytical. Finally, the 1990s have seen a shift from hospital-based to office-based education, emphasizing the real world of medicine and the need for more primary-care physicians.

A very reasonable argument can be made that the revolutions in medicine are a lot of bunk. True, there have been marked changes in the science and organization of health care. However, compared to forty years ago, the physicians of today are probably just as (un)humanistic, (un)scientific, and (im)practical as they have ever been. The medical profession, you will soon learn, is a trade, and like masonry and carpentry, the practice may change, but the principles are still the same.

If you understand that medicine is more of a trade than it is an art, then you can also understand why the principles medical education has not changed that much, and, more important, why U.S. medical schools are not that much different from each other. Ask any practicing physician and he or she will be hard-pressed to tell you whether fellow colleagues went to Harvard or East Tennessee State—even more important, he or she does not care and nor do his or her patients. So why, you may ask yourself, did I even buy this book? Why should I care where I attend school?

As an applicant, you should not wonder whether you will be a good doctor if you go to a top-ten school or be a bad doctor if you go to a bottom-ten school. The most important question you should ask yourself is: Is this school going to help me get where I want to go and become who I want to become? There are several factors that affect this decision, and you must evaluate each one of them to decide what you want and, based on your credentials, what you can have: prestige, location, curriculum, clinical training, support services, residency matching, research emphasis, degree programs, and tuition.

Prestige

U.S. News & World Report makes an enormous amount of money every year with its pseudoscientific assessment of what makes a medical school good and, conversely, bad. Curiously, this list of medical *schools* doesn't exactly correlate with its ranking of the best *hospitals*. Why is Iowa ranked by *U.S. News & World Report* as one of the top-ten medical centers but *not* one of the top-ten medical schools? Or, alternatively, Yale one of the top-ten schools but not one of the top-ten centers? This discrepancy should concern you since a school's clinical facilities have as much impact on your education as do its researchers. Who you meet in the hospital (i.e., your professional mentors) often do more to shape your career than an institution's Nobel laureates do.

It is important to use these rankings the way most colleges use SAT scores: to group schools into one of three categories (somewhere near the top, somewhere in the middle, and somewhere at the bottom). A higher ranked school will, in general, assure you of the following: students that have lofty professional aspirations, physician-mentors with lots of research money and contacts at other major medical centers, and better match statistics. Top schools tend to inbreed a lot—and thereby bolster each other's reputations, particularly on the East Coast. Prestige does not, however, guarantee some other important characteristics, such as the humanistic quality of students and physicians, opportunities for social outreach, and quality and quantity of clinical training. For example, the clinical judgment and procedural skills of some of my colleagues from the University of Southern California (a hands-on, understaffed medical center), for example, vastly exceeds that of some of my colleagues from top-five medical

schools (centers that are routinely overstaffed with doctors).

Location

Where a school is located greatly affects your life both inside and outside of school. Attending school in a large city may mean high patient volume and more procedures but may give you a more cynical view of health care and may leave less time for teaching. Similarly, it may mean more opportunities for social outreach (public education initiatives, free clinics), but less opportunity for escaping to more quiet surroundings. Remember that this is going to be your home for four years—and often more—so keep your long-term goals in mind.

Curriculum

This is probably the least variable element between schools. Virtually all schools separate education into preclinical and clinical years, and almost all schools have recently attempted to blur this distinction as much as possible. Medical education critics argued in the 1990s that patient exposure should begin as soon as possible, that the traditional basic science years do not prepare students adequately for clinical medicine, and that case-based learning is superior to lecture-based learning. Most schools have changed their curriculums to respond to these critics. Whether or not a school is making these changes, though, is less important in content than it is in style. A school that updates its curriculum is probably more progressive and

> **"A school that updates its curriculum is probably more progressive and more welcome to student input than one that is slow to make innovations."**

more welcome to student input than one that is slow to make innovations.

A more important aspect of the curriculum is grading. There is no doubt that pass/fail systems are vastly more student-friendly than letter grading systems—medical school is far more enjoyable and equally educational when it fosters cooperation rather than competition.

Clinical Training

Most applicants do not focus much on clinical training because they have little idea what it involves. In general, applicants should demand an institution that has more than one teaching facility, including preferably a Veterans Administration (VA) hospital (an excellent place to learn by doing); that encourages training in outpatient settings and outside hospitals; that has high patient volume, particularly in fields you might be interested (obstetrics, for example); and that gives students ample time for electives. Ask about the number of requirements there are beyond the standard core clerkships (medicine, surgery, psychiatry, ob/gyn, pediatrics) and whether or not students feel they have enough time to make a decision about their future careers.

Student Services

No matter how large an institution is, it may not offer medical students all the things that make student life more livable. There should be a note-taking service that is dependable (Do students prepare for exams with textbooks, syllabi, or notes?). Counselors should be available to students who are experiencing academic or personal problems (How many students have dropped out in the past year? Did they rejoin the class? How many students have committed suicide in the past five years?). Extracurricular activities should be abundant and a regular part of student life; no matter how difficult classes are, a vibrant extracurricular life speaks to a happy student body (Is there a student-run clinic, a student-run newspaper, or student-run drama production?).

> "Unlike applications for college or medical school, being the big fish in a small pond usually ensures a top match, no matter how small the pond."

Residency Match

Still a mystery to many who've been through it, the residency match is the process whereby medical students pick the hospital where they will gain their specialty training. This training will likely have a far greater impact on your education and career than your choice of a medical school. When you apply for residency, hospitals consider the reputation of your medical school, but how much this is factored in is highly variable. It is safe to say that graduates of the top five to ten schools have a distinct advantage, but, after that, it usually does not matter where you attend school. Unlike applications for college or medical school, being the big fish in a small pond usually ensures a top match, no matter how small the pond.

Primary Care

Though many students express an interest in primary care when applying, particularly now that admissions committees are looking for applicants to say this, few really understand the advantages and disadvantages of such a career until they get a chance to work in this setting. Nevertheless, if you are considering a career in family medicine, make sure your institution offers ample encouragement of such a career. Some top medical schools do not even have a formal family medicine department or clerkship experience. Ask about the percentage of students who pursue family medicine (not just primary care, which often deceptively includes ob/gyn), how politically powerful the family medicine department is, whether or not the hospital has a family medicine service (a sign of how busy and respected the department is), and what rural or inner-city (i.e., non-University–based) clinical opportunities exist.

Combined-Degree Programs

It is beyond the scope of this book to discuss all the variations on a medical school career, but suffice it to say, the opportunities are boundless. The most common advanced degree is the M.D.-Ph.D., usually pursued via the National Institutes of Health–funded Medical Scientist Training Program (MSTP). If you are considering this, remember that it is a big time commitment, a Ph.D. is not required to perform university-based research, and a number of students prematurely drop out of the program. Nevertheless, it is a powerful and prestigious degree and quite useful if you are already dedicated to a career in academic medicine. One important consideration is whether or not your program allows you to do clinical clerkships before you begin your Ph.D. studies: this is a valuable chance to expand on your research interests and to decide if you really want to work in the lab.

Other possible degree programs include Master's in Public Health (an excellent time to

pursue this is between third and fourth years), JD (for those interested in malpractice or intellectual property law), and M.B.A. (for those interested in health-care policy and economics). Ask to talk to recent graduates if you are weighing one of these options.

Tuition/Financial Aid

An unfortunate trend in the past ten years has been the increase in medical school tuition, the decrease in physician salaries, and the rescinding of unlimited residency deferments for most government loans. The net result? Most medical students graduate with a lot of debt and not a lot of money to pay it back. Since many of you will begin your family lives while in medical school or residency, the debt you incur now, though seemingly manageable, may severely limit your choice of career and location in the future. Strongly consider applying to your state's medical school, applying for scholarships even if they seem long shots, and asking each school for the average student debt.

You have a difficult decision ahead, but, believe it or not, this decision is not nearly as important as you think it is. Few people ever truly regret having gone to their medical school. What they regret more is not having the right perspective and guidance when they applied. Your goal in picking a school should be to find the best combination of prestige, location, clinical training, and cost. Keep in mind that you will have a life outside of medical school, that you do not want to limit your future by financial decisions you make now, and, most important, that everyone who graduates, even if last in the class, is a still a doctor.

HOW TO
Gain Admission to Medical School

by Ivan Oransky, M.D.

Despite declining salaries, real and proposed cutbacks in residency positions, and decreased autonomy for physicians, near-record numbers of applicants are vying for admission to medical school. It is up to the sociologists (and perhaps the psychiatrists among us) to determine why. Here are the facts: last year, according to the Association of American Medical Colleges, 41,004 people submitted 481,336 applications for 16,170 first-year U.S. medical school positions. That represents a nearly 5 percent drop from 1997 and a nearly 13 percent drop from 1996, when applicants reached a recent peak. It still indicates, however, that there are more than 2½ applicants for every first-year position.

Getting into medical school, then, remains one of the most significant challenges in professional education. It is a process that some embark on at birth, others carefully map out during college, and still others wake up at age 40 hoping to complete. Many are motivated by a desire to ease the pain and suffering of others. Some are motivated by financial concerns, some are motivated by their parents, and others may wish for a calling more

> **"Most Ph.D.'s at your college or M.D.'s at your affiliated university welcome college student research assistants who are either working on their theses or just doing independent study."**

socially redeemable than the corporate ladder. Similarly, there are those for whom medical school admission is the ultimate personal (or familial) accomplishment, and others for whom the same goal is a cakewalk.

If you belong to the latter category, you are probably Phi Beta Kappa at Harvard, have published three papers in *Science* during college, have scored a perfect 45 on the MCAT, and have single-handedly immunized all the children of the Indian subcontinent against cholera. If that's you, stop reading this, and go collect the dozens of acceptance letters waiting in your mailbox.

The rest of you should realize that, despite overwhelming odds, it is still possible to win the game. Chaos theory might offer something to those who really want to understand medical school admissions, but it is not unlike the situation at this country's elite universities: it is a crapshoot, but there are some rules and some ways to load the dice in your favor. For the most part, admission to medical school remains based on the triad (this is a word you will become used to hearing often to describe clinical phenomena; e.g., Virchow's triad) of GPA, MCAT scores, and research experience. A fault in any of these three may keep you out of Harvard and Hopkins, but stellar performances in two out of three will grant you acceptance at one or more medical schools. There are schools that are breaking away from this formula—a positive development, which should result in more humane doctors—but for now, rely on the triad. A cautionary note: the following advice doesn't condone today's med school admissions criteria. It should, however, help you get in. At the same time, keep in mind that chaos theory might have something to offer anyone who wants to really understand medical school admissions.

GPA

This one sounds obvious, but there are subtleties beyond studying hard or being naturally brilliant. The first choice is whether to choose a premed (or biology, chemistry, biochemistry, or other) major and excel in every course or to choose another area of interest that may not be as taxing and will allow you to perform at the top of your few premed classes. If you enjoy the hard sciences and can do well in them, the choice is obvious. If you want maximum time to study for those few premed classes, which consist of a year of biology, a year of inorganic chemistry, a year of organic chemistry, a year of physics, a year of math, and, usually, a year of English, then study what your heart desires. Medical school admissions committees generally break the GPA into science and nonscience GPA; if both are good, it doesn't much matter that most of your classes were in the latter category, whereas if your major is science and you do badly in it, you will have no quality grades. There are no magic numbers, although many schools routinely disregard applicants whose GPAs are below a certain figure. If your science or overall GPA is below a 3.0, try to do something—take a fifth year of college, a master's degree, or a postbaccalaureate course—to raise it.

A third option chosen by an increasing number of students is to study whatever you want to in college and worry about premed classes later. Many universities now offer this postbaccalaureate program, which allows you to focus solely on premed classes but essentially extends college by a year or two. Graduates tend to do well in medical school admissions.

The MCAT

This one is fairly straightforward. The average score of admitted students has been rising; it is now above 30 (out of 45 total) at most schools. The test is worth studying for, and the best way to prepare is to obtain as many old exam questions (many of them are out of print) as possible. Many schools and private testing companies also offers courses, which can be expensive and of questionable utility if you aren't provided with many, many practice questions. Since the only useful thing many courses offer is their published material, see if you can borrow these from a friend who has already taken the exam. It is definitely possible and even OK to take the exam more than once if you do not do well the first time. Again, there are no magic numbers, but the same basic rules apply as for GPA. For a score below 30, take the exam over if you think you can improve.

Research Experience

The jury is out on whether or not this makes you a better doctor or even a better medical student. In either case, it makes you a better medical school applicant. The research doesn't have to be wet lab (i.e., basic science) or clinical or even clinical epidemiology; it might be on plant physiology or sociology. Most Ph.D.'s at your college or M.D.'s at your affiliated university welcome college student research assistants who are either working on their theses or just doing independent study. Many foundations, such as the Arthritis Foundation, Lupus Foundation, and Pediatric AIDS Foundation, offer stipends.

Such experiences offer a few advantages. You can become close with a faculty mentor who can write a great recommendation letter. You can learn something about a given field (although chances are the itsy-bitsy part of it you study won't be of much use in clinical medicine). You can publish papers and abstracts—a huge advantage when applying. Finally, you will have something to talk about if your interviews go stale.

Candy Striping

Many applicants opt to roam hospital corridors long before medical school as volunteers, performing more specific clinical tasks. Although it is not required, candy striping is a good idea for a few reasons. First, you will get a glimpse into whether or not you like medicine. Second, admissions committees like it, and you may have experiences that you can discuss in an interview. Best of all, you may actually do some good for some patients.

The Process

Now that you have finished your premed requirements, taken the MCAT, and taken care of business in the lab, if that's your cup of tea, it is time to sit and prepare your applications. The first rule is to get everything in early. Most deadlines are rolling, but a safe bet is to have everything— the application, letters of recommendation—in by September 1, one year before you want to begin medical school. Do not procrastinate here. The process is fraught with too much stress to allow deadlines to create more. Get to know your premed adviser early, too.

For those of you who haven't already researched this, applications fall into two categories: American Medical College Admissions Service (AMCAS; 113 of 125 schools) and non-AMCAS. AMCAS applications (available at http://www.aamc.org) are usually due earlier. Contact information for individual schools is available in this book.

> **"As a result of real or perceived threats of lawsuits, nearly all letters end up saying positive things; it is the key words that matter."**

Letters of Recommendation

Again, start early. Most college advisers will only quote from or send good or glowing letters, so better to have extra time to ask for additional letters should one come in that is not so great. Request letters from faculty members with whom you have had the chance to get to know, whether or not they have given you A's. It is more important that you develop as a person in the letter. If you have done research, certainly request a letter from a research adviser. Also, if you have held an interesting job during or after college, request a letter from that person, too. Three letters is usually a minimum, and five is OK, but any more than that is not encouraged. As a result of real or perceived threats of lawsuits, nearly all letters end up saying positive things; it is the key words that matter. Try to look your letters over, if possible.

Where to Apply

Generally, students apply to anywhere from a dozen to three dozen schools, although confident students apply to fewer, and nervous students (that's the majority here) apply to as many as forty or fifty. Since a scatter-shot approach can become expensive, here are a few tips on narrowing your list. First, apply in your home state. If that means changing addresses for a home-court advantage, so be it. Most state schools, and even some private ones that receive significant funding from their states, cut residents a break. Second, be realistic. Do you really have a shot at Hopkins, Harvard, or UCSF? Also, make sure you consider osteopathic schools, especially if a more primary-care/humanist approach appeals to you. Many of their graduates end up in the same residency programs as allopathic graduates. Finally, keep in mind that you will be living wherever your med school is for at least four years, since many students stay in the same place or city for residency. Do you or you and your family really want to move to Kansas from New York? Can you afford a private school, given your already overwhelming college debt? You will graduate a doctor from any of these schools.

The Essay

For many applicants, this is the most painful of the hoops they are forced to jump through during this process. In a nutshell, be original, but not too original. Keep in mind how many thousands of essays admissions committee members must read. If possible, choose a topic you truly care about, whether or not it has to do with medicine. You will sound more genuine and human that way. Do not reiterate your resume, although creating interest in one or two key areas of your resume by mentioning particular experiences may help. Finally, have your resume read by someone whose editorial judgment you trust. Do not be ashamed to have several people critique your essay. If you are ashamed to show it to anyone, you should probably be ashamed to show it to an admissions committee.

The Interview

You have sent in the applications, run anxiously to the mailbox everyday, and been invited for several interviews. Some schools will offer to pay your travel expenses or put you up at a hotel for your interview. On the interview day, obviously, wear your best outfit. If schools let you know who will be interviewing you, find out their field of medicine or research. That may help you guess what types of questions they might ask. Be prepared to discuss your activities as well as your motivation for undertaking them. Why did you attend the college you did? Why medicine?

Overall, relax. Most schools interview about three to four times as many applicants as they accept, so your chances for acceptance are fairly good. The main purpose of the interview many say is to ensure that you have no obvious psychopathology (or that if you do, it is being properly treated). Your answers matter less than demonstrating that you have sound judgment and are a thoughtful person. Pretend your interviewer is wondering whether or not he or she would want this person caring for his or her grandmother. Finally, if the mood strikes you, write a thank-you letter. Try to be brief when writing the letter, but try to remember something you discussed in the interview. It is a nice touch, even if it may not help get you in.

With any luck, the end of this process will have you beaming with pride at medical school acceptance letters. If not, keep your chin up—many who re-apply are granted acceptance if their resumes, MCAT scores, and other credentials improve.

HOW TO
Survive Medical School

by Darshak Sanghavi, M.D.

"**I** want to help people," you've probably said to yourself or told some jaded interviewer on the road to medical school. Chances are you probably meant it. Make no bones about it—medical school is like any other rude transition from the social and intellectual coziness of college life into adulthood. You may or may not emerge with your dreams intact. Like salmon swimming upstream, some fantasies make it and some fatigue and wither. Before the first day of class, make a list of the reasons you want to be a doctor. Write them down. Be explicit. Keep the list handy, maybe on a small sheet of paper in your wallet or your purse or your jacket. Read about experiences of others, such as LeBaron's *Gentle Vengeance*, Klass's *A Not Entirely Benign Procedure*, and Rothman's *White Coat*, to name a few.

Medical school begins with the preclinical years, which are usually heavily lecture oriented and full of unfamiliar information. One can identify various personalities during the preclinical years. First are the model students, who conscientiously take detailed notes, attend all lectures, have a clear study schedule, and generally do well on exams. These individuals may lack an inborn gift for academic success but do well nonetheless. Somehow, these people are able to create a comfortable studying routine, but they do it at the

> "**Make no bones about it—medical school is like any other rude transition from the social and intellectual coziness of college life into adulthood.**"

expense of leading somewhat unexciting lives outside of school.

Next are the serious gunners, who predicate their worth on how well they compare to others. These are generally aggressive and often younger students who study to excess and often alienate their peers by their competitiveness. Their social lives are either mind-numbingly boring or convulsed by periodic sessions of release. These students occasionally achieve brilliant academic success, but they do it at the expense of learning few skills that are truly useful to healing. They are at high risk for burning out.

Then, there are the cool slackers. These are students who still believe that to be caught studying is tantamount to social suicide. For them, it's cool not to study (although they may secretly be doing so). These individuals usually tempt fate by not studying on the eves of major exams. While they lead somewhat swashbuckling lives compared to the model students, they fail to learn balance and discipline. These individuals invariably find the culture of medicine suffocating, and while they may pass medical school, they are often confused about what to do with the degree.

As in any field, one sees lost souls as well, people who chose medical school for lack of a better life plan. Pushed by domineering parents, jumping ship from a previous career, or seized by some existential crisis, these individuals are miserable because studying material uninteresting to them is destroying their souls. Lost souls usually feel out of touch with their feelings and are in serious denial. While they may escape from previous pressures for a time, they question their life plans daily. They are at high risk for social isolation, although they crave connection with others.

Finally, there are the truly gifted, who walk on water and emerge from the preclinical years unscathed. How do you know if your are one of these few? If you have to ask, you probably are not.

It is often difficult to figure out what type of student a person will be. In any event, it's key to think about your personal coping mechanisms and to be aware of them. Do you feel adequately supported? If not, why? Are you overaggressive, slipping into gunner mode? Are you out of control, like a cool slacker? Or is medicine not a good choice for your career, and are you a lost soul? Talk to your classmates for support. Most of all don't forget the dirty little secret about the preclinical years: almost everything you kill yourself memorizing is, frankly, useless for the actual practice of medicine. The advice I offer for these two years is to put them in perspective.

The clinical years, on the other hand, are critical. You'll learn real patient care. This is a good time to read Shem's *House of God* (take it with a grain of salt) and to start taking everything much more seriously. As you are acculturated into the role of doctor (a worldview that is slightly authoritarian, highly invested in scientific proof, and suspicious of any strong personal emotion), expand your exploration of the human side of medicine. Read, paint, talk to your nonmedical friends more frequently, and call your parents often. You'll appreciate their perspective.

The key lessons to take away from the clinical years are:

- It's not critical to know all the details; instead, know where to find the details.
- All people, including you and your patients, desire and require connection to your fellow humans.
- Know when you're in over your head, but don't underestimate your own abilities.
- Sleep is not a psychological construct; it is a physiological need.
- Learn how to read medical journals for useful content on a regular basis.
- Know how to use a small number of medicines and procedures well instead of knowing a lot of things superficially.
- Learn what you can and can't change about a patient's illness.
- Develop a thick skin for nonconstructive criticism.
- Remember that pain is simply pain, and nobody deserves it.
- Don't forget that common diseases are common, and uncommon presentations of common disease are more common than common presentations of uncommon diseases.
- Talk to your patients every day, and try to learn at least one nonmedical lesson from each one.

It is never too early to begin contemplating your future. Although it's not true that you need to enter medical school knowing what field you wish to enter, it's disingenuous to counsel students that you'll figure out what you want to do in your own time. Be proactive; speak to many practicing doctors (in and outside academia) early on, and envision yourself in their shoes. Be honest with yourself. For example, if you really hate dealing with stools, gastroenterology is probably not for you, despite what your preceptor thinks. The other reason to think early is for planning purposes. Getting involved in, say, a pediatric epidemiology project (if you're interested in pediatrics) makes you a much more attractive applicant to pediatrics programs than if you just worked out all summer after second year. In this way, you also come into contact with your medical school's departments, which are usually willing to mentor students who enjoy their fields. Obviously (as in anything else), don't go overboard. There's no need to wake up for Sunday morning surgery conference every week as a first-year student just to impress the department heads.

Thoreau counseled us to all "live deep and suck out all the marrow of life." That's hard when you're a sleep-deprived mess trying to study for USMLE Step I. Ultimately, medical school opens the way to a fascinating and profoundly rewarding profession. Just don't lose yourself en route.

THE WORLD
After Medical School

by Eric J. Poulsen, M.D.

Introduction

For most students, medical school is not an end in itself but a stepping-stone to a career. Medical school is also a nice way to delay having to find a real job. Few attend medical school simply for enrichment—it is simply too strenuous. Consequently, the medical school you choose needs to get you where you want to go. Yet when applying, most premedical student have no clear idea about the world after medical school (they are focused just on being accepted).

    The situation reminds me of Alice in Wonderland, when a wandering Alice meets up with the Cheshire Cat:

    " 'Would you tell me, please, which way I ought to walk from here?'

    'That depends a good deal on where you want to get to,' said the Cat.

    'I don't care where,' said Alice.

    'Then it doesn't matter which way you walk,' said the Cat."

    This article offers an overview of the world ahead to help premedical students gain a concept of what destinations lie ahead. Most medical students proceed from medical school directly to residency training and from there they enter clinical practice. A small number of medical school graduates forgo residency to pursue other careers. This chapter surveys, in general terms, the types of residencies, eventual practice scenarios, and nonclinical professional opportunities.

> **"More and more, M.D.'s are popping up in politics, even being elected to Congress."**

Residency Training

The first thing all prospective medical students should know is that the type of residency they complete is far more important in determining the complexion of their careers than the medical school they attend. So the medical school you choose now should lead you to the residency program you desire. Different schools tend to lead their students into certain types of residencies, both in terms of specialty and location.

    Let me begin by defining some terms. Residency refers to supervised training after one has graduated from medical school, which is analogous to an apprenticeship. Resident physicians are also known as house officers or house staff, the house referring to the hospital where they live. The fully trained physicians who supervise the residents are called attending physicians or attendings. The match refers to the process of landing a residency position. After medical students and residency programs have interviewed each other (it really should be a two-way experience), each party creates a list that ranks the programs they would like to attend (or applicants who the programs would like to attract) in order of preference. Each party then submits its list to a central processing agency that enters the lists into a computer. A complicated algorithm matches medical students to their highest choice that has an opening.

Internship refers to one's first year of clinical training after medical school. Some internships are simply the first year of a particular residency (e.g., internal medicine and pediatrics); other internships are independent one-year programs that prepare students for a separate residency that requires at least one year of post–medical school training before entry (e.g., dermatology and ophthalmology). Salaries for residencies vary from region to region but are typically disappointing for anyone just finishing eight or more years of rigorous college work. The first-year salary is currently $30,000–$35,000, and each subsequent year another couple thousand dollars is added. The length of residencies varies from three to six or more years, depending on the specialty.

Most states require at least one year of supervised training (i.e., an internship) in order to obtain a medical license. After that single year, a physician could legally secure a medical license and hang up a shingle as a general practitioner. It is very rare for a physician to do this today, however. Completion of a full residency is required for a physician to become eligible for board certification in a particular specialty such as internal medicine, general surgery, family practice, obstetrics/gynecology, and so on. Note that even family practice and general internal medicine are considered specialties.

Residencies can be categorized in a few ways. Usually, they are thought of in terms of specialty (e.g., internal medicine). A residency's

> **"Training to become a physician is a long haul, so settle in, enjoy the ride, and take the long view."**

specialty determines its length in years, but residencies can also be divided into what can be called academic or community based.

Academic residency programs are those associated with large university hospitals. Support staff/services at these institutions are extremely variable, and house officers may have to do things such as draw their patients' blood and transport patients to get X-rays or other tests. (Mundane yet time-consuming tasks like these are collectively known as scut work.) Most attending physicians hold academic posts, tend to publish journal articles, and are involved in teaching at their medical school. Exposure to private-practice settings is variable but often minimal. Residents at these programs see a wide variety of medical problems, including rare entities they may never see again. Academic programs tend to emphasize specialization, and graduates from these programs are more likely to pursue further subspecialization, such as postresidency fellowships, and careers in academic medicine. In fact, residencies in certain specialties, such as nuclear medicine or neurosurgery, can only be found at academic centers. Academic residency programs often have requirements and resources for residents to complete research projects of varying involvement—the project could mean a few weekends a year or an entire year of exclusive research.

Community-based residencies are those offered at community hospitals, which may or may not be affiliated with a medical school. These hospitals tend to have excellent ancillary staff and support services, which minimizes the amount of scut work for residents. Salaries are typically higher than at academic centers, and the benefits are usually better. These programs tend to emphasize proficiency in the mainstream medical problems. Exposure to rare diseases or surgical procedures is less than in academic residencies and research is usually not emphasized. Attending physicians are usually in private practice, and residents gain more exposure to the real world of medical practice compared to residents in the academic setting.

In order to successfully enter certain fields or break into tight marketplaces, a fellowship may be helpful. A fellowship is further poorly or unpaid supervised training in a subspecialty of one's chosen specialty. For example, to become a cardiologist, one first completes an internal medicine residency (three years) and then completes a fellowship in cardiology (three more years). Most fellowships are sponsored by large university medical centers.

Residency is more important in determining the complexion of one's medical career than medical school. But the right medical school can lead you to the right residency. What right means depends on you and your ultimate career objectives. While medical school prepares one to choose and to enter a field of medicine, it also prepares one to actually practice that field and may also help establish connections that lead to job opportunities.

Medical Practice

After surviving residency (and sometimes fellowship as well), it is finally time to get a job. Choosing a specialty is the biggest variable that shapes one's career. Many other factors must also be considered when it comes to actually entering into practice, no matter what the field. Physicians practice medicine in several different practice situations, which, like residencies, can be broadly categorized as academic or community (private) practice.

Academic physicians are usually employed by a medical center that is affiliated with a medical school, although sometimes academic physicians form group practices that are technically similar to private group practices. Academic physicians may be generalists (e.g., a family practitioner) but more often are specialists or subspecialists (e.g., a pediatric cardiothoracic surgeon). In fact, certain specialties can only be found in academics. They are actively involved in research of some kind, whether clinical or in the laboratory, and part of their pay may come from research rather than clinical work. They typically have teaching responsibilities for medical students and residents.

Physicians in community practice primarily see patients (rather than do research) and function in a variety of different business entities. These can be classified in terms of size (i.e., solo, small-group, or large-group practice), specialty mix, or reimbursement scheme (traditional fee-for-service, managed care, single payer). The trend over the last few years has been a shift from solo and small-group specialty practices toward large multispecialty group practices. The driving force for this change is economics—in order to streamline overhead and improve physicians' bargaining power with managed-care insurers.

The Business of Medicine

Currently, most practices in the U.S. are a mixture of fee-for-service and managed care. The balance between the two reimbursement schemes varies considerably from region to region. In Sacramento, San Diego, and Minneapolis, for example, managed care dominates; in other places, particularly more rural locations, fee-for-service is more common. Single-payer systems are essentially government paid health care for everyone. One example of such a system can be seen in Canada.

In managed care, a medical practice contracts with the insurer to cover certain aspects of care (as dictated by the practice's specialty) for a given population for a flat rate per enrollee. The practice receives the same payment no matter what care (surgery, lab tests, CT scans, etc.) are or are not done. In theory, this system encourages preventive and fiscally responsible medical practice. In reality, the name of the game here is to limit patients' access to expensive tests and procedures such as surgery or MRIs—less is more. In some managed-care contracts, capitation is used as further incentive to do less—if a physician scrimps on how much money each patient uses, the physician reeives a bonus at the end of the year.

In a fee-for-service system, a medical practice simply bills for whatever services it provides for the patient. Prior approval from the insurance companies is sometime required, and insurers do not always pay the full amount they are billed. Nonetheless, in this system, more is more. Physicians have incentive to offer more procedures and have less reason to hesitate before ordering expensive laboratory or radiology studies. Prior to widespread managed care, this system lead to unjustifiable spending in some areas, and, as a result, the managed-care movement has lead to more cost-consciousness, even in fee-for-service practice settings.

Nonmedical Opportunities

In 1994, 10 percent of M.D.'s had careers that did not involve patient care. Some doctors go straight from medical school into another profession; others diverge from clinical medicine after some period in practice. What are these folks doing? Some attend law school and end up practicing malpractice law or medical patent law. Some become hospital or medical practice administrators. Some head to Wall Street and use their education for investing insight. More and more, M.D.'s are popping up in politics, even being elected to Congress. But the largest number of physicians not entering clinical practice join biotechnology and pharmaceutical companies. The advantages of joining one of these companies often revolve around lifestyle issues. These jobs may provide regular hours, excellent salary (even entry-level positions) with stock options and bonuses, and travel opportunities. Acording to the *Journal of the American Medical Association* Vol. 279, pp. 1398–1401, May 6, 1998, the disadvantages of this are missing out on being a real doctor, bureaucracy, and the notion of ethics being subverted for profits.

Final Thoughts

Training to become a physician is a long haul, so settle in, enjoy the ride, and take the long view. Life will probably not get easier after medical school, particularly during residency. Start with some concept of your destination, but be flexible to modify your course along the way. Let me reemphasize: residency is the single most profound stage in shaping one's career in medicine, in terms of specialty, geographical location, and professional relationships. However, medical school is the critical place where a specialty is chosen and the pathway is paved to residency and beyond.

U.S. MEDICAL SCHOOLS—
A to Z

ALBANY MEDICAL COLLEGE

Albany, New York

Students Receiving Financial Aid: 41%
Applications: 9,687
Size of Entering Class: 132
Total Number of Women Students: 279 (51%)
Total Number of Men Students: 263 (49%)
World Wide Web: www.amc.edu/html/ medical_college.html

Contact: Sara J. Kremer, Director of Admissions and Registrar
47 New Scotland Avenue
Albany, NY 12208-3479
518-262-5523

Founded in 1839, Albany Medical College (Albany Med) is one of the nation's oldest private medical colleges. The school prides itself on providing rigorous medical training in an intimate and collegial environment that fosters humane values. However, Albany Med is no blue-plate special at $29,330 per year.

Albany, the state capital, is located in upstate New York. As most students attest, the winters are too long, springs too rainy, and summers too short. While not Alaska, Albany's winters are not for the weak of heart.

The Admissions Committee at Albany Med strives to select 124 diverse, well-rounded individuals. Admission is not based solely on MCAT scores. Instead, strong consideration is given to prior academic performance, the personal essay, letters of recommendation, and interviews. Typically, selected candidates are interviewed by two faculty members and one fourth-year student. At Albany Med, the interview is an attempt to learn more about the candidate's interests, not an oral examination on the finer points of the Krebs cycle. The mean undergraduate GPA and MCAT scores for the class of 2002 were 3.4 and 32, respectively.

Of the 124 students Albany Med matriculates, approximately forty are from combined undergraduate-M.D. degree programs with RPI, Union College, and Siena College. While New York State residents comprise roughly 40 percent of the student body, Californians are second at 20 percent. In 1998, 50 percent of the incoming students were women. Minority students account for approximately 30 percent of the class. Albany Med's Office of Minority Affairs actively recruits well-qualified underrepresented students.

Students at Albany Med range in age from 19 to 40. Student backgrounds are both diverse and impressive. The student body includes mothers, fathers, professional musicians, lawyers, Ph.D.'s, pharmacologists, and public health administrators. Students at Albany Med are as intelligent as they are diverse, supportive, caring, and actively involved in the community.

Preclinical Years

The first two years are organized into conceptual or organ system modules. During the first year, students learn normal physiology, histology, and anatomy, while the second year concentrates on the abnormal, the pathophysiology of disease processes. Grading is based on a modified Pass/Fail system. After each theme, a multiple-choice exam is administered. The grade of that exam determines a student's grade for the theme. Grades range from Honors to Unsatisfactory.

For many, the first two years are the most grueling. The days are long (sitting in lecture halls from 9 a.m. to 5 p.m.), the material highly detailed (some days dedicated solely to zinc fingers), and patient contact scarce. The college is revising its curriculum to include more patient contact during the preclinical years. The class of 2003 was the first to have clinical skills introduced during the first year. Still, most of the clinical exposure during the first year comes from patient presentations. Patients are brought into the lecture hall, and they discuss the symptoms that lead them to seek medical attention.

During second year, students are divided into groups of four and assigned a clinical preceptor. The students meet with their preceptor once or twice a month during the first half of the year to learn a specific aspect of the physical exam (i.e., the abdominal exam). Once all systems have been covered, the students perform history and physical exams (H&P) on actual patients in the hospital under the supervision of their preceptor. The preceptor reviews each H&P to identify weaknesses/strengths. In addition, students' clinical skills are tested using standardized or, as students call them, fake patients. Basically, students perform a history and physical exam on healthy people pretending to have some disease—not the highlight of our medical education, to say the least. Classes end in early May, which gives students three weeks off to study for the USMLE Step I.

Between the second and third years, each student is assigned to a two-week Orientation Clerkship designed to instruct students on the skills necessary to begin third year. During this time, students are instructed on how to start IVs, draw blood, apply casts, suture, perform CPR, and write progress notes. Once again, the fake patients rear their heads so that students can practice H&Ps before struggling with real patients.

Most students complain about suchthings as long days, little clinical exposure, and that preceptors are fourth-year medical students rather than attending physicians. However, students also have a number of perks, including dedicated faculty members and a student body that fosters cooperation and supports each other.

Clinical Years

Just when you don't think you can take one more minute of sitting in the hard plastic swivel chairs, SMILE, it's third year! Time to put on that white coat and pretend that you really know how to use that ophthalmoscope. All students rotate through internal medicine, pediatrics, family practice, surgery obstetrics/gynecology, and psychiatry, but in different chronology. Clinical rotations are divided among Albany Medical College Hospital (AMCH) and the College's affiliates—Stratton Veterans Affairs Medical Center, St. Peter's Hospital, Ellis Hospital, and Capital District Psychiatric Center. Most students spend the majority of their rotations at Albany Medical Center. Adjacent to the medical college, AMCH is one of the largest general hospitals in New York. It is the only

academic health science center in twenty-five counties of eastern New York and western New England. A Level I regional trauma center, Level III regional perinatal care center, and recipient of Top 100 Hospitals, AMCH houses 651 beds and averages 23,000 admissions annually.

Grading during both third and fourth years is based on clinical performance (clinical skills and judgment, knowledge, interpersonal skills, personal attributes, and dedication). Residents and attendings (i.e., those with whom you work) complete the evaluations. Grades range from Honors to Unsatisfactory.

While all third-year rotations must be completed at AMCH or one of its affiliates, fourth year offers more freedom. Fourth years consists of ten periods (one of which is vacation), each four weeks long. Five are required rotations (intensive care, general surgery acting internship, primary care acting internship, neurology, and emergency medicine). Special arrangements must be made to do required rotations away from AMCH. Having five required clerkships is a major source of contention, as most schools have fewer or none.

Clinical exposure is reasonably broad, as AMCH draws from an area of more than 2 million people. In addition to the Level I trauma center and Level III perinatal care center, AMCH is a state-designated regional AIDS treatment center, houses a Children's Hospital, and maintains a Bone Marrow Transplantation Program. Most criticism regarding clinical training is not the lack of diversity but the lack of teaching by many residents. The reality of the situation is that most residents just do not have the time; they are overburdened with hard core work. Program directors have responded to this by designating certain times for teaching. Another problem that students frequently voice is that they do not get to perform many procedures. Very few students can say that they have put in IVs or Foley catheters or have much experience drawing blood. Gripes concerning clinical years include too many required clerkships and not enough experience performing procedures. A perk about the clinical years includes working with highly trained and nationally recognized physicians and researchers, supportive/knowledgeable staff that helps coordinate away rotations, and an Academic Affairs Office that is extremely knowledgeable and supportive regarding the residency match.

Social Life

Situated in the Capital Region, Albany's geographic claim to fame is that it is 3 hours from both Boston and New York City. Initially, most students who are new to Albany complain that there's not a whole lot to do. However, these students quickly realize that Albany has enough to occupy their free time. While it is not New York City, Albany does have its share of restaurants and nightlife, bars, clubs, and theaters. Also, there are numerous shopping malls close by. For outdoor recreation, the nearby Catskill and Adirondack Mountains are ideal for hiking, camping, and skiing. Lake George, roughly an hour north, also has some great trails, beaches, and parasailing. During the summer, Saratoga, about 30 minutes away, is home to the SPAC concert series, Newport Jazz Festival, and New York City Ballet. Since it is not New York City, prices are reasonable and crime minimal. Most students live within walking distance of the college. Rents range from $300–$550 for one-bedroom apartments. The college does offer student housing on a limited basis (eighty-four students per year). Each floor is divided into four suites of six people. Each suite has a microwave and refrigerator, but there is only one stove per floor. The rooms are rather small—students can squeeze a twin mattress and desk in one—but affordable. Housing and roommate listings are available in the Student Affairs Office.

The Bottom Line

Students who graduate from Albany Medical College leave with a solid medical education, lifelong friends, and substantial debt.

BAYLOR COLLEGE OF MEDICINE

Houston, Texas

Applications: 3,897
Size of Entering Class: 167
Total Number of Women Students: 391 (47%)
Total Number of Men Students: 433 (53%)
World Wide Web: www.bcm.tmc.edu/

Contact: Dr. L. Leighton Hill, Assistant Dean
One Baylor Plaza
Houston, TX 77030-3498
713-798-4842

Baylor College of Medicine is one of the best-kept secrets in medicine—an excellent education at a relatively affordable price. It offers a rigorous basic science program with strong clinical foundations.

Admissions/Financial Aid

Baylor is a private school but has an agreement with the state of Texas to accept 70 percent of in-state students in order to get state funds that keep it the same price as the University of Texas schools. It is probably a toss-up as to which is the best school in the Texas-Oklahoma-Louisiana-Arizona area—Baylor or University of Texas Southwestern. For the past thirty years, Baylor College of Medicine has had no affiliation with Baylor University in Waco and is entirely secular. While there is no official university affiliation, there are close ties with Rice University, which is located across the street.

The class size is approximately 170 students per year, with the bulk of students coming from the University of Texas, Rice University, Texas A&M University, Baylor University, Stanford, and University of California at Berkeley. Forty percent of those who matriculated were women. Baylor interviews are unique because they typically consist of four or five interviews and include both students and faculty members. While there is less emphasis placed on numbers than on overall qualifications and personality, the average student has a GPA of 3.7 and an MCAT average of 11.

Tuition is about $8,500 for in-state residents and $21,500 for out-of-state residents. Out-of-state applicants are able to establish residency after one year if they buy property in the state, which is very affordable, and they also receive a $4,000 scholarship in the initial year. Financial aid typically consists of federally sponsored educational loans, but the College has its own scholarships that are both need-based and merit-based. If all tuition is borrowed from the beginning, the average student leaves with between $75,000 and $80,000 of debt.

Preclinical Years

One of the most unique aspects of medical education at Baylor is that all basic science is completed in 1½ years, which leaves the remaining 2½ years for clinical rotations. However, Baylor does not have a truncated schedule of academic requirements and has a rather grueling basic science course load. Students take five classes per term and have a month of summer vacation after the first term. Most students feel this is adequate and actually appreciate the condensed schedule, which leaves more time for the fun part of school: clinics.

It is difficult to say which classes are the best in the first few years, because nearly all of them are well taught, well attended, and even reasonably interesting. The standout classes tend to be those taught by the most dynamic professors and include biochemistry, histology, anatomy, and pathology. All of the classes are considered rigorous but leave one well prepared for residency and national board exams. Baylor is one of the few schools that still requires subject boards at the end of the major basic science and clinical rotations. The board exams serve as the final test in most rotations and allow the school to gauge student performance on a national level. Baylor students typically shine on these standardized tests and average about 700 (on an 800 scale) on anatomy.

The average Baylor student is competitive, though not cutthroat. Most students actually attend class every day, so there is no formal note-taking service. Each class comes with a detailed syllabus that goes through most lectures in enough detail that if you decided to take a day trip to Galveston, you wouldn't be too lost the next day. Though the subject matter of some lectures can sometimes be less than enthralling, the teachers are enthusiastic and make even biochemistry or histology come alive. Professors at Baylor take their teaching seriously and are not only leaders in their respective fields but are also extremely accessible to students.

Baylor has a clinically oriented curriculum. Students have exposure to clinical medicine as early as the first week of school and are assigned to follow a practitioner on Friday afternoons. There is also a well-integrated introduction to a clinical skills class taught by third-year students, as well as a rather rigorous history-taking class. By the time students enter clinical rotations, they are fairly well prepared and tend to founder a bit less than some students at other schools.

Grading is honors-pass-marginal pass-fail, and everything is scored on a curve so that only 10 percent of students receive honors and very few fail. The system fosters a less competitive environment than might otherwise be expected. There are formal tutors available. For those unable to keep up with the accelerated program, there is also an option to extend the basic science segment to 2½ years. However, this means an extra year of tuition.

There is time for electives even during basic sciences and these range from sports medicine to the history of medicine to nutrition to the well-received medical ethics program (taught by one of the most dynamic professors you will ever work with).

Clinical Years

Baylor's strength is the clinical experience. Baylor shares with the University of Texas at Houston the world's largest medical center and students train at one of six major hospitals, including the lavish Methodist Hospital and the busy Ben Taub County Hospital. Houston has the second-largest Veteran's Administration (VA) hospital in the country, and it is known as one of the finest among the VA hospital system. Texas Children's Hospital is the second-largest pediatric hospital in the nation and houses one of the top five pediatric residency programs. Though Dr. Michael DeBakey's continued presence often leads to the perception that Baylor is a shrine to cardiothoracic surgery, it is also well known for its pediatrics, neurology, and internal medicine. Because of the diverse population of Houston and the proximity to the

Mexican border, the variety of patients and clinical pathology is vast.

With the 2½ years Baylor students spend in clinics, there is ample time not only to explore the basics, but also to have several electives in subspecialty fields prior to choosing a residency track. Students can take electives at any time during the clinical years, which allows students who are certain that they want to go into internal medicine to take several electives as well as the core rotation before they apply for residency. There is also time to do research, without compromising the core clinical electives. Baylor has a plethora of research opportunities, and if students can't find the opportunity they are looking for at Baylor (e.g., public health), they can find it at University of Texas Houston or Rice University, both of which are within blocks of the Texas Medical Center.

The educational experience is hands-on at Baylor. As a result of working at public facilities, such as the VA and Ben Taub, students become proficient at procedures and other aspects of patient care. There is also a good balance of didactic information presented during clinical rotations, from noon conferences to academic morning reports.

Social Life

Houston is the nation's fourth-largest city, and there is usually something for everyone (except for those who like to snowboard). There's a surprisingly good cultural environment, with three art museums, a great symphony, a Tony Award–winning local theater, and a fine ballet. Though the Houston Oilers moved away, tickets can still be purchased for Astros and Rockets games. There are many fabulous restaurants, all of which are relatively affordable, and numerous clubs, bars, and cafes. Baylor is centrally located within the city and is close to the Rice Village area as well as the charming and artsy enclave of Montrose. Visitors are always surprised by the ethnic diversity in Houston, where they can get some of the best Indian, Vietnamese, and, of course, Mexican food anywhere.

Housing is cheap, with a nice one-bedroom condo for about $400 per month in condoland, which is located near the medical center. Students can purchase a two-bedroom/two-bath condo for about $35,000, which is truly a bargain for out-of-state students, who then qualify for in-state tuition. There are nearby suburban areas such as Bellaire, which are better for students with families and are still fairly affordable.

Crime is always a problem in the urban setting, and Houston is somewhat infamous for its rate of violent crime, but the dangerous parts of town are removed from the school's location. In general, it's always best to be streetwise.

The main problem with Houston is the weather: hot and humid with little natural beauty. Californians initially will be miserable, but will prob-ably get used to always having bad hair days and never seeing a hill until they go home for vacation. Baylor is not as Texan as most people imagine it to be and is a fairly cosmopolitan place.

The Bottom Line

Baylor is a good place for a great education. It's definitely intense, but the teaching is excellent, the role models are plentiful, and you'll be very well prepared for whatever residency you go into.

BOSTON UNIVERSITY SCHOOL OF MEDICINE

Boston, Massachusetts

Size of Entering Class: 150
Total Number of Women Students: 826 (53%)
Total Number of Men Students: 728 (47%)
World Wide Web: med-amsa.bu.edu/BUSM/

Contact: Dr. John F. O'Connor, Associate Dean for Admissions
Boston, MA 2215
617-638-4630

The city of Boston has the highest physician-population ratio in the country. Boston University School of Medicine (BUSM) is one of three medical schools in Boston. Students receive a strong preclinical and even stronger clinical background.

Generalist training and primary care are key missions of BU School of Medicine and the affiliated Boston Medical Center. The Center for Primary Care develops programs that establish it as a national center of excellence in primary care, general medicine, and health services research. To this end, medical students are given the exposure and experience to become leaders in the field of primary care. As early as a student's first year in medical school he or she will work one on one with a physician in internal medicine, pediatrics, or family practice, in such settings as a private practice, a community health center, or a hospital-based practice.

Boston University Medical Center has more than fifteen departments in medical and surgical subspecialties and is expanding each year to provide more space for continued biomedical research.

Admissions/Financial Aid

Lecture halls are filled with approximately 150 students per class. Approximately 25 percent of these students were offered early admission via premedical programs at the undergraduate level. The age range at matriculation is approximately 20–45, with an average age of 26. Men and women are about equal in number and the Office of Minority Affairs ensures that the classes are diverse.

Like most private schools, BUSM is expensive. In fact, it is the most expensive medical school in the eastern U.S. Unfortunately, BUSM offers little in the way of financial aid. To help defray the cost of medical education and promote primary care, there are several low-interest, primary-care loans available. BUSM does offer institutional loans at lower interest rates.

Preclinical Years

Preclinical education emphasizes the community as much as the basic sciences. A biopsychosocial model is used to emphasize the human being in society while students are dissecting the human body in gross anatomy.

The first semester is by far the toughest. Students plunge into the gross anatomy lab and get to see cells through the microscope during histology. Once students make it through the first semester, it's smooth sailing through biochemistry, physiology, and endocrinology. Immunology and genetics were added to the curriculum to keep up with the new advances in biomedical science.

Students get closer to clinical applicability during the first semester of second year. This is when they're introduced to bugs (microbiology) and drugs (pharmacology). Biology of Disease is a semester-long course taken during the second semester of second year in which students learn pathophysiology of the various organ systems in a clinical context. This is an excellent review for the students' last hurdle before they enter into third year, Step I of the USMLE.

Although most of the classes during the first two years are in large lecture halls, some are taught in a small-group setting. During the first year, Introduction to Clinical Medicine (ICM) gets students into the clinical setting to begin interviewing patients. During the second year, students are beginning to sharpen their interview and physical examination skills in preparation for their third year, when they begin to care for patients. All of this is done with actual patients in various health-care settings.

Throughout both preclinical years students also participate in Integrated Problems (IP). This is a problem-based learning experience that offers an opportunity to begin integrating the basic sciences to clinical medicine while developing skills in cooperative group learning and problem solving. (These are important skills when working on a patient-care team during the third and fourth years.)

Although other schools have moved toward a two- or three-tiered system, grading at BUSM is done on a five-tier system throughout the preclinical and clinical years. Similar to an A through F system the new system grades with honor, high pass, pass, deficiency low, and deficiency unsatisfactory (fail) levels.

Clinical Years

After passing the boards (98 percent do), students trade their books and lecture halls for stethoscopes and white coats and their late nights in the library for late nights on the ward.

If they are out in the community during their first and second years (as most of them are), they will continue their outpatient rotations at the various health centers and private practices, while their inpatient experience will be at several of the affiliated hospitals in and around Boston.

BUSM has had a longtime affiliation with the former Boston City Hospital, a beacon for the poor in Boston. Although it was renamed Boston Medical Center in 1996, it remains dedicated to serving the underserved of Boston. In recent years, the population has expanded to include an eclectic mix of immigrants from as far away as Somalia, Bosnia, Haiti, and Latin America. Students also have the unique opportunity to see patients in their own homes as part of the oldest Home Medical Service in the country.

The third year is filled with core clerkships in family medicine, internal medicine, surgery, ob/gyn, pediatrics, and psychiatry. During the fourth year, students are required to complete a subinternship (in medicine, surgery, or pediatrics) as well as rotations in radiology and neurology. The rest of the year is spent in electives, which may be done at BUSM or other institutions as students prepare for their residency.

For the last seven years, 85 percent of BUSM students have matched into the top three residencies of their choice. Approximately 30 to 40 percent of students have entered primary care (so there's still hope for the subspecialists out there).

Social Life

Students have plenty of time to experience all that Boston and New England are famous for and still have time to pass their classes. They can take a walk along the Freedom Trail to see what it was like in Boston while it was still one of the thirteen colonies. Boston is home to great restaurants. There are also a number of art museums, theaters, and the New England Aquarium. Don't forget about the Red Sox (bleacher seats for as little as $12), Bruins, and Celtics (who have recently relocated to the Fleet Center). BU (undergrad) also has one of the "winningest" hockey teams in Boston.

Not only is Boston arguably the largest college town, but it is also the center of New England. This means that students can ski and hike the premier mountains on the East Coast on weekends. This is all possible within a 2-hour drive of the city.

Boston's real estate boom in the last several years has made it a more expensive place to live. Gentrification has turned the South End into one of the most sought-after places to live. It is still livable on a student budget, probably more so with a roommate. Students may have an easier (and less expensive) time living outside of the city and commuting. There are several communities just outside of Boston that offer quieter and cheaper living.

The Bottom Line

BUSM offers an unparalleled opportunity to get into the community from day one while still offering time to enjoy Boston and New England.

BROWN UNIVERSITY SCHOOL OF MEDICINE

Providence, Rhode Island

Tuition 1996–97: $26,896 per year
Size of Entering Class: 64
Total Number of Women Students: 113 (43%)
Total Number of Men Students: 151 (57%)
World Wide Web: biomed.brown.edu/Medicine.
  html

Contact: Admissions and Financial Aid Office
1 Prospect Street
Providence, RI 02912
401-863-2149

Brown University is an Ivy League university in Providence, Rhode Island. Providence is about 1 hour south of Boston and 2½ hours east of New York City. About fifty of the sixty-five students who enter in the first year belong to the Program in Liberal Medical Education (PLME), an eight-year continuum in which students are accepted out of high school and are guaranteed seats in the medical school. Approximately fourteen of the sixty-five entering students are accepted from several postbaccalaureate programs that have an affiliation with the medical school. Occasionally, a few Brown undergraduates are granted admission to the School of Medicine. Between the preclinical and clinical years, the class size grows again with the addition of about twenty-five Dartmouth Medical School students.

With the PLME program, Brown offers many opportunities to pursue an individualized path. For example, students can enter Brown University and major in computer science. Although they may have to take the usual premedical requirements plus biochemistry, there are plenty of courses to choose from for their majors and electives and they still have all of their summers open. Because of the caliber of the undergraduate college, major corporations regularly recruit at Brown and students are able to work at some of these majors corporations. Students may also choose to spend a summer doing research at the National Institutes of Health with other Brown students and may even take a year off to work as a Howard Hughes scholar at NIH between their third and fourth years.

Preclinical Years

All medical school classes are held in the Biomedical Center, a large brick building that houses most medi-

cal research labs at Brown, the undergraduate department, and the medical school lecture halls.

One required course in the preclinical years is the Affinity Group. PLME students are assigned to an affinity group in their third undergraduate year; postbaccalaureate students are assigned when they enter the medical school. These groups meet one evening a week, usually over pizza, and take on projects, from describing cross-cultural beliefs in medicine to exploring the incidence of childhood lead poisoning in Providence.

Classes in the preclinical years are graded as pass, fail, and honors. The particular proportion of honors grades assigned varies per course. Although the curriculum is fixed, students desire, they can take any undergraduate or graduate school course as an elective. In addition, students in the PLME can take medical school courses while still undergraduates.

Anatomy is taught in the typical fashion, with the addition of computer-based tutorials. First-year students are taught skills in interviewing patients, and, in the second year, students learn physical diagnosis in one of the affiliated hospitals.

The summer between the first and second years is free for any activities. All students take the USMLE Step I exam at the end of the second year, after which students are free until the start of third-year clerkships. Passing USMLE Step II is required to graduate from the Brown University School of Medicine.

Clinical Years

Brown students are required to pass core clerkships in medicine, surgery, pediatrics, obstetrics/gynecology, psychiatry, and family medicine. Brown is affiliated with most of the surrounding hospitals. Rhode Island Hospital is the largest hospital in Rhode Island and includes the new Hasboro Children's Hospital. All core clerkships except family medicine can be done here. Next door is Women and Infant's Hospital, a maternity hospital with inpatient and surgical obstetrics. Students taking electives in pediatric subspecialties such as neonatal intensive-care unit work here. Rhode Island Hospital and Women and Infant's Hospital are only a few miles from the main Brown campus. Other affiliated hospitals include Memorial Hospital in Pawtucket (just north of Providence), Miriam Hospital in Providence (a large community hospital with medicine and surgery clerkships), Butler psychiatric hospital, Bradley children's psychiatric hospital, and the Providence VA hospital (for medicine and surgery). Although the usual hospital mergers also take place in Providence and Rhode Island, these have not affected Brown students, since there is only one medical school in the state.

In addition to the core clerkships, Brown students are required to pass a longitudinal or continuity-of-care experience. There are many clinics and practices where students do this. Medical students are also free to take any course from the undergraduate curriculum.

Social Life

Providence has plenty of inexpensive housing, from newly constructed apartments in Cranston to Brown-owned off-campus housing in Providence. Monthly rents range from $300–$700, depending on comforts. Dormitory housing is also available, but the majority of students live off the main campus. Many exotic and chain restaurants are very close to the main campus and are near Providence and the hospitals. Students will need a car for their clerkship years but not for the first two years.

The Bottom Line

Brown is a great medical school. Certainly, the student body is nationally competitive, since around 60 percent of students get their first choice for residency selection, and many of those choices include residencies at the best programs in the country. Yet the student body works together, and there is a remarkably cooperative spirit here. This may have to do with the fact that most of the students in the medical school have known each other since their undergraduate years; however, new students are welcomed quickly into study groups and circles of friends. It's an Ivy League medical school that has not forgotten that students learn best when helping each other.

CASE WESTERN RESERVE UNIVERSITY SCHOOL OF MEDICINE

Cleveland, Ohio

Size of Entering Class: 145
World Wide Web: mediswww.meds.cwru.edu/
Contact: Dr. Nathan A. Berger, Dean

10900 Euclid Avenue
Cleveland, OH 44106

Located on the shores of what the locals call America's North Coast (you guessed it: Lake Erie), the School of Medicine at Case Western has the feel of a 150-year-old work in progress. It's a place where the traditional in medical education is combined with the state-of-the-art. There's no dearth of ideas and educational experimentation at Case Western; some of it is screwy, some brilliant, all of it an earnest attempt to find better ways to fashion excellent physicians for the new century. You may sometimes feel like a guinea pig, but Case Westerm makes students doctors.

Preclinical Years

Like other medical schools, the first two years consist of sitting in a single lecture hall and mastering the fundamental underpinnings of medicine. Unlike other places, classes are held six days a week, 4 hours each day, leaving the afternoons free for studying either medicine or the exhibits at the Rock and Roll Hall of Fame. Subjects are taught in large, loose themes, including, for example, the Biological Basis of Disease (otherwise known as "bugs and drugs"). Each student is given a laptop computer upon entering his or her first year, and the School tries hard to integrate high-tech teaching modalities with the old-fashioned mind-numbing lectures. Some students type their lecture notes directly into the laptop, and most classes organize a note-sharing service to minimize all the scribbling (and typing). Most tests are multiple choice, and grading is blinded by an elaborate system of numeric codes designed to be fair and minimize student competition. If you do poorly on a test, the test code is deciphered. This is known (in ominous and Orwellian fashion) as being "identified," ostensibly so that the student can be tutored and brought up to speed. Best not to be identified at all; at Case Western, anonymity is success.

In response to student desire to have some early clinical experiences, a patient-based program that runs parallel to the classroom didactics during years one and two was established. Each student is paired with a pregnant woman and follows her through her prenatal care. After students have helped deliver the baby, they participate in each of the infant's pediatric clinic visits. This has proved to be a popular component of the first two years and will remind you why you wanted to go to medical school in the first place. It wasn't the Krebs cycle.

In addition to the core lecture series and the patient-based program, case-based teaching has been integrated into the program, and there are additional weekly small group sessions that deal with the ethical and sociopolitical aspects of medicine. A wide variety of electives are available to fill the afternoon, from acupuncture to bench research to working in STD clinics to flying with the emergency physicians of the LifeFlight helicopter.

Clinical Years

Third year is devoted to each of the major disciplines (pediatrics, surgery, etc.) and is spent mostly at University hospitals (a large complex of once-separate general women's and children's hospitals adjacent to the medical school) and MetroHealth Medical Center, the former county hospital. Less time is spent at the Veteran's Administration, Mt. Sinai, and St. Luke's, all a short drive from the school. (The Cleveland Clinic Hospital has an affiliation with another medical school, so only the rare elective is done there.) The diversity of the patient population is great and includes the demographics particular to the area, including a large Eastern European population as well as the Amish.

An alternative primary-care track was established in 1994 for students who are certain that this is their interest. It involves curricular differences in all years (earlier courses on physical diagnosis, for instance) but mostly differs in the clinical years, when the traditional in-patient rotations are integrated with a greater amount of ambulatory care medicine. Fourth year is somewhat less harried for all students and is devoted largely to electives and to applying and interviewing for residency. Students do well at the match in general: 90 percent match at a residency in the top three on their list.

Social Life

Cleveland continues to be the butt of many jokes, but the "mistake on the lake" is a nice enough city. Its citizens are justifiably proud of its cultural resources, which include the new Rock and Roll Hall of Fame and Jacob's Field, the home of the Cleveland Indians, as well as lovely museums of art and natural history. The world-famous Cleveland Orchestra performs a block from the medical school in University Circle. More raucous celebrations take place downtown and in The Flats, a cluster of restaurants and clubs in the old wharf and warehouse district on the banks of the Cuyahoga River. Of the events put on by the medical school, the best attended include an annual talent show ("Doc Opera") and a lavish banquet known as the Hippocrates Ball. Of course, there are more frequent and informal coffeehouses and parties each year.

With regard to the student body, about half of each 130-person class is from Ohio, with the rest from around the country. Each class consists of roughly 40 to 50 percent women and usually about a third nonwhite. Most students live a short walk or drive to school, many in the nearby leafy suburbs of Cleveland Heights and Shaker Heights. Rent is cheapest in the neighborhoods just adjacent to the medical school, such as Cleveland's Little Italy, but, in general, housing is not as expensive as in other cities.

The Bottom Line

Case Western is an excellent school with something for everyone. It has a long history of being friendly to those who have taken an unconventional route to medical school and is a place where innovation and new ideas are greeted with genuine enthusiasm.

COLUMBIA UNIVERSITY COLLEGE OF PHYSICIANS AND SURGEONS

New York, New York

Tuition 1996–97: $28,008 per year
Size of Entering Class: 150
Total Number of Women Students: 596 (50%)
Total Number of Men Students: 607 (50%)
World Wide Web: cpmcnet.columbia.edu/dept/ps/

Contact: Dr. Herbert Pardes, Dean, Faculty of
Medicine
116th Street and Broadway
New York, NY 10027

Since awarding its first doctoral degree in 1767, Columbia University's medical school has been known quaintly as the College of Physicians and Surgeons. Today, the school, referred to affectionately as P&S, maintains a reputation for academic excellence and rigor. Applicants often ask about the school's location in Washington Heights, which is some sixty blocks uptown from the main campus of the university. Although the neighborhood has a reputation for a lack of safety, the crime rate citywide has dropped significantly in recent years and security around the hospital and affiliated buildings is quite good. Thanks to New York City's legendary subway system, the medical school remains accessible to the social and cultural resources for which New York is famous.

Preclinical Years

The first year starts off with a weeklong orientation run by second-year students. During this week, students meet their new classmates, see what may be their first Broadway show, and begin to realize that Columbia students are incredibly happy. The following week, classes begin in the form of lectures from 9 a.m. to noon or 1 p.m. The classes include Science Basic to the Practice of Medicine (SBPM), an integrated biochemistry and physiology course; Clinical Practice, which addresses the social, political, and economic aspects of medicine; Neuroscience; Neuroanatomy; and Human Development. In addition to lectures, there are small-group sessions that meet for a few hours two afternoons per week.

About six weeks into the term, anatomy begins. Lectures take place each Monday and Thursday and are followed by a 4-hour lab scheduled until 5 p.m.

Because anatomy groups, which consist of five students per cadaver, are free to work at their own pace, most people are out of lab early. The set-up allows for instructors to be present to assist students who want to stay, while those who prefer to study on their own are not stuck in lab.

Even after anatomy begins, students generally have Friday afternoons and one other afternoon per week off. For part of the year, this second afternoon is used to begin student exposure to clinical medicine through a clinical selective. These experiences allow students to work with a doctor in a chosen specialty. First-year students also begin to develop interview skills through a class in psychiatric medicine.

The stress level for the first year runs in cycles with peaks that coincide with the weeklong exam blocks that occur about every six weeks. Although an honors/pass/fail grading system is now in place, the administration is exploring the possibility of instituting a simple pass/fail system. As the school has continued to attract stronger students, the atmosphere has become somewhat more competitive. Still, most exam preparation is done in small informal groups, and students often prepare study sheets and voluntarily put them on reserve in the library for the rest of the class. The Student Success Network (SSN) is a group of second-year students that offers review classes in SBPM. Anatomy and neuroscience are also available for free one-on-one tutoring.

Study space includes an aging four-level library and an entire floor of the medical school building. Computer facilities at Columbia have improved significantly over the past few years, and most students take advantage of the computer resources to help prepare for exams—and of course, check their e-mail.

Students can choose from a number of options for spending the three-month break between first and second year. Funding is available for research, but some students opt for nonmedical experiences while they get to know New York. Others travel to different areas of the country or abroad for exposure to clinical medicine.

The second-year class schedule is lighter than the first. One afternoon per week is spent in the popular physical diagnosis class. Instead of a week of exams like the first year, there is an exam each Monday in a different class. The stress level does creep up toward the end of the year when students begin thinking about USMLE Step I and the block of final exams that determine second-semester grades. This exam block is only about a week prior to the USMLE. This turns out to be a blessing because it obviates the need for intensive review of those subjects. Columbia students traditionally shatter the national average for Step I.

Clinical Years

Despite the recent merger of Columbia-Presbyterian Hospital with the New York Hospital (Cornell University Medical School's major affiliate), the medical schools remain completely separate, and Columbia students rotate through the same hospitals now as they did prior to the merger. According to the administration, this is unlikely to change. In addition to the hospitals located at the 168th Street campus of the Columbia-Presbyterian Medical Center (CPMC), the main affiliates are the Allen Pavilion (212th and Broadway), Harlem Hospital (506 Lenox Avenue), St. Luke's Hospital (West 114th Street), and Roosevelt Hospital (West 59th Street).

Columbia maintains a fixed schedule of required rotations for the third year and a completely elective fourth year. Groups of fifteen students rotate through ten 5-week specialty blocks. Rotations at CPMC are generally considered to be more rigorous than those at other sites. Clinical teaching is generally strong at all sites, with the exception of Harlem Hospital, which tends to be understaffed. Shuttles and New York's superior subway system make travel between sites relatively easy. One unique offering at Columbia is the opportunity during the third-year primary-care rotation to work on an Indian reservation in either New Mexico or Arizona. The psychiatry, neurology, and neurosurgery departments are especially strong, while primary-care and family medicine are especially weak.

Fourth year consists of a back-to-the-classroom month, a subinternship, and six other one-month electives. This leaves two full months of vacation, which most students use to schedule residency interviews. The flexibility of the fourth year and the many fully funded international opportunities offered at Columbia combine to form one of the school's strengths. There are affiliated hospitals in London, Paris, Moscow, and Istanbul. In addition, the Society and Medicine Program and the Infectious Disease Department send more than a dozen students to perform rotations at sites in Asia, Africa, and South America.

Social Life

Extracurricular opportunities abound at Columbia. The admissions office makes an effort to put together a diverse class of people who not only are interested in nonmedical pursuits, but also excel in these areas. Once at Columbia, students can explore their extracurricular interests and discover new ones through the P&S Club, an umbrella organization that oversees more than thirty-five groups that sponsor activities in music, art, athletics, and drama and cultural, philanthropic, and academic interests.

The benefit of living in Washington Heights is the relatively inexpensive housing. Most single first-year students live in the dorm-style Bard Hall. One-room singles at Bard (sink included) are less than $500 per month. In the Bard basement is the well-equipped Bard Athletic Center, of which all students are automatic members. By second year, about half of the students move into two-, three-, or four-bedroom apartments in the nearby Towers. Rent is slightly more than $500 per person per month for spacious rooms, two full bathrooms, and beautiful views of the city. Couples with or without children generally move directly into the Towers at the start of first year.

The Bottom Line

Columbia offers students the opportunity to receive a top-tier medical education while they enjoy New York City and explore interests outside of medicine.

CORNELL UNIVERSITY WEILL MEDICAL COLLEGE

New York, New York

World Wide Web: www.med.cornell.edu/
Contact: Antonio Gotto, Dean

445 East 69th Street
New York, NY 10021

Recently renamed for generous benefactor Sanford Weill, head of CitiGroup, the Weill Medical College of Cornell University celebrated its centennial in 1998. The school and its associated medical center enjoy a well-earned reputation in New York and around the world for first-class health care as well as academic prowess. Overlooking the East River, Cornell is located in one of New York's most exclusive neighborhoods, and patients at New York Hospital, the main teaching affiliate, tend to reflect this demographic.

Preclinical Years

Classes start most mornings at 8 a.m., and a student's absence will be noted, since many classes are small. The flip side is that with classes ending by 1 p.m., many students find enough time to pursue nonmedical activities during their afternoons. Except for gross anatomy, all basic science courses are taught in the state-of-the-art Weill Education Center, which encompasses 20,000 square feet and was completed in 1996. The center is close to the Samuel J. Wood Library and the C. V. Starr Biomedical Information Center. Professors are universally dedicated and caring and promote as much of a stress-free atmosphere as possible.

The first year consists of three months of Molecules to Cells, 3½ months of Human Structure and Function, one month of Genetics, and a month and a half of Immunology. Molecules to Cells is a well-integrated study of cell biology, biochemistry, and molecular biology, while Genetics is thought to be poorly organized.

Human Structure and Function incorporates basic anatomy, physiology, histology, embryology, and radiology in one course. Although physiology is taught quite well, the kidney gets only one week. Anatomy labs, assisted by fourth-year students, are taught side-by-side with a well-run radiology section, which allows students to better visualize anatomy much better and offers an edge later on clinical rotations. Some say

histology is taught by the best professor of the year. There is no point, however, in going to embryology lectures. Overall, the ambitious Human Structure and Function course is felt to be stuffed into too short a time frame; many feel that anatomy could have been taught in more depth.

Throughout the year, problem-based sessions are scheduled on Monday, Wednesday, and Friday mornings. Students enjoy the sessions and say that making presentations on the fictional cases allows a good understanding of disease mechanisms, clinical presentations, and differential diagnoses. Lectures, which are usually followed by half-hour question-and-answer sessions, range from excellent and clear to obtuse and boring, but the majority are well organized and useful. The week is rounded out by up to three problem-set work sessions, one multiple-choice quiz, a student-run journal club, and labs during the appropriate courses. A sometimes harrowing, but always educational, experience is the Triple Jump, in which a student receives a case and must determine which tests to order and hypothesize a diagnosis and mechanisms of disease—all without any help from sources or other students.

In the second year, courses include the popular Brain and Mind, which incorporates neurology, neuroanatomy, psychiatry, and pathology. Medicine, Patients and Society, which begins in the first year, continues. Each Thursday, students meet for one or two lectures, a discussion section, and several hours in a doctor's office. The material in this course changes with each unit, starting with ethics and empathy and then moving into examination skills, biostatistics, epidemiology, and then clinical diagnosis.

Clinical Years

Cornell students rotate through several hospitals, including the Upper East Side's New York Hospital, Queens-New York Hospital, Manhassett's North Shore University Hospital (shared with New York

University) and the Westchester County psychiatry division. Noticeably, there are no public hospitals on this roster, which can at times limit the amount of independence and hands-on training available to students. At the same time, New York Hospital (recently merged with Presbyterian Hospital, which does not affect medical students) is a renowned clinical facility that draws patients with rare diseases from around the world. In addition, the medical school maintains major affiliations with Memorial Sloan-Kettering Cancer Center and the Hospital for Special Surgery.

Grading in the clinical years is honors/high pass/pass. Students give mixed grades to the internal medicine rotation, which requires one month at New York Hospital, one month at an off-campus site, and one month of outpatient medicine. Perennial complaints are that the didactic schedule lacks organization and lacks a steady curriculum. The subinternship in medicine, however, is an outstanding experience.

Surgery varies from location to location. At New York Hospital, students have ample opportunity to get to know faculty members, which is especially useful for those interested in surgical residencies. North Shore's surgery rotation stands out for superior teaching, many conferences, and leniency in grading.

Students say that pediatrics, because of its excellent structure, is a terrific rotation. Psychiatry at the Westchester campus also receives high marks. Obstetrics and gynecology, however, is known as a particularly malignant rotation.

The clinical experience is rounded out by traditional electives, such as dermatology and anesthesiology, and the public health elective, which in recent years has sponsored unusual trips such as going out with New York City's rat patrol.

Social Life

Students at Cornell tend to be a tight-knit group, socializing often together. Happy hours in Olin Hall, on campus, are popular. The New York metropolitan area is well represented. The school's location offers access not only to the Upper East Side, popular among young 20- and 30-somethings, but also to the entire city.

About 90 percent of students opt to live in campus dorms. During the first year, rent is $350 per month. Starting in the second year, rent becomes a great deal, with students sharing two- and three-bedroom apartments for $520 per student per month.

The Bottom Line

Staffed by professors who care deeply about teaching, research and clinical medicine, Cornell is a top-ten medical school from which students can go anywhere.

CREIGHTON UNIVERSITY SCHOOL OF MEDICINE

Omaha, Nebraska

Tuition 1996–97: $26,550 per year
Students Receiving Financial Aid: 85%
Size of Entering Class: 112
Total Number of Women Students: 187 (36%)
Total Number of Men Students: 335 (64%)
World Wide Web: medicine.creighton.edu/

Contact: Dr. Henry Nipper, Assistant Dean for
Admissions
2500 California Plaza
Omaha, NE 68178-1
402-280-2799

Creighton University (est. 1878) is one of twenty-eight Jesuit-operated colleges and universities in the United States and one of four Jesuit colleges/universities that have medical schools. The Jesuit tradition places a strong emphasis on service to humanity as well as education.

The theme for the past three to four years in the medical school is aptly described by an old Bob Dylan title, "The Times They Are a Changin'." A new dean of the School of Medicine was recently appointed. A new curriculum has been incorporated that places less emphasis on the traditional lecture format and focuses on organ- and disease-based learning. More emphasis is being placed on clinical problem solving and clinical experience earlier in the curriculum. In addition, the grading system has been changed from a strict percentile/class ranking to an honors/pass/fail system. The change in grading policy was meant to further decrease competition between students, although frankly, the environment was not hostile or overly competitive under the previous system. Creighton predominantly emphasizes clinical training and provides solid clinical preparation for an internship/residency and a career. Research has generally not been a major priority for most students, although opportunities are available.

The majority of students are from Nebraska and California, with large numbers from predominantly Midwestern and Western states. Data covering the last five years show students coming from nearly every state, with the Southeast being the least represented. The high number of Western applicants likely reflects the relative paucity of medical schools in the West. Applicants from Western states who aren't accepted into their state school frequently also apply to private schools, of which Creighton is closer to home than East Coast alternatives. The difference between in-state tu-ition at a public school and private tuition is the reason why some might prefer a state school as a first option.

Admissions/Financial Aid

Tuition is $25,000 per year at Creighton, which is near the lower end of the range for private schools. The education at most places is likely comparable, but the disparity in tuition is large. However, the vast majority of students (96 percent) obtain financial aid packages to cover the cost of tuition and living expenses. The medical school has its own helpful financial aid adviser.

Preclinical Years

Four years ago, the didactic curriculum was changed from the traditional two years of core science courses to an organ- and disease-based approach. The new approach was designed to allow the integration of more clinical information into the basic science years. The goal is to transition from passive learning and rote recall to problem-solving and analytical skills. The new design is based on case discussions in small-group sessions as well as computer-assisted instruction. First-year students take a physical diagnosis course and are assigned to work in a clinic, which they continue one half day per week for the entire four years. Some students would rather have the time to study for exams than spend time in the clinic practicing physical diagnosis. However, the early clinical knowledge and patient interaction is probably worthwhile; it provides at least a basic clinical introduction that eases the transition into clinical clerkships. The strongest, most organized preclinical courses have traditionally been Gross Anatomy, Pathology, Microbiology, and Pharmacology. The weakest have been Biochemistry and Genetics. The first year ends in May, with the second not beginning until mid-August. This allows for a nice long break.

This new curriculum is starting to emphasize more research during this time, but most students have used it as vacation/personal time. The second year ends in mid- to late May, which leaves about three weeks to prepare for USMLE Step I, which is required before moving on to the clinical years.

Clinical Years

St. Joseph Hospital, a 400-bed facility located in downtown Omaha across the street from the medical school, is the primary hospital affiliated with Creighton University. St. Joseph Hospital is one of two trauma centers in the Omaha area. As part of certain clerkships, students may also rotate through the Omaha Veterans Administration (VA) Medical Center, Bergan Mercy Medical Center, Omaha Children's Hospital, St. Joseph Center for Mental Health, and Clarkson Medical Center. Clerkships begin on July 1, which allows for a couple of weeks of vacation between the USMLE Step I and starting clinical rotations. The third-year clerkships are all eight-week rotations, which include inpatient internal medicine, surgery, ob/gyn, pediatrics, psychiatry, and primary care. The fourth year allows significant time for electives but requires clerkships in critical care and surgery and a subinternship.

The most organized, best taught, and most well-liked rotations have been ob/gyn, internal medicine, and surgery. Pediatrics and psychiatry are spread among several hospitals and can be either very good or suboptimal, depending on location. For the most part, students receive very good clinical experience during the clerkships. Creighton strikes a nice balance between having enough patients and enough heterogeneity to learn how to manage a variety of illnesses without being so busy that the residents and attendings have no time to teach. Interaction between the attendings, residents, and students has traditionally been superb. The atmosphere for clinical training is very good, and there is less scut work for the students than there is at many other teaching hospitals.

One drawback is that students don't perform a lot of procedures. The popular emergency room rotation, however, provides the opportunity to develop some procedural skills.

Matching for residency becomes important in the fourth year. According to Creighton's published data over the past five years, 93 percent of Creighton graduates were matched with their first-choice specialty in one of their top four choices of location; 55 percent were matched with their first choice in both specialty and location. As with many other schools, there has been a trend toward primary care as a specialty choice. In 1997, 61 percent of Creighton graduates went into primary care. This partially explains the high rate of students matching at one of their top choices, as primary-care positions are, realistically, not as competitive as some other specialties. Nonetheless, Creighton students have done very well in obtaining residency positions.

One caveat here is that high-profile academic centers across the country tend to take students from other big-name programs. Each year, a handful of Creighton students match at such programs, but the reality is that a student must be extremely competitive, both in class performance (i.e., honors) and USMLE Step I score, to vie for positions at the elite programs. This is true for any smaller, regionally oriented school, not just Creighton.

Social Life

Omaha is a city of 350,000, with a surrounding total population of about 500,000. Some folks say that it's a great place to attend medical school because there's nothing else to do besides study. You won't confuse it with New York City, Los Angeles, or Chicago, to be sure, but that's what a lot of people like about Omaha. It's big enough to provide some extracurricular activities but has no traffic/transportation problems, relatively little crime, and a reasonable cost of living (many students and residents buy homes in Omaha).

Omaha has the world-class Henry Doorly Zoo, AAA minor-league baseball (Omaha Royals), the College World Series, minor-league hockey, plenty of nice and reasonably priced public golf courses, a lot of great restaurants for a city its size, and the Omaha Community Playhouse. Those who like to play the odds can cross the state line into Iowa (which is about 5 minutes away) and visit the casinos and/or the greyhound races. Sites for outdoor activities (e.g., mountains, lakes, and beaches) are slim in the vicinity. Another negative is the cold Midwestern winters, which last from about the end of October through March.

The Bottom Line

Creighton University provides a strong clinical education that serves graduates well in both residency and practice, but at a private tuition cost. Most Creighton students are happy with their training and with life in general during medical school. But bundle up for some cold winters.

DARTMOUTH COLLEGE DARTMOUTH MEDICAL SCHOOL

Hanover, New Hampshire

Tuition 1996–97: $24,860 per year
Students Receiving Financial Aid: 81%
Applications: 7,136
Size of Entering Class: 77
Total Number of Women Students: 141 (46%)
Total Number of Men Students: 167 (54%)

World Wide Web: www.dartmouth.edu/dms/
Contact: Andrew G. Welch, Director of
    Admissions
    Hanover, NH 03755
    603-650-1505

Dartmouth Medical School is as close to a liberal arts medical school as is possible. The School has small class sizes and, correspondingly, one of the lowest acceptance rates in the nation, so faculty members get to know the students personally. While the School has a reputation as a primary-care school, this is somewhat unfounded. Many Dartmouth students tend to pursue careers in specialties from neurosurgery to emergency medicine to dermatology. Despite the School's smallness, research endeavors are extremely active; the number of grant dollars brought in per researcher ranks very high nationally. Dartmouth Medical School fosters a student's individual interests and goals, whether those goals and interests are to become an academician sorting out the most esoteric of riddles or to become a family practitioner laboring in the trenches of rural Maine.

Preclinical Years

The preclinical years at Dartmouth are among the most humane in the country. Since implementing a program called New Directions five years ago, first- and second-year students are out of class by lunchtime on most days (an ideal setup for students with families). Grades during the preclinical years are honors/pass/fail. Grading curves are such that everyone can theoretically receive honors and no one need fail. This creates a cooperative and amicable environment in which students study in groups and create and distribute helpful study materials to classmates. The collegial, noncompetitive spirit makes Dartmouth a very lonely place for gunners (students who are aggressive and competitive in their approach to medical school).

The first-year curriculum is designed to give students the tools needed to be good medical scientists. Teaching modalities include lecture and small-group sessions. Students say the strongest courses are physiology, microbiology, and anatomy. Because embryology is taught as part of the anatomy course, many students feel that embryology is overshadowed by anatomy. Likewise, students report that metabolism is not emphasized at Dartmouth.

Quizzes are given every two weeks during the first year. This is exhausting, but students like the fact that their grades are not solely determined by their performance on final exams. During the summer between the first and second years, students are encouraged (and funded) to explore the field of medicine, from doing "bench" research to seeing patients in a physician's office.

The second-year curriculum is designed to provide the scientific background needed to be a capable physician. The curriculum is dominated by the Scientific Basis of Medicine. The course consists of integrated approaches to the pathology, pathophysiology, and pharmacology of discrete organ systems. Second-year lectures and small groups are primarily led by attending physicians from the Dartmouth-Hitchcock Medical Center (DHMC), called "the Hitch" by students. Students find the second year to be a vast improvement over the first year since the classes are all extremely clinically relevant and, therefore, more interesting to future physicians. Most Dartmouth medical students take the first part of the boards after their second year, although the School does not require that they do so. The typical Dartmouth student outscores the national average on the USMLE Step I.

Clinical Years

The third and fourth years at Dartmouth are fairly traditional. Students perform their clerkships at the new and beautiful Hitch and the Veterans Administration (VA) hospital in adjacent White River Junction,

Vermont. The Hitch has been ranked by *U.S. News & World Report* as one of the nation's best hospitals in a number of medical and surgical specialties. Although their location is rural, the hospitals serve a large geographic area, with a patient base as large as many urban areas. In addition to these hospitals, students are expected to rotate through various clinical sites in New Hampshire and Vermont (if the sites are more than a 40-minute drive away, the School provides housing). Grading during the clinical years is honors/high pass/pass/fail. As in the preclinical years, a noncompetitive attitude predominates among students.

The third-year curriculum requires eight-week rotations in surgery, psychiatry, inpatient internal medicine, and family practice and four-week rotations in outpatient internal medicine, outpatient pediatrics, inpatient pediatrics, and obstetrics and gynecology. Third-year students get two weeks of vacation and a special class to prepare them for residency interviews.

The fourth-year curriculum has fewer requirements. Students must take four weeks each of neurology, women's health, and a subinternship in a specialty of their choice. Other than that, students are free to pick electives in whatever interests them.

On average, Dartmouth attendings and house staff members are considered to be able and enthusiastic teachers. No clerkships are thought to be weak, but wise advice is to do enough key rotations at DHMC or the VA so that you can become known to faculty members who are big names in an intended area of specialization. One potential area of concern is that due to the nationwide decrease in funding for veterans' hospitals, some spots for students to learn inpatient surgery at the VA might be in jeopardy. However, the School has recently waged a successful battle to retain these spots for the near future. Dartmouth Medical School graduates do well in the match, with generally more than 90 percent getting one of their top three residency choices.

Social Life

Dartmouth students come from all over the country and world and represent diverse ethnic groups, backgrounds, and life experiences. About 10 percent of any given class is married, and the average Dartmouth student is in his or her mid-20s. The overwhelming majority of students are involved in extracurricular and community-service groups. Students tend to be exercise-conscious and take advantage of the School's

location between the Green and White Mountains and along the Connecticut River for a variety of outdoor activities, from mountain biking to cross-country skiing. The remoteness of the School makes a car an absolute necessity.

Its rural setting makes Dartmouth ideal for outdoor-type students who enjoy small-town life or those who just want to have a brief exposure to rural life before racing back to a city for the long term. Interview day at Dartmouth is low-stress—interviewees may begin with a conversation with a generalist physician over breakfast of fresh baked goods and coffee.

The town of Hanover is insular but not provincial, thanks in large part to Dartmouth College. The isolation that Hanover affords can be wonderful—there are few distractions for students. The College does bring cultural events (e.g., dance troupes, musicians, film series) to its Hopkins Center, so the area is not as devoid of diversion as it otherwise might be. A number of stores and restaurants cater to the more urbane and expensive tastes brought to town by the steady stream of visiting Dartmouth alumni and parents.

Another benefit of Dartmouth's rural locale is that it is eminently safe. Crime is mostly limited to isolated incidents of petty theft, and many people don't bother to lock their doors. Rent is reasonable ($500–$600 per month for a one-bedroom apartment) and becomes increasingly cheap as one gets farther away from the campus. No on-campus housing is available for medical students, but the College does offer housing for married students. For those who find the slow pace of rural life infuriating, the cultural opportunities too limited, or the ethnic homogeneity of the region dull, escape is easy: Boston, Montreal, and New York are 2, 3, and 5 hours away, respectively.

The Bottom Line

Dartmouth Medical School offers students an Ivy League educational experience while they are part of a small, cooperative, and intimate group with extraordinary faculty access. The price one pays for this is a hefty tuition and four years of relative seclusion in rural New England. Dartmouth engenders a fierce and unique loyalty among its students that stands as a testament to the excellent and humane training the School provides.

DUKE UNIVERSITY SCHOOL OF MEDICINE

Durham, North Carolina

Tuition 1996–97: $26,700 per year
Applications: 6,549
Size of Entering Class: 100
Total Number of Women Students: 172 (43%)
Total Number of Men Students: 229 (57%)

World Wide Web: www2.mc.duke.edu/som/
Contact: Dr. Brenda Armstrong, Director of
Admissions
Durham, NC 27708-0586
919-684-2985

Established in 1925, Duke has been ranked consistently among the top medical schools in the country. The year of scholarly work has been the centerpiece of Duke's medical curriculum for more than thirty years and provides an excellent opportunity for in-depth learning in almost any field of interest. While a few students choose to earn a master's degree (M.P.H., M.P.P., or even an M.B.A.), most undertake extensive basic science or clinical research. Students with a Ph.D. can skip this year entirely.

Preclinical Years

First year at Duke is designed to get students out of the classroom and into the clinics as quickly as possible. This may sound intimidating, but the year is actually quite reasonable. Although embryology is notably missing and gross anatomy is only eight weeks long, the honors/pass/fail curriculum is remarkably complete, with little time wasted on irrelevant details. Students emerge with a solid foundation of basic science and medical knowledge and perform exceptionally well on the USMLE Step I.

Professors provide lecture notes and are generally available for questions. In addition, there are a student note-taking service and videotapes of the lectures. Computer-based learning is increasingly integrated into the curriculum. Most importantly, students' notebook computers (compliments of first-year fees) plug right into the network connections at each seat in the lecture hall and lab rooms.

First year is broken into five blocks, each roughly corresponding to a semester in a traditional curriculum. Like a well-paced workout, the first block (biochemistry, genetics, and cell biology) starts manageably, with a couple of short days each week (most students are home by 2 p.m.) and exams every two or three weeks. Block 2 (physiology, microanatomy, and gross anatomy) is the toughest of

the year, with almost no afternoons off and a grueling stretch of weekly exams. After a much-welcomed holiday break, Block 3 (devoted entirely to neurobiology) slows down a bit, with only the final exam to worry about. Blocks 4 and 5 (immunology, microbiology, pathology, and pharmacology), which focus more on clinical topics, are less intense than Block 2. Friday afternoons are free during these blocks, but most students are ecstatic when the single classroom year is over.

Clinical Years

While clinical rotations don't start until second year, clinical experience begins early in first year with the two-year practice course, where students cover everything from examination skills to health-care economics. With practice comes the first clinical exposure—Tuesday afternoons are spent shadowing a primary-care preceptor. However, many students dislike the specialty bashing of the practice course and jokingly refer to it as Duke's (futile) attempt to get more students into primary care.

After a brief three-week summer vacation, second year begins. Most rotations are performed at Duke Hospital or across the street at the Durham Veterans Administration Medical Center. These two hospitals offer plenty of exposure to patients with common diagnoses and some unusual diseases, which gives students some unique learning opportunities and plenty of tales to tell. Many students have subrotations at other hospitals and clinics, and everybody spends the monthlong Family Medicine rotation in clinics all over North Carolina.

Internal medicine is almost universally enjoyed, with strong teaching by high-quality residents and faculty members. Obstetrics/gynecology, by contrast, is not as favored among students because of department personalities. Surgery features excellent teaching, with a variable amount of hands-on experience. Pediatrics is also enjoyed by many, with opportunities for community experience and the new Children's Hospital soon to be completed.

Make no mistake, the first, second, and fourth years at Duke already provide an excellent, well-rounded medical education. But it's the third year that makes the Duke experience one of a kind.

The centerpiece of Duke's curriculum is the third year, which is composed of nine to twelve months of scholarly work. For most, this means medical research, but many pursue other options. The breadth of research covers everything from novel gene therapy to cutting-edge laser vision correction and allows students to do anything from bench-top pipetting to performing surgical procedures. Alternatives include earning a master's degree in public policy, public health, or even business administration (the last requiring an extra year). In addition, many students spend the year studying at other institutions such as at the Howard Hughes Medical Institute/National Institutes of Health Research Scholars Program ("The Cloisters"). Select students also receive other research grants and fellowships that are awarded on a national level.

Coming after a tough year of clinical rotations, the third year is the perfect time to reflect on directions for residency. Don't worry about your medical knowledge getting rusty—most students take USMLE Step I at the end of third year (because there's plenty of time to study), and this prepares them for fourth year. Don't forget, students who already have (or are in the process of earning) the letters Ph.D. after their name are exempt from the third year altogether and finish medical school in just three years.

Fourth year is different from second year, as it is composed entirely of clinical electives. Subinternships and intensive-care unit rotations are the most demanding but offer the greatest learning opportunities. Up to two months may be performed away from Duke; many students choose to rotate through hospitals of possible residency interest, and a number study abroad each year.

Social Life

Nestled in the beautiful green forests of the North Carolina Piedmont, Durham is less than a 3-hour drive from the Appalachian highlands and the Atlantic coast. With plenty of lakes, parks, and trails, this area is perfect for outdoor activities. The Sarah P. Duke Gardens, a 55-acre landscaped and wooded gardens adorned with more than 1,500 types of plants, is located just adjacent to the main campus.

As a private school, Duke draws about 80 percent of its students from outside of North Carolina (perhaps encouraged in part by the regional interview option for applicants). Duke has a diverse mix of students, not only in gender and ethnicity but also in background and interests. There are always a few Ph.D.'s in each class, and plenty of people are straight out of college. A small fraction of students are married upon matriculation, and that number increases rapidly over the four years.

Rent is cheap in Durham, so almost all students live in apartment complexes or houses around Duke. For less than $600 a month, students can rent an older two-bedroom apartment within walking distance of Duke. However, $750 a month fetches a spacious two-bedroom apartment in a nicer part of town, with only a 5- to 10-minute drive to campus. A car is essentially required.

Durham is no big city when it comes to nightlife and entertainment, but there are a few choice places. Many students like to hang out at Satisfactions, a local sports bar with great pizza. Ninth Street is Duke's diminutive version of a college strip, so many prefer the excitement of University of North Carolina's (UNC) Franklin Street in nearby Chapel Hill. Of course, UNC is also known for its fierce basketball rivalry with Duke, where interest in NCAA basketball borders on obsession. Recreational sports with classmates are always popular, and there are year-round intramural sports with the undergraduates. As far as professional teams, the hometown Durham Bulls is the professional baseball club made famous by the 1987 blockbuster *Bull Durham*. Other professional teams in the region include the NBA's Charlotte Hornets, NFL's Carolina Panthers, and NHL's Carolina Hurricanes.

The Bottom Line

A perennial top-five school, Duke offers only one year in the classroom, outstanding clinical training, and a unique bonus year of scholarly work, allowing time to chalk up research experience with internationally known faculty members.

EAST CAROLINA UNIVERSITY SCHOOL OF MEDICINE

Greenville, North Carolina

Size of Entering Class: 72
Total Number of Women Students: 165 (48%)
Total Number of Men Students: 182 (52%)
World Wide Web: www.med.ecu.edu/
Contact: Dr. Sam Pennington, Associate Dean for
Research and Graduate Studies

East Fifth Street
Greenville, NC 27858-4353
252-816-2827

Set in the heart of eastern North Carolina tobacco country, this humble medical school packs quite a punch. What began as a one-year program at a small rural county hospital in 1972 has now blossomed into a twenty-one-year-old fully accredited four-year medical school at a major tertiary-care center. East Carolina University (ECU) has earned its reputation for rural health and family medicine from its mission to produce primary-care physicians to care for the underserved populations of eastern North Carolina. ECU attracts North Carolinians of all types. The University has a large contingent of nontraditional students and students who are members of minority groups, and its students are graduates of colleges and universities from all over the country. No matter what a student's background, ECU fosters an environment of teamwork and camaraderie. This is exemplified by the infamous annual water-gun fight between the first- and second-year students that occurs in spite of the administration's threats to prevent it. Perhaps it is the small class size or perhaps it is the dedication of the faculty that makes this medical school such a nurturing environment. However, there's something about ECU that makes it a fun and exciting setting for medical school education.

Admissions/Financial Aid

For those sweating the cost of medical school, financial aid is available in the form of federal loans. However, few students are awarded need-based scholarships due to the already-low cost of tuition and living at ECU.

Preclinical Years

Preclinical years are almost a misnomer for the first two years at ECU. Anatomy, biochemistry, physiology,

pathology, and pharmacology are all strong, which leaves little else lacking in preparation for the boards. In the midst of building a strong foundation in the basic sciences, clinical training begins. One afternoon a week for the entire two years is spent learning clinical skills. This time is spent not only working with standardized patients but also practicing history and physical diagnostic skills on patients in the adjacent Pitt County Memorial Hospital. Students also serve as guinea pigs for a prototypical standardized patient exam destined to join the national licensing board exam. Because ECU is a relatively new school, one of its strengths is its facilities: labs and classrooms are state-of-the-art. The newly renovated student lounge comes complete with couches, billiards, Foosball, and a wide-screen TV, making study breaks perhaps a little too tempting. Faculty members at ECU are also outstanding. They have been known to arrange extra help sessions early in the morning before class or to roam the halls in the wee hours of the night before exams in case a desperate student is in need of last-minute tutoring. Where else would you see bouquets of handpicked flowers set beside specimens during a neuroanatomy practical exam? In fact, the students are so enamored with the faculty that they choose to end each semester with a large potluck before exams in honor of their professors.

Although ECU is not known for being a research institution, there are plenty of research opportunities for the summer between first and second year. Other popular summer opportunities in addition to research include rural health programs, clinical externships, tutoring medical school prep courses, and travel.

Clinical Years

It should come as no surprise that the clinical years at ECU place greater emphasis on family medicine than do most medical schools across the country. Third year is divided into eight-week blocks of internal medicine, ob/gyn, psychiatry, family medicine, pediatrics, and surgery. Time not spent at Pitt County Memorial Hospital is spent in the surrounding rural counties during the psychiatry, family medicine, and pediatric clerkships. Do not fret about a lack of breadth at ECU during the clinical years—hands-on opportunities abound at this tertiary-care center. Pitt County Memorial Hospital draws from a wide referral base that spans I-95 to the coast of North Carolina, offering its pupils plenty of pathology to add to their repertoire. On inpatient services, no medical student is made to feel like a wallflower. Students are an integral part of the team and are encouraged to take on as much responsibility as they are comfortable taking. The ob/gyn and surgery clerkships are especially known for offering hands-on experience. Rural sites also serve as excellent opportunities for learning procedures without competing with residents for experience.

After weathering the trials and tribulations of third year, students are rewarded with a year of electives. In keeping with ECU's primary-care mission, two primary-care requirements must be fulfilled from dozens of choices. For those with a more adventuresome side, the administration is flexible in helping create individually designed electives, including travel abroad or research projects. Foremost on most fourth-year students' minds, however, is how to spend the four weeks of vacation allowed anytime throughout the year. While most spend at least part of this time interviewing for residency programs, there are no stipulations against using it for, say, honeymoons, cruises, or studying for Step II of the boards. Senior medical students are equally preoccupied with the infamous Match Day. Every year, 56 percent of ECU students choose a career in primary care, including family medicine, internal medicine, and pediatrics. ECU also has its share of aspiring surgeons (including neurosurgery, ophthalmology, and urology), dermatologists, and obstetricians/gynecologists. In the past several years, approximately three quarters of the graduating class has matched in one of their top three choices in programs across the country.

Social Life

Believe it or not, there is time at ECU to spend outside of the classrooms, labs, clinics, and hospital to have a life. City slickers need not despair. Greenville, with a population of approximately 55,000, has plenty of cultural events and shopping (at least there are a Barnes & Noble and a Gap) to offer. The University has an excellent fine arts program that presents the community with theater, concerts, and symphonies. Even the Vienna Boys' Choir has made its way to this quaint oasis. Of course, the rural location offers outdoor activities that range from hunting to mountain biking. When you feel the need to get away from the daily grind, North Carolina's beautiful beaches are within a 2-hour drive, as is the more metropolitan Raleigh/Durham/Chapel Hill area, with the Appalachian Mountains 5 to 6 hours away. The low cost of living in Greenville, where one- or two-bedroom apartments are available for $300–$600 per month, is hard to beat.

The School has its mission to thank for the rich diversity in its medical student body; ECU was commissioned, in part, to provide opportunities to minority and disadvantaged students. The student body ranges from 20 to 50 years old, with a high percentage of minority students, and the School recently graduated the first congenitally hard-of-hearing doctor. Don't let ECU's small size fool you. The average class size at ECU averages 72 students. ECU houses very strong chapters in national medical organizations, including the American Medical Association (awarded national chapter of the month in January 1998), the American Medical Women's Association, the Student National Medical Association (serving minority communities), and the American Medical Student Association. ECU also coordinates several local community outreach programs, such as working in the local homeless shelter clinic. On a lighter note, the small class size affords strong camaraderie within and between classes, with practical jokes galore to break the tension during exam time.

The Bottom Line

ECU is definitely not a big-name school that turns heads, but it is a bargain. With the cheapest in-state tuition in the country, one of the lowest costs of living, and a first-class medical education, the deal that ECU offers its students cannot be beat. Although students are well educated in all aspects of medicine, this is the place for those seeking rich rural or primary-care experiences.

EAST TENNESSEE STATE UNIVERSITY JAMES H. QUILLEN COLLEGE OF MEDICINE

Johnson City, Tennessee

Tuition 1996–97: $19,258 per year
Size of Entering Class: 60
Total Number of Women Students: 124 (43%)
Total Number of Men Students: 164 (57%)
World Wide Web: qcom.etsu.edu/

Contact: Edwin D. Taylor, Assistant Dean for
Admissions and Records
Box 70734
Johnson City, TN 37614-0734
423-439-6221

Set at the foot of the Appalachian Mountains in northeast Tennessee, a fairly rural, lower socioeconomic area, the James H. Quillen College of Medicine has, since its founding in 1978, taken pride in producing high-quality primary-care physicians. Consistently more than 60 percent of graduates choose residencies in primary care, and many of these physicians practice in a rural setting. This focused commitment has allowed Quillen to become a national leader in the training of primary-care physicians, illustrated by *U.S. News & World Report* ranking Quillen sixth in the nation for programs in rural medicine.

The Rural Primary Care Track (RPCT) is a unique opportunity for students to be intimately involved in rural medicine throughout the four years of medical school. The W. K. Kellogg Foundation granted $6 million to Quillen for this program, of which about 15 percent of students take advantage. Still, many graduates do not choose primary care, and students are encouraged to pursue whatever field of medicine they choose.

Preclinical Years

One of the strengths of Quillen is the collegial responsibility taken by each student to assist classmates. It is not uncommon for students to make copies of helpful articles or of charts they've compiled for every student, then distribute the copies anonymously in student mailboxes.

Quillen's schedule the first two years is traditional. Gross anatomy, biochemistry, histology, physiology, and neurology are taught the first year, while pathology, pharmacology, microbiology, and psychiatry are taught the second year. Each course holds four to five tests per semester, which are grouped in blocks of two to three days.

Grading is letter ranked, and B's are given generously. Two to four students in each class must typically repeat a year.

In general, students give high marks to gross anatomy, microbiology, and pathology because the course directors have the ability to make material relevant to patient care—this in spite of the fact that many students' only clinical exposure during the first two years is during Christmas break, when relatives ask them to take a look at "this funny rash." Professors and attendings are friends as well as educators and make themselves readily available at almost any hour.

Students bemoan two shortcomings in the first two years: a lack of electives and a lack of research opportunities. Although research projects are available, options are limited. Similarly, while free time should be available for electives, students are kept busy in Practicing Medicine, a course that spends many hours per week teaching skills that could be acquired in a fraction of the time.

In the summer between first and second year, students may perform research projects, mostly clinical research or epidemiology-based projects. Lab work is difficult to find.

A few recent improvements include many new computers with Internet access in the student lounge, and the new medical education building scheduled for completion in the spring of 2. Both of these were sorely needed and represent the support of Quillen by the community and the state government.

The RPCT is a unique program spanning all four years. RPCT students attend didactic and clinical courses in a rural hospital and clinic one day per week for the first two years. The day RPCT students attend the clinic, traditional-track students have a clinical skills course and lectures in medical specialties. During the third year, RPCT students spend four months in a rural setting and rotate in family medicine and internal medicine. While no financial benefits are offered for choosing this path, many RPCT students sign contracts with local hospitals to pay back one year of postresidency service for one year's tuition.

Clinical Years

With a formal affiliation with five area teaching hospitals that provide access to more than 2,300 patient beds, students are afforded a great deal of patient contact. Residents or attendings are on hand to provide guidance and to educate, sometimes resulting in minimal individual initiative. One exception is the Mountain Home Veterans Affairs Hospital, in the middle of Johnson City. Students are treated with respect and trust by an excellent faculty that is dedicated to education.

Surgery is one of the better rotations. Pediatrics and family medicine also are well organized. The weakest rotation is obstetrics and gynecology, where students have chronically complained of subpar teaching and organization. Psychiatry also leaves something to be desired. In both of these rotations, students spend varying amounts of time in different hospitals, which alters experiences.

Social Life

The population of Johnson City, located at the base of Great Smoky Mountains National Park, is 55,000, although two other cities are within 20 miles, bringing the nearby population to 450,000. Because of the great natural beauty surrounding this area, outdoor activities abound. Several state parks, including the Blue Ridge Parkway, and five Tennessee Valley Authority lakes provide spectacular mountain biking, hiking, fishing, snow skiing and waterskiing, sailing, and world-class white-water rafting and kayaking.

Housing is very affordable. A one-bedroom apartment runs about $350 to $450 per month. Many students choose to buy a condominium; a new two-bedroom is about $70,000. Housing close to the hospital and the school is readily available. All housing options have a wonderful view of the surrounding mountains as well.

Living in the midst of miles of natural beauty makes for a limited nightlife. While bars and clubs exist, many nights are spent at individuals' parties. The area is quite homogeneous, with the population made up of mostly white Protestants.

The Bottom Line

The James H. Quillen College of Medicine, while weak in a few areas, provides a high-quality medical education in a nurturing environment.

EASTERN VIRGINIA MEDICAL SCHOOL

Norfolk, Virginia

Students Receiving Financial Aid: 85%
Applications: 5,655
Size of Entering Class: 100
Total Number of Women Students: 177 (44%)
Total Number of Men Students: 228 (56%)

World Wide Web: www.evms.edu/
Contact: Susan Castora, Director of Admissions
Box 1980
Norfolk, VA 23501-1980
757-446-5812

Eastern Virginia Medical School (EVMS) does an excellent job at introducing, guiding, and, ultimately, preparing a student for the years of residency. It fosters a noncompetitive environment and provides opportunities for research and community involvement for anyone from the minimally motivated student to the basic overachiever. Medical school is more about what students make of it than where they go, but it is critically important to receive the necessary tools to move toward the next phase of training.

Admissions/Financial Aid

As it is a state-supported school, many of the entering medical students at EVMS are residents of the state of Virginia. In recent years, about 30 percent of students have been from other states. The mean age among entering students in the last couple of years has been between 25 and 27, with many of them having advanced degrees.

EVMS receives about 4,000 to 6,000 applications per year. About 10 percent of the applicants are interviewed to arrive at a class size of 100. Qualities such as a strong academic background and intelligence are important, but equally important are commitment and compassion. The admissions committee is composed of basic science professors, clinical faculty members, and two members of each class. Those medical students not on the committee are encouraged to participate in the interviews and give input regarding the ultimate acceptance of the prospective applicant.

The annual tuition for a resident and a nonresident are $14,500 and $26,000, respectively. Numerous loans (both School-administered and federal subsidized and nonsubsidized) are available. All students applying for financial aid are required to submit parental tax information so that a packet of aid can be determined. In addition, special scholar-

ships are available for students who desire to work in underserved areas upon the completion of their residency.

Of special note, EVMS is committed to the recruitment and retention of minority students. The office of minority affairs serves as a contact source and also makes recommendations for interviews and awards scholarships. Premed students may take part in the summer enrichment program. This program is a six- to eight-week mini-medical school session that allows college students to experience what medical school is all about. Students take similar courses (e.g., biochemistry and gross anatomy) as well as work with a member of the clinical faculty once a week. They even participate in mock exams held by members of the admissions committee. Once enrolled, minority students may take advantage of the number of resources provided, including textbooks and tutorial services.

Preclinical Years

Classes in the first year usually start at 8 or 9 a.m. and finish around 3 or 4 p.m. Most of the course instructors hand out syllabi (which tend to be thick) and, for the most part, test questions are directly from that information. Most of the faculty members are supportive and are available for questions or additional assistance. A student progress committee is notified if a student is not performing well, and special arrangements are made with a faculty member for tutorial sessions. Exams are given approximately every three to four weeks and the majority are multiple choice. The grading system works in a honors/high pass/pass/marginal/fail system. The top third of students achieve a high pass and the top 5 percent receive honors.

During the summer months between the first and second years, students are afforded numerous opportunities that range from research to summer jobs to taking part in community service activities.

Some of the research projects provide monetary compensation and may include working in such areas as the Diabetes Institute, the Jones Institute, and the Pediatric Research Institute. For those less inclined to scholastic endeavors, daily visits to Virginia Beach are possible, which is located within 25 minutes of the campus.

Before students realize it, that twelve-week break passes with alarming speed and second-year classes begin. This time, many of the classes are year-round, and those nice complete syllabi are no longer available. The material is not quite as familiar, and much of the burden to extract the information from the text is the student's. The positive side is that students finally feel as if the material is relevant and they enjoy learning. Also, working with actual patients is increased and classes in diagnosis and physical exam skills are emphasized. When classes finally end in May, students are given approximately five weeks off. Three to four of these weeks should be for studying for USMLE. Students may study independently or take a review course. There is a nominal fee ($700), and classes are six days per week, typically from 8 a.m. to 5 p.m. In recent years, the pass rate has been 95 percent.

Clinical Years

The clinical years begin with a two-week orientation that reviews such issues as what to expect from each required clerkship, patient care, medical records/charting, and ACLS certification. The rotations are divided into two blocks (i.e., pediatrics/surgery/obstetrics and gynecology and family/internal/psych). Students have a choice in selecting their rotations, but they must be taken within the designated blocks (e.g., if surgery was the first rotation, it cannot be followed by family medicine). It is not generally possible to do a fourth-year elective before completing a core. The various hospital settings include community, private, military, and veterans' hospitals. For the most part, the clinical experience received is excellent.

The fourth year of medical school is a time to celebrate. Much of the work has already been done. Students' only job is to pick a specialty and proceed with the task of finding employment in July. While you still have to take rotations, many of them are what students choose to do. The only stipulations are that every student has to do one week of substance abuse prevention, two weeks of geriatric, two 2-week blocks of surgical subspecialty, and eight weeks off. Excellent rotations include trauma and emergency medicine.

Social Life

The city of Norfolk is one of seven cities that make up the area known as Hampton Roads. Norfolk does not attract students in the same capacity as some of the larger cities like New York or Atlanta. However, upon closer inspection, students realize its more notable qualities. In celebrating its nautical heritage, there are a number of summer festivals as well as various pop artists/symphony/opera seasonal performances. This area is strategically placed for weekend excursions to Washington, D.C., Charlottesville, or the Outer Banks of North Carolina. Each fall and spring, a three-day weekend retreat is sponsored by the Human Values Program, during which students participate in various workshops, and many students mostly enjoy basking in the sun and attending late-night parties.

Most of the students live in a section of Norfolk near the medical school known as Ghent, a charming neighborhood with Victorian homes and tree-lined streets. Across from the school is an apartment complex owned and operated by EVMS. One- and two-bedroom options are available (ranging between $475 and $650 per month). Other housing options in the area range from $350 to $1,000 per month (depending on individual tastes). There are usually cheaper options in Virginia Beach or Portsmouth, but students then have to contend with traffic. Many affordable restaurants/bars/coffee shops (First Coffee Colony and margaritas at Colley Cantina are not to be missed) are in the area within walking distance. By exercising safety precautions and some degree of intelligence, most students don't have any problems with crime.

On campus, EVMS students have almost unlimited opportunities to design organizations and associations according to the changing interests of the student body. The surgery club, operation smile, yearbook club, AMSA, and women in medicine club are only a few of the activities in which EVMS students can become involved. Climate may range from humid summer days with temperatures higher than 100 to cold (even snowy) days with temperatures in the teens.

The Bottom Line

Because of its youth, EVMS sometimes struggles to compete with more established medical schools in the neighboring area. Nonetheless, it provides a noncompetitive environment and a firm educational foundation. While an EVMS degree may not bring about immediate fame and recognition, students continue to have equal opportunities in obtaining competitive residencies.

EMORY UNIVERSITY SCHOOL OF MEDICINE

Atlanta, Georgia

Tuition 1996–97: $25,770 per year
Size of Entering Class: 111
World Wide Web: www.emory.edu/WHSC/MED
Contact: Dr. John Stone, Associate Dean and
Director of Admissions

Atlanta, GA 30322-1100
404-727-5660

Located adjacent to the U.S. Centers for Disease Control and Prevention and the national headquarters for the American Cancer Society in what is arguably the most scenic area of Atlanta, Emory University School of Medicine is on a mission to become the premier medical school of the Southeast. Emory continues to attract and cultivate leaders in the field of medicine (and build new hospitals at an astounding rate).

In 1997, Emory received 7,765 applications for positions in the first-year medical school class. From this pool, approximately 10 percent were interviewed and 3 percent accepted. In addition to one-on-one interviews, Emory continues to use a panel interview (three applicants on one side of the table and three interviewers on the other). Approximately 40 percent of the students are women, and 15 percent are described as minority. The average Emory student scored 30.6 on the MCAT and graduated with a 3.64 grade point average from their undergraduate institution.

Since Emory is a private school, everybody pays the same tuition: $25,770, plus $400 in fees. Tuition rates for entering classes are frozen for all four years. Students feel that the financial aid department is approachable and attentive to their needs. In fact, the financial aid office often sponsors lunches, during which students can voice concerns or offer praise. Roughly three fourths of the students receive financial aid, with 64 percent receiving some form of scholarship or grant, including seven students each year who receive full scholarships through the merit-based Woodruff Scholarship Program. The average indebtedness for Emory's 1998 graduates who received financial aid was $84,695.

Preclinical Years

Emory's preclinical curriculum is a series of full- and half-year courses in anatomy, biochemistry, pathology, physiology, pathophysiology, cell biology, and neuroanatomy. First-year students are tested only three times during the year; second-year students enjoy a fourth test. These joint exams cover all subjects and usually last all day. Students say they loathe these joint exams, but most agree the long testing period prepares them well for the USMLE exams. Emory's average USMLE Step I score has consistently been in the 90th percentile nationwide.

Legend has it that Emory students used to climb trees outside the anatomy lab on the night before exams in an attempt to see the topics on which the professors would be testing them. A frustrated professor found out and chopped all the trees down in the courtyard. While students generally do not feel they go to such lengths for grades, they have to work hard. Professors have stopped wielding axes, but they certainly do not make their courses easy. The bar is set very high, and A's are difficult to come by. Despite this challenging environment, students work together, studying and sharing materials, and are not competitive toward each other.

Only one preclinical elective is offered during the second year. Students choose from more than thirty courses, including Reading Chest Films, Medical Spanish, Medical Literature, and Cardiology Examination.

Approximately 60 percent of Emory medical students choose to work on a research project during their training, with 20 percent participating in an international project. Every year, the administration publishes a guide for students who wish to perform research. The guide lists clinical and laboratory researchers interested in taking on students. Many students use the time between their first and second year to work on a project. More than 40 percent of Emory students submit or publish a paper before they graduate.

Clinical Years

With more than eighty hospitals located in the Atlanta area, Emory medical students train at large and varied hospitals and specialty clinics, including Emory University Hospital (587 beds), Atlanta Veterans Administration Hospital (321 beds), Grady Memorial Hospital (1,050 beds), Crawford Long Hospital (583 beds), Egleston Children's Hospital/Scottish Rite (235 beds), Hughes Spalding Children's Hospital (72 beds), and Wesley Woods Geriatric Center (100 beds).

Letter grades are issued during the clerkship years. Most required rotations (medicine, surgery, pediatrics, psychiatry, ob/gyn, neurology) rely heavily on the national miniboard shelf exam for students' grades. Students who receive excellent ward evaluations and score well above the national average on the miniboard may be frustrated when they receive a B for the clerkship because so many classmates scored well above the national average.

The strong classroom and clinical training makes Emory students competitive in the match, and, every year, Emory matches students with some of the country's most competitive residency programs. Approximately 90 percent of Emory's students match at one of their top three choices and 65–70 percent match at their top choice.

Social Life

Emory students are very social. The celebrations that followed joint exams became so big that the administration finally decided that having classes the day after joints was useless, so they canceled the classes. In addition, there are Halloween parties, Christmas parties, and a formal Cadaver Ball that is held every spring.

Beyond Emory, Atlanta has a lot to offer. The Atlanta Braves offer their fans a wide range of ticket prices. The Atlanta Falcons have enjoyed much success as of late on the football field, and construction is under way on a new basketball arena for the Atlanta Hawks. In addition, Atlanta has recently acquired a professional hockey franchise.

Other sites of interest include the High Museum of Art, which features a modest permanent collection but features fabulous touring exhibits. The Fox Theater and several outdoor amphitheaters provide excellent venues for concerts and visiting Broadway productions. Students have a wide variety of restaurants and bars to choose from.

Most students choose to live near Emory's campus. One bedroom apartments range from $750 to $900 per month. Rent for two-bedroom apartments usually exceeds $1,000 per month. Many students rent houses together in one of Atlanta's trendiest areas, the Virginia Highlands, located only a few miles from Emory.

The Bottom Line

Emory University School of Medicine is a terrific school in a city that caters to a young population. Emory's strengths are staggering resources, outstanding preparation for the boards, and in-the-trenches training at Grady Hospital.

FINCH UNIVERSITY OF HEALTH SCIENCES/THE CHICAGO MEDICAL SCHOOL

North Chicago, Illinois

Tuition 1996–97: $32,270 per year
Applications: 11,211
Size of Entering Class: 150
Total Number of Women Students: 297 (39%)
Total Number of Men Students: 461 (61%)
World Wide Web: www.finchcms.edu/

Contact: Kristine Jones, Director of Admissions
and Records
3333 Green Bay Road
North Chicago, IL 60064-3095
847-578-3204

Finch University of Health Sciences/The Chicago Medical School (FUHS/CMS) has the distinction of having as one of its major clinical sites Cook County Hospital, the location on which the television show *E.R.* is based. Although the School is located in North Chicago, a 45-minute drive from downtown Chicago, many students live in Chicago itself, and the School serves a diverse population of patients in Chicago, North Chicago, and other surrounding suburbs.

Preclinical Years

Classes begin at a snail's pace. Most students take advantage of the start of first semester to go downtown, explore Chicago, party, and collect their thoughts. About three weeks into the academic year, gross anatomy starts, with 5 to 6 hours of class a day. Fortunately, most CMS departments prepare class notes that are distributed at the beginning of each semester. A student-run transcript service is also usually available for those classes without department notes. The combination makes most classes optional.

The new Student Learning Resource Center has an impressive library and computer facility, which many first-year classes use to provide additional study material such as histology and neuroscience slides. Professors maintain an open-door policy and heed student concerns. Because CMS emphasizes education over research, students are never overlooked. Classes are graded on a scale of A, B, C, and F, which fosters competition. Students are usually given a day between each different subject exam.

An integral part of the first- and second-year curriculum is the Introduction to Clinical Medicine (ICM). This class uses the classroom and outside

physician preceptors to teach students the proper techniques of history taking and physical examination at various hospital sites and offices. Students own a stethoscope and a sphygmomanometer. More important, they learn that sphygmomanometer is a fancy word for blood pressure cuff and they learn how to use it. In the second year, students examine real patients in preparation for third-year clerkships.

During the summer between first and second year, some students choose to vacation, while others seek employment to offset mounting debt. Students can do research on a CMS summer research fellowship, serve as a teaching assistant for gross anatomy, work toward a master's in pathology, shadow a physician, or observe the emergency room at Mount Sinai Hospital, a Level I trauma center for the city of Chicago.

The second year is much like the first, but most students find it far more interesting because pharmacology, pathology, and microbiology become more patient oriented. One strength at CMS is pathology, which is taught by the coauthors of the *Board Review Series for Pathology* (Williams & Wilkins). In addition, CMS emphasizes teaching that prepares students for board exams. Students are also given three to four weeks off to study before the USMLE Step I.

Clinical Years

Third and fourth year is when FUHS/CMS shines. Students draw blood, start IVs, place central lines, place arterial lines, close at the end of surgical procedures, reduce fractures, place and remove chest tubes, and intubate patients, all accompanied by a commitment to teaching from attendings and residents.

Required third-year rotations are emergency medicine, family medicine, medicine, medicine core, obstetrics and gynecology, pediatrics, psychiatry, surgery, neurology, and ambulatory care. Teaching hospital affiliations include Cook County Hospital, Illinois Masonic Medical Center, Edward Hines Veterans Administration Medical Center, Lutheran General Hospital, Mount Sinai Hospital and Medical Center, North Chicago Veterans Administration Medical Center, Norwalk Hospital (a private hospital in Connecticut), Swedish Covenant Hospital, and Henry Ford Hospital. Students can apply to spend several rotations or the entire third year at Henry Ford, which is located in Detroit, Michigan.

Surgery is an outstanding rotation at all sites, although the experience varies between sites, as it does for all clerkships. For example, students who complete surgery at Lutheran General Hospital miss out on trauma experience, but they also escape call responsibilities.

Emergency medicine is a standout rotation. Students rotate through the Cook County emergency room or the Mount Sinai Hospital emergency room, both Level I trauma centers, for four weeks during their third year. "See one, do one, teach one" is the prevailing educational philosophy here.

Fourth year is very flexible and allows students to prepare for USMLE Step II and gather their materials for residency applications. Students are required to take a four-week medical subinternship and four weeks in a primary-care setting. Fourteen weeks are designated for electives at CMS-affiliated hospitals, while another fourteen weeks are also allowed for externships and electives at other sites. Sports medicine, urogynecology, and surgical critical care are only a few of the electives offered at CMS. The Office for Student Affairs (OSA) makes counseling students and preparing them for the match a priority throughout the first three years.

Social Life

Students at FUHS/CMS are graduates of a wide array of undergraduate institutions. The class of 2002 comprises sixty-eight women and 112 men, who range in age from 20 to 56 and come from twenty-five different states.

Living for four years in the Chicago area allows students the opportunity to take advantage of the city's rich cultural diversity, including its museums, theater, and historic sites. Chicago is filled with young professionals, and there are plenty of clubs, bars, and sporting events. A student-run intramural sports league is also popular. The FUHS/CMS Student Council provides guidance and structure for more than twenty-five student-run clubs and organizations.

Most students live in the Woodlands, an apartment complex adjacent to the School. One-bedroom apartments range from $749 to $889 and two-bedrooms range from $849 to $1039. Others live in Chicago or Evanston, all within convenient driving distances.

The Bottom Line

CMS, despite the hefty price tag, turns well-rounded students into well-rounded physicians, thanks to extensive hands-on training and outstanding clinical exposure.

GEORGETOWN UNIVERSITY SCHOOL OF MEDICINE

Washington, District of Columbia

Tuition 1996–97: $28,650 per year
Size of Entering Class: 185
Total Number of Women Students: 288 (40%)
Total Number of Men Students: 439 (60%)
World Wide Web: www.dml.georgetown.edu/schmed

Contact: Karen Pfordresher, Assistant Dean for Admissions
37th and O Street, NW
Washington, DC 20057
202-687-1154

Georgetown University is the oldest Jesuit institution in the United States. Education is a Jesuit tradition, and the education you will receive at Georgetown is excellent but rigorous. On your first visit as an applicant to Georgetown, you will meet Ms. Sullivan, the admissions adviser, who introduces you to the school and its traditions. Even more important, she tells applicants the specifics about medical school, and she tells it like it is. Some people think this is offsetting. Others appreciate that she doesn't sugarcoat what is likely to be the toughest four years of your life.

Preclinical Years

Students begin their training with anatomy, including gross anatomy, microanatomy, and embryology. Though there is an attempt to integrate these classes, there is often just enough disconnection to leave you confused. The curriculum tends to become more symbiotic after that, however, when classes are taught in large blocks, including biochemistry, physiology, endocrinology, and neuroanatomy.

Georgetown has incorporated problem-based learning (PBL) into the curriculum. Each session consists of eight students and a preceptor working through a clinical case. The cases focus on the specific block being taught. Students are given new data during each session and are asked to perform research on their specific topic prior to the next session. The actual quality of instruction depends quite heavily on how involved the students are and the background of the instructor. At the very least, however, students do tend to become experts at effective library search techniques. The groups and instructors are assigned randomly, but this helps you meet students you might not otherwise meet.

In addition to the basic science/PBL curriculum, students must also learn about the social dynamics of medicine and health care, including biostatistics, epidemiology, and introduction to patient care. Students begin to see patients during the second semester, when they follow a primary-care physician in his or her clinic one day a week. Students usually like this first taste of clinical medicine.

Between the first and second years, students are given two months off. Many perform research at Georgetown or the nearby National Institutes of Health. The second year covers disease processes. Classes are taken concurrently and cover immunology, microbiology, pharmacology, and pathology. Georgetown has one of the longest pharmacology classes (three quarters) and pathology classes ($3\frac{1}{2}$ quarters) of any medical school in the United States. Students find this extended curriculum useful when taking their boards. In addition, students continue ambulatory care, usually with a different primary-care physician. In their second year, students usually take a more active role in the clinic. In addition, special opportunities, such as emergency room or hospice, are available. Students have a physical diagnosis class taught by the affable Dr. Tsou. The first half of this course has students learning the basics of the physical exam. The second half has students gaining hands-on experience in the hospital by taking complete histories and performing complete physicals on patients. A problem-solving course covers various topics, including hematology, dermatology, sexuality, and electives. Lectures and discussions in bioethics are given in the fourth quarter.

Nurses and graduate students join medical students in the first two years. Most notable of these are the students who are pursuing a masters degree in physiology (Physios). These usually are students who are trying to improve their medical school application by showing that they can succeed in first-year medical school classes. Needless to say, these students can be competitive. Their competitive streak, however, does not always rub off on the rest of the class. Classes are graded honors (top 10 percent), high pass (next greater than 10 percent), pass-low pass (bottom 10 percent), and fail (two standard deviations below the mean). Grades are derived mainly from multiple-choice examinations. There has been some discussion about switching the courses, especially the first-year courses, to pass/fail.

A student-run Medical Note Taking Service (MNTS) transcribes most lectures. The student note-takers are paid well, so the notes produced are usually of high quality and include graphs and detailed explanations.

Clinical Years

Third year is pretty inflexible. All students take four weeks each of neurology, psychiatry, and family practice; six weeks each of pediatrics and ob/gyn; twelve weeks of medicine; and twelve weeks of surgery. The majority of the third year is spent at Georgetown; however, students also rotate through Arlington Hospital, Fairfax Hospital, Walter Reed Army Medical Center, Bethesda Naval Medical Center, and the Veterans Administration. The teaching at Georgetown and Walter Reed is outstanding. Fairfax and Arlington are more community-based hospitals, so the patient volume is greater. Except for family practice, the majority of time is spent with the house staff (residents). However, all rotations have scheduled lectures by attendings. At the end of each rotation, a multiple-choice boards-type exam is given. You need a car to get to all the hospitals. Parking at all of the hospitals, except Georgetown, is free. Georgetown is $6 per day, except for weekends.

Dean Robinowitz likes to say that fourth year is as flexible as third year is inflexible. Students are required to do a six-week acting internship (AI) in

medicine and surgery, four weeks in ER, and two 4-week blocks of primary care. That leaves five monthlong blocks to take electives and one month for vacation. Electives can be taken at any hospital in the U.S., and international electives are also available. Students are treated like interns on the AIs, including being responsible for cross-covering other patients. These are tough rotations, but they help prove to fourth years that they really do know what to do when the pager goes off, and that means intern year is less intimidating. There is discussion of breaking the AIs down to three blocks of four weeks: a month on medicine, a month on surgery, and a month in your anticipated specialty.

Social Life

The high cost of education tends to bring together a certain subset of students who are able to bear the financial burden of one of the more expensive schools in the nation. Students tend to be young and single. A fair number are also on military scholarships.

Washington, D.C., is a great place to go to school, and you will find that four years is probably not enough to do everything there is to do. There are plenty of outdoor activities, including many trails for biking or jogging. Nightlife is also plentiful, with most first-year students haunting Georgetown at night, then migrating to the Adams Morgan and Dupont Circle areas as they tire of the college bar scene. Most first and second years live near the medical school in either Foxhall or Glover Park. There are group homes and apartments here within easy walking distance of the School. Rent is average for a big city (about $400 to $500 per roommate per month), and the School has an extensive network for helping students find roommates. Single basement apartments are a little more expensive. Third- and fourth-year students tend to move out to Virginia.

The Bottom Line

The price is steep, but the rewards tend to be many: an exciting city, a rich academic tradition, and a social student body.

GEORGE WASHINGTON UNIVERSITY SCHOOL OF MEDICINE AND HEALTH SCIENCES

Washington, District of Columbia

Size of Entering Class: 153
World Wide Web: www.gwumc.edu/edu
Contact: Dr. Allan B. Weingold, Vice President for Academic Affairs

Washington, DC 20052

George Washington University (GWU) offers students many perks, but they come at a high price. Students who graduate from GWU leave with memories of studying on the National Mall, shopping and playing in Georgetown, and listening to congressional debates. Ironically enough for a school located in the nation's capital, though, GWU gets no federal funding, making the school's tuition one of the highest in the country. Students need to seriously consider how in debt they want to be if they want to attend GWU.

Admissions/Financial Aid

The class size averages about 150. Student ages range from 21 to the 40's. For the class of 2001, the range was 20 to 39, with an average age of 24. GWU is proud to accept nontraditional students, and, as a result, many students are older with families. There are always cliques but these tend to disintegrate during the third and fourth years when students are placed on rotations in random order.

The financial aid office is small but makes a concerted effort to know all the students in the class. There are mandatory sessions held yearly to help counsel students about their cumulative debt burden. The office also distributes periodic notices to inform students about new loan opportunities and alternative sources of funding.

Preclinical Years

The first two years recently have been altered to integrate the various disciplines better as well as to increase the amount of group problem-solving time. The lectures tend to be standard fare, but the Practice of Medicine (POM) program introduced in fall 1993 has helped keep the education a bit more up to date with the recent changes in medical education. The program lasts for all four years of medical school, and, in the first two years, focuses on patient interviewing,

physical diagnosis, and problem-based learning. Early on, the class was rife with problems, but the administration has been duly responsive to student criticism; of primary importance, the amount of additional lecture time was scaled back. Though students still complain about the utility of the small group discussions, many find later on that they learned valuable clinical problem-solving skills. The most useful part of POM is the primary-care apprenticeship that links students from the beginning with a clinic in pediatrics, internal medicine, or family practice.

The traditional classes are taught based on systems. The first semester is based on the cell and the second on organ systems. One of the most difficult parts is biochemistry, though the professor offers clear lectures and extra question-and-answer sessions to help students master the material. Gross anatomy begins in the middle of the year and is well taught. Second year includes pharmacology, pathology, and microbiology. The quality of teaching tends to vary from subject to subject, with renal as one of the more difficult subjects to master (and, apparently, to teach).

In general, lecture hours are long, with classes from 9 a.m. to 2 p.m. in the second year. The note service tends to allow students to skip classes they tire of, though the quality of notes can vary depending on the student contracted for the job (the previous year's notes, however, are often for sale as well). Grading is honors/pass/fail and competitiveness is generally frowned upon. One area of unfortunate conflict is in the introduction to clinical medicine classes. Medical students are taught alongside physician assistant and nurse practitioner students. However, because the testing and grading of medical students is much more strict, there tends to be some tension between the two groups. This becomes particularly apparent when there are discussions about future jobs. At the same time, medical students are able to learn from the experience of the nurses, and this is a rare opportunity to meet their future nonphysician colleagues.

Students have off during the summer between the first and second years and many take extended vacations or pursue research. There are opportunities to become involved in research at National Institutes of Health and the Food and Drug Administration, politics with the Committee of Health Policy (founded at George Washington) and Congress, international health with the World Health Organization, and free medical services with several homeless clinics.

Clinical Years

Students at GWU get a wide range of clinical experiences from public inner-city hospitals to suburban clinics. There have been a number of recent changes involving the main university hospital. It was purchased by a for-profit health care corporation two years ago. The initial result was the exodus of some teaching faculty members, but much of the tumult has now resolved and the prospects for the hospital have increased considerably. The new operators of the hospital have agreed to continue all residency and student teaching programs as before, and many now feel that hospital is better off, noting a rising census and more stable financial picture. The company also plans to build a new, more modern hospital across the street from the present structure, with an estimated completion date 2001.

Students are required to do all third-year rotations in D.C.: pediatrics, obstetrics ad gynecology, medicine, primary care, surgery, and psychiatry. All of the rotations are eight weeks long, except for primary care, which is six weeks. The fourth year is primarily for electives, though there are a few specific requirements. Students must do an acting internship in medicine, family practice, or pediatrics and must do a rotation in anesthesiology, the primary goal of which is to learn how to intubate. POM continues during the final two years and incorporates basic science review and nonclinical topics—it's usually an ideal time to socialize with friends given the hectic schedule of third and fourth years.

There are twelve area hospitals at which GWU students train. Students are lucky that most of the pediatrics is done at Children's National Medical Center. It is a world-renowned hospital and the education students receive there is amazing. In 1993, the pediatrics clerkship was named best in the nation. GWU Hospital is always busy and filled with a lot of indigent care patients, as opposed to Holy Cross Hospital with mostly private patients. The Veteran's Administration and St. Elizabeth's Psychiatric Institute are full of work, especially scut work. Fairfax Hospital is one of the busiest obstetric units in the country, so students have numerous opportunities to deliver babies. The ED at GW is a level one trauma center and anything can walk in the door. The major drawback is the tiny size. Students may see patients in the hallway if it is busy. Primary care is emphasized, with clinics located across the street from the hospital, staffed by University-affiliated attendings and residents. More than 50 percent of GWU graduates enter primary-care residencies.

Social Life

No medical school has everything, but Washington, D.C., gives students the option of some of the best theaters, museums, and nightlife in the country. In addition to that, each class sponsors parties and semiformal dances after each exam. Every year there is Medical School Follies, a musical comedy show staged by each class. It is always a sentimental affair for the graduating students but the main purpose is to lampoon the School and faculty. The Follies band is made up of students, faculty, and staff and provides the music. Every other year, during Follies weekend, is Day in the Life of a Medical Student, otherwise known as parent's weekend.

Students can live in Virginia, Maryland, or D.C. Living near campus is expensive but convenient to the school and hospital. There is a metro stop directly in front of the medical school, making it a good option for those who choose to live in other parts of the metropolitan area. Because there are so many hospitals, however, third-year students need to have a car.

There is no campus housing for graduate students. Parking is expensive, and the only price break is for third and fourth year students. Students with families tend to live farther out where they can find bigger homes and better school districts. Crime can be a problem if students are not careful and forget that they are in a major city. GWU has its own security force that works in close contact with Metro Police, Secret Service, and Capitol Police.

The Bottom Line

GWU offers students a well-balanced education. More than 80 percent of graduates match at one of their top-three choices, with almost 50 percent getting their first choice.

HARVARD UNIVERSITY, HARVARD MEDICAL SCHOOL

Cambridge, Massachusetts

Tuition 1996–97: $26,000 per year
Size of Entering Class: 165
Total Number of Women Students: 348 (48%)
Total Number of Men Students: 373 (52%)

World Wide Web: www.med.harvard.edu/
Contact: Dr. Joseph Martin, Dean
    Cambridge, MA 02138

Harvard Medical School (HMS) is one of the oldest and most respected medical schools in the country. It has been ranked the number one medical school in the country for several years in a row. HMS receives more money for research than any other medical school. For those with interests in research, the finances and the facilities can be found to do almost anything.

Admissions/Financial Aid

HMS has recently joined the AMCAS application process. This makes applying to Harvard easier than it has been in the past. Of the 3,500 applicants, only 165 enter the freshman class. The average GPA of enrolling HMS students is 3.7, and the average MCAT scores are verbal reasoning, 10.9; physical science, 11.7; and basic science, 12.0. Interviews are held with one faculty member and with one medical student or with two faculty members. Interviews generally carry a light tone. Students are chosen based on their achievements outside of medicine as much as their achievements in the scientific field. This leads to an interesting mix of students.

Tuition is currently $26,000 per year. Estimated yearly costs at HMS are $42,000–$43,000. Financial aid packages are available through the financial aid office. Up to $20,000 is offered through Stafford Loans ($8,500 subsidized, $11,500 unsubsidized). Students can apply for an HMS scholarship for the remainder of their balance. HMS scholarships are offered based on need. The financial aid office also directs students to independent loaners that offer aid to Harvard Medical School students.

Preclinical Years

HMS offers several programs for perspective students. For a medical doctor degree, 80 percent of the students are enrolled in the New Pathway system. The New Pathway comprises traditional medical lectures and case-based tutorials. Two to three mornings per week students gather in small group sessions to dissect real medical cases. Students receive 1 to 2 pages per session and develop extensive differential diagnosises. Each student picks a topic to research based on the tutorial discussions and presents the findings the next session. A physician moderates the discussion but does not teach. As more pages are received, the differential is refined and the pathology and pathophysiology are discussed. This allows students to better incorporate classroom teaching with clinical scenarios. It also helps students develop the skills to find data pertinent to medical cases. Most cases are useful in teaching basic medical concepts. Cases work well in blocks like physiology, endocrinology, or biochemistry. However, in certain blocks cases are useless.

Lectures follow the tutorial session and classes usually finish between noon and 1 p.m. This allows students to vigorously pursue interests out of the classroom. Lectures at Harvard often focus on cutting-edge research. Although interesting, topics may be too esoteric for first- and second-year students. This means free time is often used for reading the basic lecture materials and text books. During the preclinical years, grades are all pass/fail. A striking feature in the classroom is the lack of competition among students. Classmates frequently help one another. This environment fosters camaraderie and facilitates learning.

New Pathway students are involved in a patient/doctor program for the first three years of medical school. New Pathway students meet with preceptors one afternoon a week and learn the skills of history taking and physical exam.

Twenty percent of HMS students are enrolled in the joint Harvard/MIT system called Health Sciences and Technology (HST). This curriculum is traditional in nature. The majority of teaching is through lecture and lab. HST students learn medicine through basic sciences and take classes at MIT as well as Harvard.

HMS also has an M.D./Ph.D. program sponsored by NIH. The average time to completion is seven years. Tuition is paid for through scholarship funds, and students are also offered a stipend for living expenses. M.D./Ph.D. students can enroll in either the New Pathway or the HST system and may choose to complete their Ph.D. at Harvard or MIT.

Clinical Years

The clinical years at Harvard are a rude awakening for many students. The many hours of free time in the first and second years are replaced with long, hard hours in the hospital. In most rotations, students are expected to take overnight call. The pass/fail system is replaced with a four-grade system. Students also receive written evaluations for each rotation. Rotations are selected from some of the top teaching programs in the country. Core rotations include four months of medicine, three months of surgery, 1½ months of pediatrics, 1½ months of obstetrics/gynecology, one month of radiology, one month of psychiatry, one month of basic science, and several months of elective time.

Social Life

Harvard students represent a diverse and fascinating group of students. Forty to 50 percent of the classes are women, and 15 to 25 percent of the students are underrepresented minority groups. The social life in the Medical School is active. HMS students are frequently invited to social functions at other Harvard graduate programs and have many social functions of their own. As the years progresses, many people find themselves moving to the surrounding towns. The focus of social life changes from the Medical School to the city.

The Bottom Line

Harvard is a wonderful place to attend medical school. The facilities are second to none. Teaching is self-directed and especially good for those who are motivated. Those used to more structure may find the informal method of teaching hard to adjust to. Harvard prides itself in molding students who will be the leaders in the medical field and has succeeded in doing so. Graduating with a degree from Harvard allows most graduates the opportunity to go anywhere in the country.

HOWARD UNIVERSITY COLLEGE OF MEDICINE

Washington, District of Columbia

Size of Entering Class: 100
World Wide Web: www.med.howard.edu/
Contact: Ann Finney, Admissions Officer

2400 Sixth Street, NW
Washington, DC 20059-2
202-806-6270

Outsiders usually have the idea that the Howard University College of Medicine is disproportionately African American. All it takes, however, is a personal visit to debunk that notion. When you step into a classroom, you are immediately surprised by the diversity of cultures. It is almost an academic United Nations. No matter what ethnicity you are, you are not likely to feel out of place in the Howard environment. The classroom atmosphere is friendly, though a subtle tinge of competition is there if you seek it.

Admissions/Financial Aid

Applicants are required to submit two letters of recommendation from science instructors or from the students' undergraduate premedical committee. Interviews are conducted by a lecturer or clinicians from the Howard University Hospital. Since the school's goal is to train primary-care physicians for underserved areas, much of the interview focuses on discussing your motivation for becoming a physician, your interest in Howard, and your awareness of current health issues. It is also a time to explain any gaps in your transcript; the interviewer gives you a chance to explain the C you received in organic chemistry or why the 9 on your physics MCAT doesn't reflect the A you earned in college.

Tuition for the first year is $17,348, though with living expenses, the total bill usually exceeds $30,000 per year. The average financial aid package is $27,000–$30,000 per year. Most of this is government loans, but the school usually grants $3,000 per year to students in addition to their loan package. A number of scholarships are also available for students who qualify based on academic excellence, state of origin, or future medical specialty. The average level of indebtedness for the class of 1998 was $85,000.

Preclinical Years

The College of Medicine is a traditional school, and the first two years are devoted to the basic sciences.

The first semester consists primarily of anatomy and biochemistry. Because the volume of information required is so great, anatomy consumes most of a student's time. This can be a problem for those who find themselves strapped trying to learn biochemistry in between anatomy laboratory. This is probably the peak time for medical student stress, and students are rapidly forced to develop time-management skills and a skill for deciding what is really important to learn.

Students begin their training in clinical medicine in the first semester. In Introduction to Patient Care, students shadow a veteran clinician and learn how to perform a history and physical for 2 hours a week. The class also has a required lecture series, which, unfortunately, is not nearly as interesting as the clinical end. Throughout the basic science years, lecturers make an effort to integrate clinical scenarios, and a special class is offered to help students hone their problem-solving skills. Most students would prefer that more of this would be offered.

The second semester begins with an unusual Howard creation, the "minimester" of neurosciences. For the first four weeks of the second semester, students are thoroughly immersed in neurosciences from 8 a.m. to 5 p.m., Monday to Friday, with exams once a week. The only relief during the day is a 2-hour break. Thankfully, the class is taught by one of the school's most remarkable professors, Dr. Trouth. Lively and interesting, Dr. Trouth is skilled at presenting complex physiology in an organized and clear manner. He also makes a point of highlighting the most important facts (i.e., most likely to be on a test) for an often-overwhelmed class. The only downside to his lectures is his penchant for calling on students off the class roster to answer questions, forcing them to keep up-to-date with the required reading. Students get a four-day break after the minimester, then proceed to microbiology, physiology, immunology, and psychiatry for the rest of the year. Students begin pathology and pharmacology in the second year, which continues until April. The entire month of May is free for students to study for USMLE Step I. The school is also now incorporating a special boards-review class for second years.

Clinical Years

In their third and fourth years, students rotate through their required rotations at a number of hospitals in the Washington, D.C., metropolitan area. Because of the city's diverse economy and culture, students are exposed to a wide range of clinical problems through rotations at D.C. General Hospital, Saint Elizabeth's Hospital, Veterans Administration Hospital, Prince George's Hospital, and Washington Hospital. Rotations at the main University Hospital tend to be the most highly sought after, given that they offer the most familiar surroundings, most active social life, and, often, the most interesting cases. Students tend to have the highest praise for the surgery rotation, finding the professors highly knowledgeable and eager to teach. Fourth year consists of required rotations in internal medicine and surgery, as well as some time for electives.

Social Life

Located in the nation's capital, Washington, D.C., and smack-dab between Maryland and Virginia, there is no shortage of extracurricular activities. Concerts, theater, shops, movies, parks, restaurants, and clubs are abundant and varied. The real question students often ask is: "What not to do?" Students tend to be quite social, and many explore the city for nightlife or cultural events. Students from Africa, the Caribbean, Central and South America, and Asia tend to assimilate well together, particularly since Washington, D.C., offers so many culturally diverse activities and restaurants.

Class-specific activities include midsemester trips to other cities and Student National Medical Association conferences. During the month of March, the school hosts the Smoker, an annual event in which students from all classes roast the school and its professors. The Smoker includes student-performed skits and singing and allows the entire medical school to laugh at itself together.

The Bottom Line

Howard offers an opportunity for students to learn medicine in a traditional curriculum while being exposed to a wide variety of cultures both in the classroom and in the city.

INDIANA UNIVERSITY SCHOOL OF MEDICINE

Indianapolis, Indiana

Applications: 3,134
Size of Entering Class: 280
Total Number of Women Students: 511 (40%)
Total Number of Men Students: 770 (60%)
World Wide Web: www.iupui.edu/it/medschl/ home.html

Contact: Dr. Robert W. Holden, Dean
355 North Lansing
Indianapolis, IN 46202-2896

Indiana University's Medical Center (IUMC) comprises the Schools of Medicine, Nursing, Dentistry, and Allied Health Sciences and Purdue University Indianapolis. IUMC, the other schools that make up Indiana University, and Purdue University Indianapolis comprise Indiana University—Purdue University Indianapolis. The payoff of this three-way combination is that IUMC students have the benefit of rubbing academic shoulders with Purdue students who concentrate not only on science, engineering, and high technology but also on the arts, business, and humanities.

As for its own strengths, IUMC is noted for studies in cancer, cardiology, gastroenterology, gynecology, neurology, otolaryngology, rheumatology, and urology. An additional clinical program in endocrinology has recently brought added recognition, while the medical school's graduate program receives accolades for its primary-care focus.

Even though there is plenty of academic excitement for students at the Indianapolis campus, the medical center is spread throughout the entire state. The School of Medicine at Indianapolis is just one of a network of nine campuses that make up the medical school. The Indianapolis campus is the hub, from which eight regional Centers for Medical Education radiate—Indiana University Bloomington, Lafayette Center at Purdue, University of Notre Dame, Ball State University, Indiana State University, University of Evansville, Indiana University Northwest, and Fort Wayne Center for Medical Education at Purdue.

Admissions/Financial Aid

Because the medical school's stated purpose is to fulfill the health-care needs of Indiana residents, the admis-

sions office is aware that its graduates work with patients from widely diverse social and economic backgrounds. For that reason, the admissions office wants to ensure that applicants have a strong background in the humanities and in the social and behavioral sciences. As can be expected of a state school, Indiana residents are given preference in each year's class of 280. About 95 percent of students come from the state, while 6 percent are members of underrepresented minorities. Of these, most are African Americans.

The medical school makes a concerted effort to recruit minorities with programs at the college level and at the high school level for underrepresented and disadvantaged students who show an interest in health-care careers. The medical school's support does not end with matriculation. Tutorial assistance is offered as a two-week program that students can take prior to the beginning of the first-year student orientation. In addition, another program gives to disadvantaged and minority students who demonstrate potential the chance to prepare for the competitive environment of medical school.

Research at IUMC is responsible for earning a large amount of the resources that make the institution a major academic center. Cancer research at IU, for instance, just brought in a $7.2-million award from the National Cancer Institute. Diabetes is another research focal point. The medical school is one of six research centers chosen by the Centers for Disease Control and Prevention to undertake a five-year study in managed-care environments for diabetics. Other groundbreaking research thrusts include an Alcohol Research Center, an Alzheimer's and Related Diseases Center, an Arthritis Center, and the unique

Adolescent Sexually Transmitted Diseases Center, which is the only one in the country that focuses solely on this age group. It, too, received a $7-million grant from the National Institutes of Health.

Preclinical Years

Students may choose one of the eight Medical Education Centers in the state as the site in which to begin their education. Though these centers are all under the same academic umbrella, each offers a slightly different curriculum focus. For instance, the Northwest Center for Medical Education's Regional Center offers case-based learning. Students at this center, in particular, are exposed to problem-based learning and tutorial sessions. However, this brand of medical education is not necessarily confined to just one or two centers. As of 1998, the entire curriculum is undergoing revision and is taking a highly interdisciplinary turn.

At all of the centers, first- and second-year students receive a core of basic science courses and are exposed early on to clinical situations through Introduction to Clinical Medicine, a multidisciplinary course taken for the first two years.

First-year students take anatomy, histology, biochemistry, physiology, microbiology, neurobiology, patient/doctor relationship, and concepts of health and disease, in which they learn how to apply courses to the real world of clinical problems.

During the second year, practical experience intensifies as students join hospital medical teams and participate in labs. Courses include biostatistics, pharmacology, pathology, clinical medicine, and medical genetics.

Clinical Years

The third year of medical school for all students is spent at the Indianapolis campus, at which the curriculum covers family medicine, internal medicine, surgery, obstetrics and gynecology, pediatrics, and psychiatry. A twelve-month rotating clinical clerkship is also required.

There are many hospitals from which to choose. IUMC has a reputation for high-quality hospital care since 1914, when the Indiana Medical College opened a hospital next to a cornfield and a city dump. Even at its start it was dubbed one of the best-planned and best-equipped hospitals in the country. With the variety of hospitals in proximity to the Indianapolis

campus and the several thousand patients statewide who are referred to these facilities, IUMC students see a multitude of cases.

Fourth-year students have required clerkships in surgical subspecialties, neurology, and radiology. Electives, which take up most of a fourth-year student's time, can be chosen from institutions throughout Indiana as well as in other states and countries, pending faculty member permission. A biomedical research paper is obligatory during the fourth year.

One of the best-known hospitals at IUMC is Riley Hospital for Children, which has its own impressive list of kudos. It is Indiana's only comprehensive pediatric hospital and is the largest intensive care children's hospital in the nation. It has the only pediatric burn unit in Indiana and is the only hospital in the state that provides organ transplants. Recently, a pediatric bone marrow transplant unit was added to treat children with cancer and blood-related disorders. The Indiana University Hospital and Outpatient Center is the only facility in the state with a high-technology imaging center that offers positron emission tomography (PET), CT, and magnetic resonance imaging (MRI) modalities.

Another facility, Indiana Health Care, has also gained recognition as a center for primary-care group practice and specializes in pediatrics, family practice, obstetrics and gynecology, and internal medicine. The Indiana University Methodist Family Practice Center—a comprehensive-care facility for the entire family—was recently opened, which adds yet another training facility for IU medical students.

With the numerous opportunities it offers in family practice and pediatrics and the stress it places on family practice as a career option, IUMC is one of forty-six medical schools honored by the American Academy of Family Physicians.

Social Life

Most people associate Indianapolis with race cars; however, that's not all there is in the city, which is right in the middle of the state and yet not too far from Chicago and Cincinnati. While the Indy 500 and NASCAR racing might dominate the big sports picture, the Indiana Pacers basketball and Indianapolis Colts football teams rival for a close second in local sports fans' hearts. Professional baseball, hockey, soccer, and tennis to the roster are also accessible.

Over a period of twenty years, the Indiana Sports Corporation has created a strategy to attract major amateur sporting events to Indianapolis. In late 1999 or early 2 the NCAA will move 500 miles from Kansas City to its new Michael Graves–designed headquarters just across the street from the IU campus. This will coincide with the return of the NCAA Men's Basketball Final Four championships to the RCA Dome for the third time in ten years.

IU students have to go only a few blocks from their campus in White River State Park to enjoy all that this twelfth-largest city in the nation has. They can check out the $320-million Circle Centre Mall and then move on to the restaurants, clubs, and entertainment, from movies to touring Broadway shows. Although everything is a relatively short stroll from IU, there is plenty going on at the campus to keep any serious medical student thoroughly distracted. A Hog Wild Weekend, male and female beauty contests, a winter formal, Mardi Gras, and a bike race are a few of the top contenders.

Living and eating are usually two big budget busters, but not for IU students. Nearby city restaurants feature student staples such as sandwiches and burgers along with blues bands. Some restaurants are great places to kick back, watch a movie, and eat and drink enexpensively, including a bottomless soft drink. As for student living arrangements, IU has gone out of its way to offer affordable on-campus housing for about 60 percent of its full-time day students.

The Bottom Line

Indiana University's Medical Center is all business when it comes to educating physicians. IUMC students are not only geographically in the center of the state and of a city, they're also in proximity to other institutions, which puts them in contact with an educational and cultural mix, from cutting-edge technical devices designed at Purdue to the latest business trends from Indiana University. With physicians getting into both of these areas in addition to the practice of medicine, IUMC is a stimulating place to be.

JOHNS HOPKINS UNIVERSITY SCHOOL OF MEDICINE

Baltimore, Maryland

Tuition 1996–97: $25,000 per year
Size of Entering Class: 120
Total Number of Women Students: 388 (45%)
Total Number of Men Students: 480 (55%)
World Wide Web: infonet.welch.jhu.edu/som/

Contact: Dr. Leon Gordis, Associate Dean of
Admissions
3400 North Charles Street
Baltimore, MD 21218-2699
410-955-3182

Johns Hopkins University School of Medicine is an institution steeped in tradition and respect for tradition. Hopkins has been voted America's Best Hospital five years in a row by *U.S. News & World Report* and advertises this rating with a large banner at the main hospital entrance. Hopkins students are continuously reminded that they are one of a very select group.

Admissions/Financial Aid

It is difficult to gain admission. Of the 3,800 students who apply to Hopkins each year, about 700 are interviewed, and 120 students are admitted. Last year, 53 percent of the admitted class was female. Underrepresented minority applicants are invited for a welcoming weekend organized by minority medical student groups and are admitted according to special criteria.

Although Hopkins is a private school with total costs of more than $30,000 per year, financial aid can relieve the financial worry. Eighty percent of students receive financial aid, and the average indebtedness is about $55,000. Tuition is locked in and inflation-proof at matriculation, the unit loan is fully fundable through deferred-interest loans, and grant money is amazingly available (the average grant is $13,000). Informal polls of students reveal that Hopkins gave them outright grants three to twelve times as large as those offered by competing East Coast schools. Last year, the medical school dean even toyed with the idea of abolishing tuition completely.

Preclinical Years

Four years ago, the Hopkins faculty received a multimillion-dollar grant from the Robert Wood Johnson Foundation to revise the medical school curriculum. Many changes have occurred since the School received the grant. During first year, classes are over by 1:00 and students have up to 3 hours of small-group attention daily from full-fledged professors,

even Nobel Prize hopefuls. Instead of having multiple classes (histology, cell biology, molecular biology, etc.) that have their own tests, the entire education occurs one class at a time. Therefore, there's one test every two to three weeks.

Surprisingly, tests are open book (except in anatomy). This leads to a collegial atmosphere where one can actually enjoy medical school and classmates. Every fortnight, students observe a clinician one-on-one and sometimes participate in care (one first-year student even helped deliver a baby). Although Hopkins still has a letter grade system, almost 75 percent receive B's in their classes, making for a somewhat mellow atmosphere. Students often quip, "C=M.D." Hopkins has also launched a much-ballyhooed Physician and Society class to humanize student-doctors, but students generally consider this feeble.

An almost three-month vacation follows first year, during which students can get funding to do almost anything (they have traveled to Australia, worked on Indian reservations, and even written computer programs over that summer). However, Hopkins becomes a lot less fun during the second year. Students should get ready to write off this year of their life. Instead of the big-picture approach, second year is details, details, and details. Gone are open-book tests and all but one to two free afternoons, and class becomes an exercise in endurance. Students have plenty of time to ponder the universe from 8 am to 5 p.m. every day. Unfortunately, they have the added burden of volumes upon volumes of additional reading (at Hopkins, all professors are required to furnish complete notes of each lecture). But there is a good side: students finally learn medications and dosing, pathophysiology (the study of failing organ systems), and pathology (the study of failing tissues).

Clinical Years

Hopkins begins clinical training right after spring break of the second year, almost three months earlier than other schools. Unlike other medical schools, Hopkins doesn't require national board exams before beginning clinical training (students can take them any time before graduation). Managed care has not penetrated Maryland yet, so students do not learn office medicine as they would in California. While Johns Hopkins is the prime hospital, affiliated hospitals include Hopkins Bayview, Sinai, St. Agnes, Franklin Square, Good Samaritan, and others.

The tradition of Hopkins excellence is clear during weekly Medical Grand Rounds, which are a veritable who's who of world-famous clinicians discussing the latest advances in medicine. The Johns Hopkins Hospital is renowned for its stellar departments in medicine, pediatrics, surgery, ophthalmology, neurology, and almost every other specialty (notably, however, Hopkins lacks a family practice department). During clinical years, students carry patients, order labs, work with world-class attendings, and present to their floor team. They are pimped (asked tough questions they probably don't know the answer to), but end up strong (the ultimate compliment given by house staff). Hopkins surgery is said to be more hands-off than other schools (students almost never do anything but stitch occasionally), but it is very well organized. Heart transplants, Whipple procedures, and knee replacements—students see them all at Hopkins. Pediatrics is strong as well, but it is in transition and currently has no chairperson. Students are more hesitant to recommend psychiatry and ob/gyn because of their poor teaching and department personalities.

Because clerkships begin early and can be taken in any order, students have great freedom to explore (they can take orthopedics, pediatric oncology, or anything else in the fall of third year). Specialty clerkships (about half of a medical education) are tops, with world-class attendings in cardiology, infectious diseases, surgical subspecialties, geriatrics, rheumatology, and more. If anything negative can be said, it is that the emphasis on new knowledge and research excites more students to pursue academic careers and specialization rather than routine primary care. In fact, almost 15 percent of students seek out fellowships so they can take a year off during medical school and pursue research. However, the School is considering requiring a primary-care clerkship for future classes.

At the end of clinical training, students are highly marketable to residencies and even fellowships.

The Dean writes letters on behalf of all students applying to residencies, and truly facilitates the process.

Social Life

Hopkins attracts students from almost all fifty states, with a good representation of sexes and ethnicities. About 10 percent are married, and most are in their early 20s (although students range to age 40). With so much free time first year, school is very social with dinners, dancing, and parties galore. This peters out somewhat as the years go on (small social groups inevitably form), but Schoolwide activities such as the annual Monte Carlo Night formal, Mardi Gras party, and winter satire show still draw many students. Most first-year students live in Reed Hall, a mouse-filled but fun dorm situated in East Baltimore, and some nights they are sure they hear machine-gun fire. Because of incidents four years ago, security has been beefed up, without similar incidents in the past three years. Because rent is so cheap in Baltimore ($800 per month can get students a three-bedroom apartment in the nice parts of town) and the East Baltimore area is so dangerous, upperclassmen generally move to genteel Mt. Washington, hip Mt. Vernon, or raucous Fells Point.

A car is almost mandatory, and students can get away to rural Maryland for biking, vineyard tours, or autumn pumpkin picking in about 20 minutes. While Baltimore has gotten a bad rap for safety, it is an eminently accessible city. Orioles baseball games at Camden Yards are awesome, subscriptions to the historic CenterStage Theater are only $39 per year, and even the finest restaurants are affordable. Students often congregate in bar-packed Fells Point for dancing or drink beers in the more refined Mt. Washington Tavern. Sailors can rent boats for only $20 a day in the Baltimore harbor, and sea watchers can relax and watch them in the nicely redeveloped Inner Harbor with its museums and shops. Washington, D.C., is an hour's drive or train ride away. Climate ranges from sultry summers to moderate winters with occasional snow.

The Bottom Line

Hopkins offers maximum prestige and outstanding resources, but at the cost of a private school tuition rate and four years in a mediocre city. However, even years and years after graduation, graduates are known as a "Hopkins" woman or man. Where graduates choose to go afterward is limited only by their imagination.

KIRKSVILLE COLLEGE OF OSTEOPATHIC MEDICINE

Kirksville, Missouri

Students Receiving Financial Aid: 88%
Applications: 4,157
Total Number of Women Students: 158 (27%)
Total Number of Men Students: 419 (73%)
World Wide Web: www.kcom.edu

Contact: Lori Haxton, Director of Admissions
800 West Jefferson Street
Kirksville, MO 63501
816-626-2237

Kirksville College of Osteopathic Medicine (KCOM) is the founding school of osteopathic medicine. In fact, some say the ghost of A. T. Still, the father of osteopathy, still roams the campus preaching the values of his creation. In Kirksville, Missouri—fondly referred to as "the Ville"—isolation is key. With few distractions to compete for studying time, students can concentrate on passing the courses needed to complete medical school.

Preclinical Years

The seclusion of Kirksville allows students to survive anatomy's average of 20 lab hours a week and mandatory bilateral dissections. This schedule may change, however, as the faculty recently petitioned the administration to lengthen the anatomy lecture/lab course from its current thirteen weeks to span a year or more, integrating it with other basic science and clinical courses.

A new addition to the first-year curriculum is the Complete Doctor course, which covers everything from physical exam skills to caring for the terminally ill. Most students enjoy the physical exam skills portion but complain that the accompanying lectures, which address topics from the history of osteopathy to psychological theories, are unnecessarily drawn out and repetitive.

Although the majority of full-time faculty members are involved in research at some level, teaching comes first. Lectures are usually practical, simple, and thorough. The practicing physicians who teach the clinical classes are somewhat less adept at organizing and delivering lucid presentations. While these lectures are replete with interesting clinical pictures and scenarios, lecture transcriptions ($100 per year) are a must for structuring the information down the road. These

clinicians often bring patients to accompany lectures in subjects like dermatology and neurology.

KCOM provides a moderate degree of clinical exposure in the first two years. A two-week preceptorship between the first and second years with a primary-care physician in rural Missouri serves as the principal clinical experience. Depending on students' assertiveness and their assigned preceptor, they may place their first suture, deliver their first baby, or learn how to sleep with their our eyes open. All students are required to perform one history and physical during the two weeks. The majority of students report positive, but inconsistent, experiences. In addition to the preceptorship, students perform histories and physicals on standardized patients and later review these on videotape with peers.

KCOM has made considerable efforts to keep up with technology. The lecture halls are equipped with network outlets and Internet access at each seat. Many students bring laptops to lectures. Students who own computers say they've been helpful, but not necessary, since the school library owns twenty computers complete with basic software and Internet access.

At the end of the first two years, students have just over a week to prepare for the COMLEX Level I. Despite the short preparation time, which is the source of widespread complaints among students, KCOM usually performs above the average. In 1998, 98 percent of KCOM students passed the COMLEX Level I, compared with a national average of 93 percent.

For those who don't get enough academica the first time around, KCOM offers one-year fellowship programs in anatomy, research, and osteopathic theory and methods between the third and fourth years. Starting in fall 1999, KCOM will offer master's degrees in public health, health administration, and geriatrics.

KCOM medical students will be eligible to enroll in these programs at a reduced cost. After completing minimal classroom work in Kirksville during the preclinical years, students finish their degrees over the following years through a distance learning program.

Clinical Years

KCOM provides students with numerous opportunities for clinical rotation at sites that include Missouri (St. Francis Medical Center, Southeast Missouri Hospital, Capital Regional Medical Center, Freeman Health Systems, Northeast Regional Medical Center, Phelps County Regional Medical Center, and Deaconess Medical Center/West), Michigan (St. John Detroit Riverview Hospital, Genesys Regional Medical Center, St. John Health System Oakland Hospital, and Riverside Osteopathic Hospital/Henry Ford), Ohio (Cuyahoga Falls General Hospital, Doctors Hospital of Stark County, Mount Sinai Medical Center East, St. Joseph Health Center, and Meridia South Pointe Hospital), Arizona (Thunderbird Samaritan Regional Medical Center, Mesa General Hospital, and John C. Lincoln), Utah, and Colorado, with an additional fourth year option in New York, Georgia, or Texas. Utah and Colorado are pilot sites and may not necessarily be offered in the future.

Arizona, Utah, and Colorado provide more individual, preceptor-based rotations with minimal didactics, while the other sites consist of more hospital-based rotations and offer more didactics. However, all regions provide a monthly education day for students to discuss journal articles, present cases, or attend lectures. Geographical considerations aside, most students interested in primary care choose Arizona or Missouri, while those with interests in specialties choose among the remaining states. The selection process for the class of 2001, based on a lottery-by-preference system, resulted in 85 percent of the students attending their first-choice site.

Typically, the more rural sites, found mostly in Missouri and smaller suburban hospitals, allow plenty of hands-on experience but lack a broad range of pathology. The larger hospitals, such as Genesys Regional Medical Center, may expose students to a greater variety of patients, but the pecking order of resident, intern, and student can sometimes limit the opportunities to perform procedures. One exception to this general rule is St. John Detroit Riverview Hospital, where students encounter the pathology of an inner-city patient base while also playing a more direct role in patient care and treatment.

KCOM's commitment to technology continues throughout the clinical years. KCOM requires that all hospitals house a KCOM-owned computer with Internet access. This allows all KCOM students, regardless of location, to periodically submit evaluations of their clinical rotations via e-mail to the Medical Education Department in Kirksville. Additionally, students use the Internet as a resource for current research articles or to collaborate with colleagues in other states.

Social Life

A rural town of 20,000 in northern Missouri, Kirksville is 3 hours away from a real airport and an hour away from any city with a population greater than 100,000. The location fosters a close-knit family atmosphere among students. Not only do studetns spend most of the day together at school, but also they're bound to run into classmates virtually every time they go to the grocery store or the one movie theater in town. The family atmosphere is comfortable for students, nearly 30 percent of whom are married, many with children.

When cabin fever hits "the Ville," most students head 90 miles south to Columbia, home to the University of Missouri (Mizzou). In addition to the larger college-town atmosphere of Mizzou, Columbia provides the only real shopping within reasonable driving distance.

The cost of living is very low: $400 a month will rent a nice two-bedroom house, and $700 will provide for a small palace. While KCOM student housing offers a fun social environment, it is no cheaper than other available options. Nearly all housing—as well as everything else in town—is within a 10-minute drive. Also within a short drive is Thousand Hills State Park, complete with a lake, biking and hiking trails, and picnic areas. Students often bike the forested perimeter of the lake, as well as several other trails within northern Missouri.

The Bottom Line

KCOM is a student-friendly school that remains true to its historical roots while progressively incorporating new ideas and technology. If applicants thrive on urban living and question their small-town stamina, however, KCOM may not be the place for them.

LAKE ERIE COLLEGE OF OSTEOPATHIC MEDICINE

Erie, Pennsylvania

Applications: 3,781
World Wide Web: www.lecom.edu
Contact: Elaine Morse, Admissions Coordinator

1858 West Grandview Boulevard
Erie, PA 16509-1025
814-866-6641

One of the newest medical schools in the country, Lake Erie College of Medicine (LECOM) opened its doors in 1993 and has since grown to be a valuable source for primary-care physicians in western Pennsylvania. LECOM's mission is to prepare students to become primary-care osteopathic physicians in the state of Pennsylvania and in surrounding areas. Most students fulfill this ideal, but they are not prevented from exploring other options.

Admissions/Financial Aid

LECOM draws most of its students from Pennsylvania, Ohio, and New York. About half of the student body entered medical school directly out of college. The average age of first-year students falls between 23 and 25. If students think shorts and a T-shirt are adequate attire for attending class, they need to think again if they're considering LECOM. The school has a dress code that requires students to convey a professional appearance whenever on College grounds.

Admission is competitive, only one in seven applicants receives an interview. LECOM participates in the AACOMAS application service; the application deadline is March 15. Each student invited to interview has one interview with two or three faculty members in a relatively relaxed atmosphere. The school offers very little financial aid, and most students rely on government loans to pay for tuition and living expenses. Tuition is far from cheap, and, unless students are independently wealthy, they need to be prepared to budget their money wisely to carry them through the summer months until the next loan check arrives.

Preclinical Years

The preclinical years consist of one semester of core science courses, followed by three semesters of systems-based education. Anatomy dominates the first semester, followed by biochemistry, microbiology, and pathology. Osteopathic manipulative medicine is taught throughout the first two years, and students are evaluated with both written and practical exams.

Favorite teachers include Dr. Krueger, whose animated style of teaching in anatomy and embryology makes dry topics more palatable. Dr. Ziegler is also a favorite for his ability to combine lectures in pathology with commentary on politics. He also admonishes students to enjoy their vacation before the beginning of the second year, as it will be their last.

Exposure to clinical medicine begins in the second semester with the introduction of systems-based teaching. The bulk of the lectures are handled by clinicians who lecture on systems appropriate to their specialty.

Also in the second semester, students begin the Osteopathic Preceptor Education Project (OPEP), in which they are paired with a clinician and spend several afternoons in an office or clinic gaining hands-on experience. This project is continued in the second year as Clinical Osteopathic Diagnostic Applications (CODA). Students are graded based on their performance on multiple-choice exams and receive a letter grade at the conclusion of each course. There is an unavoidable air of competition among students, and rankings are provided along with test results. Between the first and second years, students can take advantage of programs such as Bridging the Gaps, in which students carry out projects in the community and are compensated with a stipend. Some students opt for a monthlong international medical education experience in countries such as Poland and South Africa.

Clinical Years

During the third and fourth years, students are required to complete twenty-four clinical clerkships.

Each of the twenty-four rotations is for a period of four weeks. Students may rotate through any of the more than thirty sites currently affiliated with LECOM. Among the more popular rotation sites is West Penn Hospital in Pittsburgh. The rotations are as valuable as the student makes them. An aggressive attitude and eagerness to learn procedures or techniques are valuable tools and help one make the most of the rotation years.

Students are allowed sixteen weeks of electives, which are very flexible, and are able to negotiate rotation opportunities with physicians or clinics, pending approval by the Dean of Clinical education. Third- and fourth-year students experience the full range of medical education, including primary care, specialty fields, and managed care. Four weeks of vacation are offered during both the third and fourth years, which allows students ample time for residency applications and interviews. Students are counseled throughout the process of application for residency and the match. Ninety-eight percent of LECOM students match with their first choice of residency location.

Social Life

Erie is not the most ideal place to go to school, but if lounging on the beach during the warm months or skiing during the winter sound enjoyable, there is plenty to do. Presque Isle is one of the largest expanses of lakeside beaches in the region and offers plenty of outdoor activities that range from fishing and hiking to canoeing or in-line skating. The beaches stretch for miles, and there are countless trails that are open to exploration. During the cold months, excellent skiing is within a 2-hour drive of Erie. Buffalo, Cleveland, and Pittsburgh are all within a 2-hour drive.

Among the most popular activities for students and faculty is the Wednesday night bowling league. Nightlife in Erie is limited, but there are a fair number of dance clubs and pubs. Housing is cheap, and crime is not a serious problem. A two-bedroom apartment will run less than $400, depending on the area.

The Bottom Line

LECOM offers students a traditional lecture-based curriculum and a diverse number of clinical settings to learn osteopathic medicine. Graduates look back bitterly at the school's regimented atmosphere, 8 a.m. to 5 p.m. classes, and dress code, but most believe that the discipline it taught them made them better physicians.

LOMA LINDA UNIVERSITY SCHOOL OF MEDICINE

Loma Linda, California

Tuition 1996–97: $26,088 per year
Applications: 4,284
Total Number of Women Students: 272 (41%)
Total Number of Men Students: 390 (59%)

World Wide Web: www.llu.edu/llu/medicine/
Contact: Dr. Brian Bull, Dean
Loma Linda, CA 92350

Loma Linda University School of Medicine (LLUSM) was founded in 1905 in southern California to train medical missionaries. While the School still maintains close ties to the Seventh-Day Adventist Church and many medical students and graduates still spend time overseas, Loma Linda has risen to prominence in other areas, particularly as a national leader in pediatric cardiac surgery. Remember Baby Fae and her baboon heart? Students have the opportunity, for example, to fly across the country in Lear jets to harvest hearts for the pediatric transplant candidates in Loma Linda's state-of-the-art pediatric cardiac-care unit.

But LLUSM's greatest strengths lie in a solid medical education delivered by a caring faculty that aims to produce physicians dedicated to the concept of whole-person care: treating the patient as an individual, not just as a disease process.

Preclinical Years

One of the major drawbacks of the first year is the twenty-week-long first quarter, during which students are thrown into, with little preparation, an arduous schedule of biochemistry, gross anatomy, embryology, and histology. Fortunately, the second and third quarters require somewhat less mental stamina, and students actually have time to emerge, blinking myopically in the bright California sunshine, from their study dungeons to have some fun. Multiple attempts are constantly made to integrate clinical experience in the first two years with the basic sciences. Though the physical diagnosis course is well taught and small-group, case-based sessions are held one afternoon per week, students have few opportunities to apply their clinical skills.

Second-year courses are much better taught, much more clinically relevant, and much more fun. Pathology review sessions feature group stretch breaks and an unlimited supply of snacks, compliments of LLUSM students' favorite professor. Introduction to Clinical Medicine provides a first-rate segue into the clinical years.

LLUSM's roots show through in one requirement: religion courses. While many are initially skeptical and even annoyed by these courses, they usually find them extremely pertinent and thought provoking. The classes provide a humanities-oriented Christian focus in otherwise basic science–dominated years. They also are helpful in answering ethics questions on national board exams.

Unfortunately, students are ranked according to their academic performance. This system does increase the stress level but, surprisingly, does not create an atmosphere of cutthroat competition. Students are required to pass Step I of the national boards in order to advance to the clinical years and must pass Step II in order to graduate.

Clinical Years

One of the foremost advantages of the LLUSM experience is the opportunity to rotate through an incredible variety of clinical sites. In addition to the University Medical Center, the Loma Linda Veterans hospital, and two county hospitals, LLUSM is affiliated with a local community hospital, a Kaiser-Permanente medical center, and two smaller hospitals in Los Angeles. There is also a free walk-in clinic. The third-year family practice rotation can be completed in Chicago, Orlando, or Ohio.

Students are exposed to a heterogeneous patient population. The socioeconomic backgrounds in the patient spectrum vary immensely and may include a movie star's mother, a famous ice skater, a huge population of working poor, the many drug addicts in the Inland Empire (amphetamine capital of the world), and the destitute of developing nations.

Student autonomy varies with the hospital type, but the general ethic is that medical students are integral members of each clinical team. For example, at Riverside General Hospital, students are essential to a team that can admit upwards of twenty-five patients per night between a resident and two interns on the medical service.

LLUSM actively supports (logistically and financially) student rotations at a worldwide network of hospitals. First- and fourth-year students have been to Nepal, Africa, Central and South America, China, Southeast Asia, and Guinea. Others have crafted their own overseas experiences.

Unfortunately, students are not provided with much elective time. Requirements in neurology, ambulatory care, intensive care/emergency medicine, surgery, medicine, and pediatrics/obstetrics and gynecology/family medicine consume five of nine months. One of the remaining four months may be taken for vacation or interviewing. The fourth year also lacks in the counseling provided during the residency application process. Beyond the deans, there are few resources offered to students seeking advice about the match and about residency programs outside of the Loma Linda sphere. Traditionally, most students match at Loma Linda or California programs.

Social Life

The nightlife in the town of Loma Linda is about as exciting as a 3-hour histology lecture, and the surrounding area, known as the Inland Empire, faithfully lives up to its distinction as the "Armpit of Southern California." However, Loma Linda's proximity to Los Angeles, Orange County, the beach, the mountains, and the desert more than makes up for its inherent sleepiness. It is true: students can surf in the morning and ski in the afternoon. For those seeking to make an earnest but ill-advised attempt to dent their insurmountable medical school debt, Las Vegas is a short 4-hour drive at freeway speeds.

In addition, there are number of exceptional ethnic restaurants in the immediate Loma Linda vicinity. A huge (and FREE) athletic benefit to those so inclined is the recently constructed gym, known as Drayson, which rivals any state-of-the-art health club, complete with a waterslide. The Drayson Center sponsors a variety of competitive year-round intramural sporting leagues, including soccer, flag football, softball, basketball, and volleyball.

Because of its somewhat undesirable location, housing prices are more than reasonable. For example, a two-bedroom two-bath apartment with free parking is $330 per month. There is a dormitory available, although many students avoid living there at all costs. Most students choose to live in one of the many reasonably priced and conveniently located apartment complexes. There are even those who rent houses, sometimes more cheaply than apartments (approximately $250–$300 per month).

Although Loma Linda is located near a high-crime area, it is generally quite safe. Unfortunately, this leaves the Loma Linda police force ample time to enforce the stringent parking regulations.

The Bottom Line

LLUSM provides a medical education that emphasizes whole-person care, solid basic sciences, and exposure to a wide variety of clinical experiences in southern California and around the globe.

LOUISIANA STATE UNIVERSITY SCHOOL OF MEDICINE IN NEW ORLEANS

New Orleans, Louisiana

Applications: 1,226
Size of Entering Class: 167
Total Number of Women Students: 294 (41%)
Total Number of Men Students: 418 (59%)
World Wide Web: www.medschool.lsumc.edu/

Contact: Dr. S. McClugage, Assistant Dean for Admissions
433 Bolivar Street
New Orleans, LA 70112-2223
504-568-6262

Louisiana State University School of Medicine in New Orleans (LSU-NO) was established in 1931 and is the home of the state's three largest medical schools. LSU-NO represents one component of the Louisiana State University Health Sciences Center (LSUHSC), which also includes the Schools of Allied Health, Dentistry, Graduate Studies, and Nursing and trains the majority of health-care professionals in Louisiana, thereby achieving one of the institution's missions.

LSU-NO receives approximately 900 applications from Louisiana residents each year and hundreds more from nonresidents. From these, the admissions committee selects about 165 applicants to fill the first-year class. Be aware, however, that LSU-NO essentially only considers applicants who are residents of Louisiana. There is the ever-so-slight possibility that a nonresident (no doubt from a state carved out of the Louisiana Purchase) could gain admission.

Admissions/Financial Aid

Beginning in fall 1999, tuition will be $8,856 per year, a $2,030 increase over 1998. This is the first increase in tuition since 1992–93. The cost of books and supplies is estimated at $2,558. Once here, students are assigned a second-year student (big brother or big sister) to provide the inside scoop on which books and supplies are really needed and which ones only serve as large paperweights. Furthermore, students may donate or sell at greatly reduced prices all of their used books and supplies. Financial aid is widely available. Be sure to ask about scholarship opportunities specifically, in addition to government loans.

Preclinical Years

The first class on the first day is gross anatomy, and its infamous "Head and Neck Test," as it is known,

will dominate the first semester. The testing format at LSU-NO is combined, which means that all subjects are tested simultaneously on one Titanic test that is given every six or so weeks. Grades are given as honors/high pass/pass/fail (remember, P=M.D.). The grading system, along with the fact that misery loves company, keeps competition at a minimum.

By second semester, students have a better idea of how to budget their time between study and play. Physiology, biochemistry, and neuroanatomy dominate this semester. By comparison, this semester is considered one of the least taxing of the preclinical years.

The summer between first and second year affords opportunities to research, travel, or do just about anything. A lot of people choose only to get some rest and relaxation during this break after being overworked first year.

During second year, students finally begin to take courses that actually seem as if they have something to do with medicine, especially pathology and pharmacology. Microbiology, immunology, and parasitology, or MIP as it is affectionately known, is also taught second year.

A course that deserves a special mention is Introduction to Clinical Medicine (ICM). ICM actually begins in the first year, with basic life-support training, ambulance ride-alongs, and emergency-room clinical time. Second-year ICM involves lectures on physical exam techniques, signs and symptoms of disease, how to perform a medical history and physical exam, case study discussions, and similar experiences.

As second year winds to a close in early May, fear crescendos as the USMLE Step I approaches. LSU-NO requires that all students take Step I immediately following their second year and earn a passing score in order to continue uninterrupted during third year. For this reason, most students spend considerable time preparing for the exam. LSU-NO students traditionally perform well on the exam, with average scores in the range of 205 to 210.

Clinical Years

Third year begins the second phase of medical training—the clinical years. All students are required to take internal medicine (twelve weeks), general surgery, urology and otolaryngology (twelve weeks), obstetrics/gynecology (six weeks), psychiatry (six weeks), pediatrics (eight weeks), and family medicine (four weeks). Students train at a number of hospitals in the city, both public and private. Students also have the option of requesting that ssome of the clerkships be performed outside of the New Orleans area but within Louisiana at affiliated hospitals. At first, most third-year students feel so dumb that they wonder if they've actually been in medical school for two years. Things are made easier by sympathetic staff, residents, and nurses, but students will not always have that luxury. In fact, some people can be downright nasty. Don't begrudge, though. A large portion of grades during the clinical years is subjective and not based on exam scores. During the third year, an assertive student can deliver ten or more babies, learn good suturing techniques, perform a lumbar tap and thoracentesis, remove a lipoma, and possibly perform a few intubations. LSU-NO believes that the most effective way to learn medicine is by hands-on experience. After learning how to read all the abbreviations in the progress notes, where to find blankets for the bed when on call, and how to cope with the outdated facilities at the public hospitals, third year turns out to be okay.

Finally, the famed fourth year begins. This year is far and away the best year of medical school.

Although there are a few required clerkships in fourth year, what and where is up to each student. Passing the USMLE Step II exam is required to graduate.

Fourth-year students spend much of their time trying to decide what specialty to go into and where to go for residency. In the 1998 match, LSU did well—78 percent matched at their first choice and 10 percent matched at their second choice, with no one left unmatched. Except for the hassles of interviewing and the stress of the match, this year is basically a time to relax and to finally go on that trip to Acapulco you have been planning since first year.

Student Life

Founded as a French outpost 300 years ago, New Orleans is now famous for its Mardi Gras celebrations, historic Vieux Carré, gourmet Creole cuisine, zestful nightlife, and warm subtropical climate. The city has tons to offer, but students tend to either love it or hate it.

Housing in New Orleans is relatively inexpensive. Expect to shell out about $400 to $450 a month for a decent apartment in a nice area of town. A popular choice with incoming students is to live in the on-campus residence hall. The residence hall provides dormitory-style living that ranges from $723 to $794 per semester or apartment-style living at around $360 per month. The downside to living in the hall is that the rooms tend to be quite small and the waiting list to get in is very long.

The Bottom Line

LSU-NO is an inexpensive and laid-back medical school geared toward training physicians who will remain in Louisiana. What lacks in state-of-the-art facilities or a powerhouse name is made up for in a first-rate, hands-on medical education.

LOUISIANA STATE UNIVERSITY SCHOOL OF MEDICINE IN SHREVEPORT

Shreveport, Louisiana

Applications: 1,026
Size of Entering Class: 100
Total Number of Women Students: 138 (35%)
Total Number of Men Students: 261 (65%)
World Wide Web: www.sh.lsumc.edu/

Contact: Dr. F. Scott Kennedy, Assistant Dean for Student Admissions
Shreveport, LA 71130
318-675-5190

The School of Medicine in Shreveport was founded in 1968 as part of the Louisiana State University Medical Center (LSUMC) with a legislative dedication to provide a sound medical education to residents of Louisiana. Located in northwestern Louisiana on the Red River, the School offers an alternative to the urban congestion and living costs of New Orleans, where its older sister medical campus is located. LSUMC-Shreveport is a young and innovative institution, integrating the use of multimedia, Internet, and specialized computer programs into the curriculum and new facilities, such as the Biomedical Research Institution, the Children's Hospital, and the Feist-Weiller Cancer Center.

Although the curriculum is fairly traditional in structure, contact with patients begins early, and opportunities for elective study are provided during all four years. Clinical rotations include a unique two-year clerkship experience in a student-run primary-care clinic.

Admissions/Financial Aid

Approximately 80 percent of the student body obtains financial aid for tuition and living expenses in the form of loans. With scholarships and loans available, all accepted students have been able to meet their financial need.

Preclinical Years

Incoming first-year students are warmly welcomed with a courtyard Back to School Party and invitations to dinner at the homes of faculty members. They are introduced to their newly purchased laptop computers, which can access the Internet throughout the library and the core lab. Students quickly organize the note-taking service so that transcribed notes can be downloaded from the class Web site.

While the first two years are devoted to the study of the basic sciences, they are supplemented with short courses in radiology, psychiatry, genetics, epidemiology, ethics, and, of course, physical examination skills. Most courses blend didactic and case-based teaching approaches with variable computerized assistance. Many students complain of the large number of hours spent in lectures, which they are expected to attend. The comprehensive care course introduces students to the basics of doctor-patient relationships, history taking, and interviewing; it offers students their first contact with patients in the clinic. The combination of biochemistry and anatomy at the start of the year packs plenty of punch, but it is interspersed with post-test parties at the student union and frequent trips to the in-house student lounge and exercise room. The early spring courses in histology and neuroscience, enhanced by multimedia slide viewing programs, are comprehensive and well taught. One of the advantages of the smaller school atmosphere is that teachers are closely involved and often make themselves available to help outside the classroom. Several caring faculty members lead weekly mentoring groups for the first- and second-year students; these are convenient and extremely beneficial.

The second year begins with only two major classes, pathology and microbiology. With 1,600 pages of typed microbiology notes, a note-taking service is no longer needed. The pace is feverish, as the tests begin in August and continue almost every Monday until Thanksgiving. The year continues with pharmacology, psychiatry, neurology, family medicine, and physical diagnosis. The Introduction to Clinical Medicine course then pulls together much of what students learned in basic sciences and serves as a great review for the boards.

First- and second-year students have the opportunity to choose spring electives in a number of different clinical settings. A popular summer offering is the Primary Care Rural Preceptorship Program, which matches students with private practitioners throughout Louisiana for a four-week period and provides a $1,200 stipend for living expenses. Students may participate in summer research projects in the basic or clinical sciences, including neuroscience, molecular biology, and cardiovascular disease, at the recently completed Biomedical Research Institute.

Clinical Years

Most clinical rotations are held at LSU Hospital (675 beds), and additional training is held at Shreveport's Veterans Administration (VA) Hospital (450 beds) and E. A. Conway Hospital (for two weeks during obstetrics/gynecology) in nearby Monroe. The LSU Hospital includes a primary-care center with numerous outpatient clinics and a tertiary-care center for Level 1 trauma, serving a three-state region known as the Ark-La-Tex. The requirements of the third year consist of five-week blocks in surgery, surgical subspecialties, psychiatry, pediatrics, obstetrics/gynecology (two blocks), and internal medicine (two blocks). Comprehensive care (family medicine) runs throughout the year. Many rotations include nights on call. The variable amount of scut work that falls to the student is usually compensated for by the rich opportunities for patient care, while the quality of the teaching experience often depends on the student's team. Surgery and obstetrics/gynecology offer plenty of hand-on experience for motivated students (e.g., delivering six to twenty babies). In perhaps the most unique opportunity, students work two half-days each week in the Comprehensive Care Clinic serving as the patients' primary-care provider.

Student's can tailor the fourth year to meet their interests. Five 4-week rotations are required in surgery, outpatient and inpatient internal medicine, pediatrics, and neurology. Nearly half of the fourth year is elective time on campus or at other institutions, with two months available for vacation and/or interviewing for residency. Although nearly 70 percent of graduating students enter primary-care training,

including obstetrics/gynecology, a review of 1998 graduates shows those students entering a variety of other fields, including surgical subspecialties (orthopedics, otolaryngology, urology, ophthalmology), radiology, and dermatology. Of the 1998 graduates, 41 percent continued on to programs outside of the state, while 38 percent decided to remain at LSUMC-Shreveport for residency. Eighty-eight percent of participating students matched in one of their top three choices.

Student Life

Some argue that Shreveport offers few distractions from studying; however, students still find time to enjoy what the city has to offer. The weather is warm most of the year, and popular outdoor activities include golf, tennis, hunting, and fishing. Some students enjoy biking or jogging on the 375-acre Clyde Fant Parkway along the Red River. Metropolitan offerings range from sculpture by Rodin at the R. W. Norton Art Gallery to live Blues at Tommy's Place or performances like *Moon over Buffalo* at the Strand Theatre. Shreveport hosts its own hockey team, the Mudbugs, as well as plenty of tourists who come for riverboat casino gambling.

Although there is no on-campus housing, rent is cheap around Shreveport and across the Red River in Bossier City, at $350 to $500 for one- or two-bedroom apartments. A car is almost mandatory. When questions and problems about student life arise, the people in Student Affairs are firmly in the student's court, often going out of their way to help.

In addition to the class-sponsored events held after some exams, the Executive Council sponsors parties during the year, which include a Halloween Party, Christmas Party, and everybody's favorite, a Crawfish Boil. In the spring, the freshman class sponsors the Cadaver Ball, a semiformal affair with a stage show that satirizes the anatomy course. In recent years, students have worked to improve the School's AMA and AMSA chapters and have sent groups of students to Chicago and Washington, D.C., for annual meetings. Some students opt to volunteer at the Martin Luther King community health clinic or work on the school yearbook, the *Pulse*.

The Bottom Line

LSUMC in Shreveport caters exclusively to Louisiana residents and offers a small class size, innovative curriculum, solid exposure to rural and primary care, safe and casual atmosphere, and low cost.

LOYOLA UNIVERSITY CHICAGO STRITCH SCHOOL OF MEDICINE

Chicago, Illinois

Applications: 9,114
Size of Entering Class: 130
Total Number of Women Students: 234 (45%)
Total Number of Men Students: 285 (55%)
World Wide Web: www.meddean.luc.edu/

Contact: LaDonna E. Norstrom, Assistant Dean for Admissions
820 North Michigan Avenue
Chicago, IL 60611-2196
708-216-3229

Loyola University, Stritch School of Medicine is a Jesuit Medical School in Maywood, Illinois, 20 minutes east of Chicago. A new impressive medical school building, designed specifically for the integrated style of learning that the Loyola curriculum demands, was opened in fall 1998.

Preclinical Years

During a recent orientation, the Dean of Admissions announced the accomplishments of several members of Loyola's incoming class: "a professional skydiver, an explorer of Nepal, a volunteer with Mother Teresa, a nurse from Eastern Europe." Meeting other students is the best part of orientation week, but other time is consumed by exploring the nightlife of Chicago and the taverns of nearby Forest Park.

The actual work of medical school begins immediately on the first day of classes with an introduction to Structure of the Human Body. Prior to any dissection, there is a blessing of the cadavers, featuring readings by students of their own writings. For the next ten weeks, the only class scheduled is Structure, which means an hour of morning lecture followed by dissection, which may last all day. It's a jam-packed course that is difficult at best, but is over in the second week of October. A week of fall break follows, making for an ideal time to get away and relax.

Most students attend class every day, which is probably because there are typically only 2 to 3 hours of lecture, followed by a few hours of small-group case discussions. Classes almost always finish by 12:30 p.m., except on afternoons reserved for Introduction to the Practice of Medicine (IPM). Instructors write out detailed outlines and objectives of their lecture mate-

rial, leaving no need for a transcript service. Loyola fosters a friendly and cooperative atmosphere. For example, students often gather as an "Objectives Group" to aid their studying. Classes are graded honors/high pass/pass/fail (essentially A, B, C, and F), which may or may not be based on the class mean, depending on the course.

There is plenty of study space, although many students prefer the beautiful sixteen-floor Loyola Law Library that overlooks Lake Michigan in downtown Chicago. There are also plenty of computers; between the library, the dissecting lab, and the computer lab in the new building, there are fifty PCs and Macs available in addition to four PCs in each pair of learning clusters. The entire building, including the dissecting labs, features 24-hour-a-day card-key access.

Following Structure, first-year students take cell and molecular biology, host-defense (immunology), function of the human body (physiology), and Development I. Students take two to three subjects at once, with exams integrating all of the courses.

The two months off after the first year is a time to travel, visit friends and family, perform a service project, or just relax. Ministry offers an excellent program that takes students to Guatemala each summer to volunteer in optometry clinics. Other students spend their summers at Loyola or another university completing a research project to be presented at the fall St. Luke's Day poster presentation, held in celebration of the Jesuit patron saint of physicians.

Second year covers neuroscience, therapeutics (pharmacology), mechanisms of human disease (pathology), microbiology, and Development II. In addition, students are required to perform histories and physicals on patients as part of the second-year

IPM course with an assigned preceptor in a chosen specialty. Finals end in early May, leaving students plenty of time to study for the USMLE Step 1. Loyola students consistently score above the national average on the boards, with few or no failures.

Clinical Years

Clinical rotations are performed at a diverse range of area hospitals, including Loyola's Foster G. McGaw Hospital, which receives high marks for clerkships in medicine, surgery, and pediatrics. In addition, students rotate through the Hines Veterans Administration Hospital, the third-largest VA in the country and an excellent hospital for independent learning. Columbus, a downtown hospital, gives students a chance to learn from a diverse pediatric population. Finally, Alexian Brothers has its merits as a large private hospital north of the city. For family medicine, students are assigned to one of the many small Loyola-associated clinics scattered throughout the city. An adviser of the student's choice (e.g., the Internal Medicine Residency Director, or the Chief of Thoracic Surgery at Loyola) assists the students in choosing rotation sites.

In the fourth year, students have twelve weeks of required rotations: four weeks of neurology and two 4-week subinternships (four weeks in medicine or pediatrics and four weeks in critical care). Three of the rotations that comprise the rest of the thirty-four weeks of electives may be spent away from Loyola. Some students use this time to audition in locations where they see themselves doing a residency, while others take off for the Amazon, Africa, or the Loyola-sponsored St. Lucia rotation in the Caribbean. During the medicine subinternship, fourth-year students instruct the second-year students in physical exam skills as part of their IPM course. IPM continues in the third and fourth years, often composed of ethical discussions or humanities readings.

Ninety three percent of the students at Loyola received their first, second, or third residency choice in 1998. Sixty percent of the class went into primary care.

Social Life

Maywood and the nearby suburbs have a lot to offer in terms of their proximity to the city, without the hassles of city life. Most students live in the safe neighboring towns of Oak Park, Forest Park, and Riverside. Oak Park is the hometown of Frank Lloyd Wright, and touring his architecturally enchanting homes is a must for any visit from the parents. In any of these suburbs, a whole house, with room for a group of students, can be rented for about $400 per person per month. One-bedroom apartments in any of the suburbs average about $550 per month and have the added benefit of being right near the DesPlaines River Trail and the paved trail that runs through the forest preserves, both premium places for running, biking, and in-line skating. A handful of students from each class live in downtown Chicago.

An amazing amount of opportunities to play or to volunteer your time are available, only some of which are associated with school. Student organizations frequently sponsor speakers on topics that are either ignored or inadequately addressed by the curriculum. Recent speakers have covered subjects in alternative medicine, the changing role of physicians in managed care, and issues surrounding minorities in medicine. Students can also practice blood drawing, blood pressure measurement, and history taking at the nearby volunteer-staffed Maywood Clinic.

A new health and fitness center, where all students are automatically members, offers intramural sports, aerobics classes, racquetball, swimming, whirlpools, steam rooms, and saunas. The School fosters a family atmosphere with Ministry, an office where someone is always available to talk or listen and where there are always plenty of cookies and candy for the starving medical students.

The Bottom Line

Loyola University Medical Center's motto is "We also treat the human spirit," and that saying also goes for the medical school, as it moves to embrace a more independent style of learning.

MARSHALL UNIVERSITY SCHOOL OF MEDICINE

Huntington, West Virginia

Applications: 1,152
Size of Entering Class: 48
Total Number of Women Students: 95 (38%)
Total Number of Men Students: 157 (62%)
World Wide Web: musom.marshall.edu/

Contact: Cynthia A. Warren, Director of
Admissions
400 Hal Greer Boulevard
Huntington, WV 25755-2020
304-691-1738

Marshall University, a small school with forty-eight students per class nestled in the hills of West Virginia, provides a comfortable and quiet environment in which to pursue the study of medicine. Established in 1977, the School of Medicine was developed from the concept of a medical school without walls, where the needs of the community and those of the student body could be mutually addressed in a spirit of cooperation. This dialogue has fostered the School's mission, which emphasizes the development of well-rounded primary-care physicians by providing a well-balanced hands-on approach that features early clinical experience.

Preclinical Years

The support and encouragement of the faculty and staff at Marshall are invaluable to the student body. For example, it is common for professors, at the request of a group of students, to be available in the evenings or even on weekends to provide additional, more personal instruction. This type of personal attention and genuine concern is also found in the Dean of Student Affairs, the secretaries, and even in the interactions between fellow students.

Marshall strives to create a pleasant experience by providing students with a well-tended safety net. The Dean of Students monitors student progress, and, if additional help is needed, students are offered additional time with professors or senior medical students or the choice of decelerating the preclinical years into three years.

The curriculum of the preclinical years is characterized by early patient contact. In the first semester, preceptors cover the pertinent areas of the history and physical exam in conjunction with the gross anatomy and physical diagnosis courses. This rewarding approach may seem ideal to the eager

medical student who wishes to play doctor at the earliest possible moment, but the time demands on a first-year student are great, and spending several hours at the hospital the day before a large exam in gross anatomy can be inconvenient.

The grading system is a standard percentage-based letter format but does not interfere with the support and encouragement provided by fellow students. As the semesters follow one upon the other, the letter grades seem to lose their place, as the central concern becomes the main focus.

Most students find the neuroscience, pharmacology, and Introduction to Clinical Medicine courses to be the highlight of the preclinical years because of the high quality of teaching and the degree of competency that one achieves throughout the course. The nadir of the preclinical years is pathology because it is poorly taught, with sporadic lectures and exams that do not reflect the material assigned for reading and private study.

The summer after the first year leaves time for research, self-study, or travel, but the School offers minimal financial assistance and poor structure. Year two, which is marked by two to three exams per week, passes quickly with increasing patient contact. The year ends with a free comprehensive review course for USMLE Step I that features many well-known authors of board review books.

Clinical Years

The clinical years begin with a brief course that provides a transition to clinical medicine and builds confidence for the first clerkship. The rotations are performed at two community hospitals, a Veterans Administration hospital, and many rural sites located throughout the state. During the third and fourth years, four months at one or more of these rural sites is required.

Working at a rural site provides an excellent opportunity to work one-on-one with a preceptor and to gain a tremendous amount of hands-on experience by performing deliveries or being first assist on operative procedures. The absence of residents and the decreased time demands at these sites are a time of unparalleled development of confidence in the art of caring for patients. The downside of the rural experience includes less-than-deluxe accommodations, long commutes, and occasionally finding that the nearest mall or movie theater is far, far away.

The remainder of third year rotations are usually conducted at one of the two community hospitals, which provide exposure to higher acuity patients and more modern interventions. Rotations can demand a great deal of time, but the amount of scut work is kept to a minimum. Psychiatry and surgery are consistently ranked highly, but obstetrics and gynecology is considered by many to be poorly organized and far from student friendly.

The senior year provides time for electives, which range from alternative medicine, including naturopathy, aryuveda, homeopathy, and traditional Chinese medicine, to neurosurgery and pathology. The School encourages and aids those students who wish to use elective time to visit hospitals to which they are considering applying for residency.

Typically, Marshall graduates do very well in their residencies, fellowships, and practices in fields such as family practice, orthopedic surgery, and interventional radiology.

Social Life

At Marshall, a small medical school, the student body has a high degree of cohesiveness, and it is not uncommon to have staff and faculty members join the extracurricular activities. The family atmosphere that is fostered at the School is present in the surrounding community as well. Huntington provides a pleasant university-town setting that is quiet and safe—the crime rate in West Virginia is consistently one of the lowest in the nation—but still offers entertainment. Between the University downtown, the medical school, and the local bookstore/coffeehouse, it's easy to find a quiet place to nail down the finer points of the anatomy of the head and neck. Outside of Huntington, groups of students often head to nearby ski resorts or to one of the many white-water rafting areas in the state. The cost of living is low, with one- and two-bedroom apartments in the range of $375 to $575 and houses in the range of $400 to $600.

The Bottom Line

Marshall, located in a community setting where cost of living and crime are low, allows students to focus on obtaining an education that emphasizes the development of the general skills necessary to become a caring and competent physician.

MAYO MEDICAL SCHOOL

Rochester, Minnesota

Students Receiving Financial Aid: 96%
Applications: 3,621
Size of Entering Class: 43
Total Number of Women Students: 85 (51%)
Total Number of Men Students: 82 (49%)
World Wide Web: www.mayo.edu/mms/
MMS_Home_Page.html

Contact: Assistant Dean
200 First Street, SW
Rochester, MN 55905
507-284-2316

The Mayo Medical School offers a truly superb and unique opportunity for medical education. Founded in the 1800s, Mayo has become the world's largest group practice, with nearly 2,000 staff physicians and scientists, nearly half a million annual patient registrations, and three campuses (Rochester, MN; Scottsdale, AZ; and Jacksonville, FL). Rochester, home of the main campus and the Medical School, is a city full of paradoxes—a center of cutting-edge technology planted among the cornfields of the heartland.

From its inception, education has served a vital role at Mayo, and its medical students quickly discover that this emphasis has not changed. Mayo Medical School draws approximately 100 applicants for each position, permitting the admissions committee to select a diverse student body with not only exceptional academic qualifications but also demonstrated personal, social, and humanitarian interests and achievements. These select students are provided with unmatched resources, including financial assistance, a staff of renowned physicians and scientists who voluntarily and eagerly teach, and an environment that truly fosters cooperation at all levels.

Admissions/Financial Aid

The numbers may at first be intimidating: nearly 4,000 students vie for forty-two positions (six are reserved for M.D./Ph.D. applicants, and two are reserved for oral and maxillofacial surgery (OMS) applicants). Mayo accepts the standard AMCAS application but uses a telephone interview as the secondary application for candidates who meet initial screening criteria (about 600 people). Mayo tries to carefully evaluate all aspects of the application and does not just focus on

the numbers. Those "passing" the telephone interview (about 400 people) are invited for a personal interview in Rochester. Interviews are typically relaxed, even borderline enjoyable (if that's possible). Interviewers reportedly look for evidence of integrity, adaptability, maturity, leadership, and humanitarian concern. Despite the relaxed atmosphere of the interview, it is heavily weighted—be at your best!

The published tuition of $22,440 is misleading. Forty-five percent of entering students receive a full tuition scholarship, and a merit scholarship program reduces the cost by 50 percent for all other students. Residents of Minnesota, Arizona, and Florida receive an additional 50 percent off tuition and pay only $5,610. M.D./Ph.D. and OMS students receive full tuition remission and a generous stipend for the full period of training.

Preclinical Years

First-year course work begins with anatomy, histology, immunology, and molecular biology. The remainder of first year focuses around the major organ systems. Much of the learning is problem based and takes place in groups of approximately ten students. Grading for most courses is honors, high pass, pass, marginal pass, and fail. Though Mayo typically attracts bright students who create a challenging environment, the learning situation is highly cooperative.

Since early clinical exposure is a priority of Mayo Medical School, students begin patient contact within the first weeks of enrollment. First-year students are matched with a primary-care mentor, who gives a one-on-one introduction to the clinic and to patient care. Further, the Introduction to the

Patient course teaches students the fundamentals of history taking and physical examination and culminates in each student applying these skills to a Mayo patient by the end of the first year.

After a five-week break, a rigorous second year begins. An initial didactic block includes Microbiology and Infectious Disease, Introduction to Psychopathology, Introduction to Bioethics, Sexual Medicine, and Family Medicine. Following this block, students begin rotating through the clinic in the morning and attending lectures in the afternoon. Second-year clinical rotations include internal medicine, pediatrics, neurology, dermatology, musculoskeletal medicine and rehabilitation, and obstetrics and gynecology. Students typically interview and examine patients before the attending, present the case to the attending, and then observe as the attending examines the patient, all of which provides an incredible opportunity to develop and polish clinical skills.

Second-year afternoon course work is dominated by pathophysiology and pharmacology, two courses that span most of the school year and require considerable study time. Lectures end at either 3 p.m. or 5 p.m., leaving the evening hours for studying. While second year is grueling, students generally find it more rewarding than the first year. At least one objective measure, the USMLE Step I (the boards), indicates that Mayo's preclinical curriculum is more than adequate, with the following statistics from 1998: all Mayo students passed, 17 percent scored above the 99th percentile, 33 percent scored above the 95th percentile, 44 percent scored above the 90th percentile, and the class mean was in the 87th percentile.

Clinical Years

The clerkships of the third year involve working side-by-side with attendings and residents in internal medicine, obstetrics and gynecology, general surgery, neurology, pediatrics, psychiatry, and radiology. Since students have already had considerable clinical exposure during second-year rotations, they rapidly increase their level of participation in the initial care of patients as third-year students. The level of autonomy is gradually adjusted based on confidence and competence in the particular area, as well as the eagerness of the student. A lot is expected of Mayo students, but staff and residents are typically patient. Grades are based on attending and resident comments, demonstrated abilities, and written standardized examinations.

Mayo is truly a world-class health-care center and regularly attracts patients from all over the world who are seeking the advice of renowned experts in nearly every imaginable specialty. Thus, medical students have the opportunity to see and work up many zebras (very unusual cases) in addition to the extensive opportunities to practice and develop skills related to more common disease processes. Mayo serves as a primary-care provider for much of southeastern Minnesota.

Mayo firmly believes that a well-rounded physician has exposure to the importance of biomedical research. This is emphasized by the third-year research trimester, during which students conduct a biomedical research project, either with a Mayo investigator or at another institution. Students often travel to countries as remote as Botswana. Students gain the rudiments of research design, and many also author manuscripts. The research trimester frequently differentiates Mayo students during residency application.

During the fourth year, students complete a number of electives as well as a six-week internal medicine subinternship and four required clerkships (pediatrics, family medicine, internal medicine, and surgery). Students are strongly encouraged to perform at least one rotation off campus.

For the residency match for the class of 1999, 97 percent received their first, second, or third choice; 94 percent received their first or second choice; 75 percent received their first choice; and 44 percent matched in primary care.

Social Life

Rochester, with a population of approximately 80,000, has been voted the best city in which to live by *Money* magazine and is an incredible place to raise a family. The public and private grade schools are superb, crime and unemployment are low, average income is high, and housing is affordable. Despite these glowing features, many students, particularly those coming from large university cities, find Rochester a bit lackluster. The small class size generally leads to a tight-knit group of students, and there are many student-organized parties and gatherings. There are, however, limited places for students to socialize within the community. There is respite, however, students can escape to the Twin Cities, a 1½ hour drive to find a wide array of fine restaurants, cultural opportunities, nightclubs, and the mother of all megamalls.

Recreational activities are abundant in Rochester. There are several miles of bike or cross-country skiing paths. Rochester Park and Recreation offers a large variety of sports leagues, and Mayo offers a heavily subsidized membership to its own exercise facilities.

Mayo Medical School does not provide housing, but several apartments are located within walking distance of the clinic. Some students, especially M.D./Ph.D. candidates and students with families, purchase homes. Public transportation is rather limited; very few students survive without a car, especially since the winters can be brutal, with windchills dipping to 50° below zero.

The Bottom Line

Mayo offers an opportunity to train at a world-famous health-care center, replete with resources and a renowned staff dedicated to teaching. The cost of attending is minimal, while the value of training received is immeasurable.

MEDICAL COLLEGE OF GEORGIA SCHOOL OF MEDICINE

Augusta, Georgia

Tuition 1996–97: $19,448 per year
Students Receiving Financial Aid: 81%
Applications: 1,664
Size of Entering Class: 180
Total Number of Women Students: 224 (31%)
Total Number of Men Students: 493 (69%)

World Wide Web: www.mcg.edu
Contact: Dr. Mary Ella Logan, Associate Dean for
Admissions
1120 Fifteenth Street
Augusta, GA 30912
706-721-3186

Outside of Georgia, Augusta is known almost exclusively for the Master's, the world-famous golf tournament held at Augusta National. However, Augusta is also home to the Medical College of Georgia (MCG), which prides itself on its challenging, noncompetitive atmosphere, making students master medicine without working against their classmates.

Admissions/Financial Aid

The School admits about 180 people each year. Part of the University System of Georgia, the School is almost exclusively for in-state students. The yearly tuition for in-state residents is about $9,000 per year, and nine-month living expenses are usually about $9,000 per year as well. Financial aid usually is given through state and federal government loans.

Preclinical Years

Students usually begin the day of class furiously scribbling down everything professors say—until the first break of the day, when a second-year student in charge of the note-taking service lets students know they can put their pens down if they want. The first year of basic sciences focuses on learning how the healthy human body functions. Students also begin taking Physical Diagnosis, in which students practice physical exams on each other. A separate problem-based learning course teaches students how to approach problems from a clinical perspective— dissecting individual cases into a series of questions and researching the answers before the next class.

Second year is dominated by pathology and pharmacology, by far the most detail-oriented and challenging classes of the preclinical curriculum. Several smaller classes are taught during this time as well, the most notable being Clinical Medicine. Led by one of the finest instructors at MCG, Clinical Medicine gives students exposure to some of the most common clinical problems physicians face. During third year, many students find themselves wishing they had paid closer attention during this class. In Physical Diagnosis, students begin examining patients in the hospital and presenting their findings to attending physicians. The final exam for the course includes performing a complete history and physical on an unknown patient in less than an hour. Unfortunately, not everyone is always up to the challenge, and many students have been known to ramble.

Students are graded on an absolute scale, not on a curve. The School encourages students to work together, and the results usually show. Competition is virtually nonexistent, and students consistently score above the national average on the USMLE, with a failure rate of only about 2 to 3 percent.

Clinical Years

In the third year, students complete a set of core rotations, similar to those at other medical schools. This includes three months of internal medicine; six weeks each of family medicine, general surgery, pediatrics, and obstetrics/gynecology; and four weeks each of psychiatry and neurology/neurosurgery. The three local adult hospitals include MCG Hospital, the VA Hospital, and University Hospital (a private facility). Family medicine, surgery, internal medicine, and ob/gyn can be completed at facilities outside of Augusta, including those in Atlanta, Savannah, and Columbus. The pediatrics rotation has just been blessed with a new university-affiliated Children's Hospital.

Experiences vary, but rotations at MCG all emphasize hands-on training. Students must write daily notes on their patients, present to attendings, and scrub in on all surgeries. Some courses require a short paper to be written on a subject of choice. Nearly all rotations have a final exam, and the final grade includes a written report by the attending and resident physicians.

Fourth year requires at least six elective rotations and a subinternship in medicine, pediatrics, or family medicine. Students can also do rotations anywhere in the world if they are approved through the curriculum office.

Social Life

Life outside of class is filled with intramural sports and a number of School-sponsored gatherings. The student government organizes monthly TGIF parties, which are well attended by the class. Student activities are also enhanced by the presence of other allied health schools in Augusta, including a school for nursing and physical therapy.

Augusta is actively working to revive its downtown area, and new bars and restaurants are opening monthly. Of course, the town comes to a halt during the first full week in April, when Augusta becomes the center of the sporting world for the Master's golf tournament.

The Bottom Line

MCG is an exceptional value for Georgia state residents and gives students a solid education in a noncompetitive environment.

MEDICAL COLLEGE OF OHIO SCHOOL OF MEDICINE

Toledo, Ohio

Size of Entering Class: 140
Total Number of Women Students: 224 (40%)
Total Number of Men Students: 343 (60%)
World Wide Web: www.mco.edu

Contact: Dr. Almira F. Gohara, Dean
PO Box 18
Toledo, OH 43699-8

As Ohio's only stand-alone medical school, the Medical College of Ohio (MCO) in Toledo, Ohio, offers a unique, supportive, and technologically superior environment for medical education. With no undergraduate program to deter focus or funding, the students, professors, researchers, and administrators concentrate on medicine. MCO offers an approachable faculty, a collaborative learning atmosphere, and a very active student life, with more than 80 percent involvement in more than forty student organizations. MCO provides a supportive learning environment, a technologically advanced school, and a campus that is growing by leaps and bounds.

One of the most striking aspects of the MCO community is how the medical staff administrators and faculty support and listen to the students. During the first week of medical school, the Medical College Dean, Dr. Amira Gohara, invites small groups of medical students to eat lunch with her so she has an opportunity to get to know them. Every professor gives out his or her home and pager numbers. The faculty members learn the students' first names and stay long hours after class and lab to make sure concepts are understood.

MCO is also a leader in computer technology. The campus Intranet provides grade progress reports, student financial statements, and free e-mail/Internet access. The School has also thrown out the old projector slides and put together a computer curriculum, complete with class notes and labs and illustrative images on line. This has allowed the students to access class and lab material from both school and home at any hour. MCO is equipped with state-of-the-art computers throughout campus, with a computer resource lab and computer hotline for all students. It is also one of the only schools in the country that is equipped to administer the computerized USMLE on

campus. Plans for future expansion include a whole building devoted to technology.

MCO's campus continues to grow. MCO is composed of four specialized schools: the School of Medicine, School of Allied Health, School of Nursing, and Graduate School. The research institution is moving forward, with millions of dollars in grant money awarded every year. With three on-campus teaching hospitals, newly renovated classrooms, and the largest medical library in northwest Ohio, MCO has become a noteworthy teaching facility.

Admissions/Financial Aid

Admission to MCO is challenging. With 3,100 applications and 600 interviews, 135 students and five flex students (five-year program) matriculate each year. The class of 2002 consists of 37 percent women and 8 percent minority students. The admissions department opens doors to all students who are considering applying to medical school. They provide programs such as the spring visitation day to help students with their medical school decision. In conjunction with the multicultural affairs department, a minority visitation day is held to help minority students matriculate to MCO.

Tuition at MCO is about $11,000 per year. With the help of a very active financial aid department, 86 percent of the students receive financial aid. This makes attending MCO not only affordable, but also reasonable. The financial aid office is well staffed and is always available to students. The financial aid office also initiates policies that maximize benefits to students by reducing turnaround time for loan disbursements, increasing federal loan eligibility, and accommodating student needs with budget adjustments.

Preclinical Years

The class of 1998–99 was the first class at MCO to participate in the new Problem-Based Learning (PBL) curriculum. The students engage in case discussions, complete with learning objectives and exams that span a three-week period. The students receive a new case every three weeks and work in teams to learn the medical issues. The rest of the curriculum is in a block format. The first year has three blocks that consist of cellular and molecular biology, human structure and development, and neuroscience and behavioral science. The second year has two blocks that consist of immunity and infection and organ systems. students take an integrated pathophysiology course, as well as a physician, patient, and society course, that span both years. This new program is designed to lessen class time and promote both self-motivated and group learning. With the new block system, exams are given every three or four weeks and cover one subject at a time. So far, the feedback has been wonderful. Students have enjoyed the group learning method and find that the material sticks better when they have to present it to their classmates.

Classroom work is not the only type of learning required of first- and second-year medical students. In an effort to expose medical students to the clinical setting, MCO provides opportunities early on to work in groups of four, twice a month, with local physicians; students gain hands-on experience with patients through these opportunites. Not only do the students perform routine history taking and physicals, but they also work with the physician to diagnose and treat the patients. Physician mentors are also provided to the students to allow for even more clinical exposure.

Clinical Years

The driving force for many book-studying first- and second-year medical students is the clinical experience, which is finally realized at the beginning of the third year. It is the time when the hospital experience, the patient contact, and the classroom learning make their education feel like real medicine. MCO has a rigorous program for third-year students, which includes rotations in family medicine, surgery, pediatrics, internal medicine, obstetrics/gynecology, and psychiatry. The fourth-year requirements include four weeks of neurology and twenty-eight weeks of electives. The electives give fourth-year students a chance to focus on their career choice and allow time to interview for

residency programs. During the third and fourth years, students also take eight weeks of rural clinical medicine at sites throughout Ohio and Michigan (AHEC program).

MCO prides itself on being a top primary-care school, but it is strong in all specialties. For the 1999 graduating class, 94 percent received one of their top three choices and 70 percent received their first choice (with 56 percent in primary care). Clinical education is available not only through MCO's three teaching hospitals, but also through almost all the hospitals in and around Toledo. The clinical experience at MCO is full of long hours and many stressful nights, but rewarding, with a top-notch education that serves students well as physicians.

Social Life

Toledo, Ohio offers a cultural mix of activities for both single and married students. While this city is not like New York City or Boston, it has all the comforts of a big city, with the cost of living of a small Ohio town. While MCO's Office of Student Life keeps life on campus alive through dances, talent shows, and multicultural events, Toledo is also strategically located between Detroit (1 hour away), Cleveland (2 hours away), Columbus (2 hours away), and Cincinnati (3 hours away). Reaching any of those cities for a professional ball game or evening event makes for a pleasant escape from school life. In Toledo, students can buy tickets to see the Mudhens, go to the opera, catch a hockey game, or go out for a night on the town. Toledo is a great place for dining out, since it has the highest number of restaurants per capita in the world. The weather is typically mild, with relatively hot summers and cold winters (with occasional snow).

The Bottom Line

The Medical College of Ohio offers the perfect foundation for a medical education. It is a school that provides a warm environment that puts the students first. MCO has been climbing the ranks among medical schools and has earned a strong reputation for developing excellent doctors. After students become acquainted with the faculty and administration, take part in the vast technology the School has to offer, and participate in a rigorous medical curriculum, they not only grow as students but they also grow as a part of the MCO family.

MCP HAHNEMANN UNIVERSITY SCHOOL OF MEDICINE

Philadelphia, Pennsylvania

Tuition 1996–97: $25,725 per year
Applications: 11,503
Size of Entering Class: 246
Total Number of Women Students: 678 (48%)
Total Number of Men Students: 728 (52%)
World Wide Web: www.auhs.edu/homepage.html

Contact: Dr. Sue Zarro, Associate Dean for
Student Affairs and Admissions
Broad and Vine
Philadelphia, PA 19102
215-762-3063

There have been a number of significant changes at MCP Hahnemann University (MCPHU) in the last five years. In 1994 MCP, the former Women's Medical College, agreed to merge academic programs with Hahnemann University, a former institution of homeopathy, to create the country's largest private medical institution. The merger of two medical schools generated excitement as well as concerns about the future of the new university, Allegheny University of the Health Sciences, which included the medical school, a new school of public health, a school of nursing, and a school of health professions.

As the developments of this merger were unfolding, the parent organization of Allegheny University, AHERF, filed for bankruptcy in 1998. Shortly thereafter, Tenet Healthcare Corporation purchased the University and the Philadelphia hospitals in the AHERF system. As part of this sales agreement, Drexel University, a neighboring academic institution in Philadelphia, manages the University with the intention of ultimately merging with it.

In spite of these recent changes, MCP Hahnemann continues a long tradition of educating outstanding clinicians of tomorrow. Located in the East Falls section of Philadelphia, a modern educational facility provides the home campus for a diverse, energetic student body. The first combined class of MCP Hahnemann School of Medicine will graduate in 1999.

Admissions/Financial Aid

Approximately 11,000 applications are received annually. Of these, 1,000 applicants are interviewed by faculty and current students for the 250 seats in each class. The average age of the incoming class is about 24 years old, which reflects the large number of nontraditional students who have pursued other endeavors prior to applying to medical school. It is common to find students who have had previous careers as lawyers, nurses, engineers, researchers, or teachers. A significant number of the students are married, and some students have children. Every year there are several students admitted through a six-year combined program with Lehigh University.

Historically, women have comprised almost 60 percent of each class at MCP, and this commitment to women continues within MCP Hahnemann. Residents of Pennsylvania represent the largest percentage of each class, with the remainder of the students representing other regions of the country. Minorities represent about one quarter of each class, although this varies from year to year.

Tuition was $26,250 for the 1998–99 academic year. Since school-based financial aid scholarships are limited, students graduate with an average indebtedness in excess of $100,000.

Preclinical Years

Perhaps the most unique aspect of MCPHU is that there are two separate educational tracts into which students may enroll for the two-year basic science curriculum: Program for Integrated Learning (PIL) and IFM. The two curricula are separate, without academic interaction during the entire two years. As a result, it is easy to socialize among the classmates within a chosen tract, but it takes some effort to get to know the students from the other tract.

PIL is a problem-based learning curriculum, supplemented with informal lectures and labs. Students spend a significant amount of time in small groups with faculty members discussing various aspects of the case-based materials. Students are encouraged to structure their learning according to individual needs in order to foster lifelong learning habits. Clinical skills sessions and community service course work are integrated into the curriculum from the first month of medical school. At the end of the first year there is a nine-week session based in a primary-care office setting that emphasizes clinical skills and patient-focused learning. About 30 percent of the students select this tract.

The IFM curriculum has evolved from a lecture and lab format to one that integrates lectures and labs with discussion groups, case-based material, and clinical medicine. Students have scheduled sessions each week with clinical preceptors in primary care settings to develop clinical skills from the start of the first year. The majority of students select this tract.

A clinical-learning lab provides students the opportunity to learn clinical skills using standardized patients. Every session is videotaped so that you can review your performance with faculty for constructive feedback. These review sessions are enormously popular, as well as entertaining. A variety of electives are available through the medical humanities seminar series.

The grading system is honors, pass, and fail. Students are supportive and there is minimal grade competition. Most students seek to pass, but an occasional honors grade is certainly welcomed. Passing the USMLE Step I is required to advance to the clinical years.

Clinical Years

In the third year, all students rotate through medicine, surgery, obstetrics and gynecology, pediatrics, psychiatry, and family medicine, which leaves no time for electives. A significant amount of time in each rotation is spent in ambulatory settings providing primary care. There are numerous teaching hospitals in the University system, including MCP Hospital, Hahnemann Hospital, St. Christopher's Children's Hospital, Graduate Hospital, Allegheny Hospital in Pittsburgh, and many more within the Delaware Valley and beyond. There are wide range of clinical settings, patient populations, and medical specialties available at MCPHU since the merger, a clear advantage for students. At the beginning of the year, students select a clinical pathway that will offer career counseling as well as guidance in course selection. This recent addition has been overwhelmingly popular.

During the fourth year, all students must complete neurology, a medicine subinternship, a pathway subinternship, and six electives. The delay in

elective time is a distinct disadvantage, especially for those interested in specialties beyond the core areas covered in the third year. There are two months of vacation time to schedule residency interviews. Students have been successful in the residency match, with 82 percent of last year's class matching at one of their top three choices. A passing grade on USMLE Step II is also required for graduation.

Social Life

There is a network of support services for students, including tutoring, mentoring, minority issues, and more. Student interest and community outreach activities groups are plentiful. Despite busy academic schedules, most students find time to participate in activities outside of medical school.

Philadelphia provides a diverse setting for student entertainment. Historic attractions include Independence Hall, the Liberty Bell, the Betsy Ross house, and the Franklin Institute. Cultural activities are readily available and affordable at locations like the Philadelphia Museum of Art or the Academy of Music. Outings to Fairmount Park and Penn's Landing are easily accessible within the city limits. Popular entertainment venues include South Street, Manayunk, and Delaware Avenue. New York City, Washington, D.C., Atlantic City, Lancaster, and the Pocono Mountains are easily accessible and are within a few hours' drive.

There is no on-campus housing, but there is plenty of housing in the surrounding neighborhoods for students. Rents in these neighborhoods are very reasonable for shared apartments and houses and run from $600–$800 per month ($200–$400 per person). Of course, there are endless options for housing in the city of Philadelphia, but prices can be quite high for the more desirable locations.

The Bottom Line

Despite the recent turmoil, MCPHU has emerged as a larger, more dynamic medical school. There are endless opportunities for students in the classroom, in the research labs, and on the wards. Despite the class size, the atmosphere remains friendly and collegial. The faculty has been and continues to be committed to helping students achieve their personal and professional goals. The emphasis at MCPHU is clearly placed on graduating caring physicians with appropriate skills to become the successful clinicians of tomorrow.

MEDICAL COLLEGE OF WISCONSIN

Milwaukee, Wisconsin

Tuition 1996–97: $26,355 per year
Size of Entering Class: 200
World Wide Web: www.mcw.edu
Contact: Lesley A. Mack, Registrar

8701 Watertown Plank Road
Milwaukee, WI 53226-0509
414-456-8733

The Medical College of Wisconsin (MCW), located in Milwaukee, Wisconsin, has its roots in the 1890s, when two private medical schools were formed in the city. There were various historical twists and turns until 1970, when the school took its current name. MCW moved into a brand-new building on the grounds of the Milwaukee Regional Medical Center, its current campus in west suburban Milwaukee, in 1978. In 1998, a new 170,000-square-foot addition, the Health Research Center, opened with a spacious new library and plenty of study space.

One interesting thing about MCW is its size: classes are usually around 205 students. However, there's still a small-school feel to the College, with many students living, studying, and going out together.

Students are diverse and intelligent. About 27 percent are minorities, 36 percent are women, and 10 percent are older than 26. Consequently, a wide number of backgrounds are seen: Peace Corps, law, business, fire fighting, concert piano, and others. The average MCAT score is 10 per section, and the average overall GPA is 3.67. Surprisingly, many students are from California.

The school works hard to do what is necessary to get students through. The school provides housing, tutoring, and financial aid. There have been cases when the school actually found scholarship sources for students without the student needing to lift a finger. There are also little bonuses, like snack days during test weeks, sponsored social functions, and so on.

Concerning medical training, MCW emphasizes primary care. In fact, MCW ranks seventeenth in the nation for training in that field. Therefore, primary-care doctor production is high. It is not that the school makes it hard for a student to choose thyroidology, but there are no specialist mentors available in the mentor program for first- and second-year students. It is easy to find an adviser in any field during the third and fourth years, but students have to

plan ahead if they have a specific specialty in mind—before the first few months of the fourth year, only the summer after first year is really open to get a feel for something by doing an elective rotation in it.

Preclinical Years

The first year is spent learning biochemistry, anatomy, physiology, and the neurosciences. There is also a two-yearlong course called Clinical Continuum. This has a number of different facets to it, including mentorship; a human behavior course; a patient relationship project; short courses on epidemiology, ethics, palliative care, medical informatics, and biostatistics; and how to do a medical history and physical examination on a live patient.

Regular classes are, for the most part, good, with some outstanding teachers, especially in physiology. Classes still consist of mostly lectures, with some lab work. MCW has a fairly well-organized note service, in which participants share note-taking chores. Biochemistry easily has the highest failure rate, which can be blamed on the subject matter. The Clinical Continuum course involves running around to this clinic and that lecture. The psychiatry department, which runs the human behavior course, is often viewed as being unyielding and unpredictable.

Year two brings two semesters of pathology and one each of pharmacology, microbiology, psychiatry, and more Clinical Continuum. Pharmacology is a good course, but tests are not multiple choice, so students have to change their way of learning. Overall, pathology is a good course, but the renal pathology section can be mind-boggling and the final covers the whole year.

Clinical Years

After taking the USMLE Step I, students gather what wits they have left and do rotations at the various clinical affiliates. The Milwaukee Regional Medical Center sits on 248 acres a short drive west of downtown Milwaukee and is home to Froedert Memorial Lutheran Hospital (FMLH), Children's Hospital of Wisconsin (CHW), and the Milwaukee County Mental Health Division, among other facilities and affiliated hospitals. Milwaukee County farms out indigent care to many area hospitals, with FMLH, a Level 1 trauma center, receiving the lion's share of such cases and providing the bulk of resident and student training. CHW is the only Level 1 trauma center in the state and also provides many pediatric cases for students/residents. The mental health facility is the busiest psychiatric emergency room in the country. Also, MCW is affiliated with the nearby Veterans Administration hospital, which further widens the range of patients.

Third-year clerkships include internal medicine, anesthesiology, ophthalmology, psychiatry, surgery, ambulatory medicine, pediatrics, and obstetrics/gynecology. Internal medicine is a tough month, especially in FMLH, but it is important. Part of the internal medicine evaluation involves successfully doing a history and physical exam on a faculty member. Anesthesiology is two weeks long and is taken before or after six weeks of psychiatry. Ambulatory medicine is done in a primary-care clinic either in the area or, for a few, at some of Wisconsin's summer tourist spots, where students have been able to spend time swimming, waterskiing, hiking, and enjoying other fun outside activities.

During the fourth year, the only required rotations are a subinternship (grueling, of course) and electives in surgery and medicine (in a specialty such as cardiology or pulmonology). The rest of the year is completely up to the student. Two months are scheduled vacation months, with one probably best used for interviewing in the winter. The rest are chosen based on future plans. Advisers need to sign off on student schedules, so students need to think of good reasons for each of their choices.

Many residents who attended other medical schools comment on how much more MCW students get to do than they did: IVs, intubations, arterial lines, paracentesis, thoracentesis, suturing, small surgical procedures or small parts of big surgical procedures, and many baby deliveries. The training occurs at the above-mentioned hospitals, numerous private hospitals (at least six), and clinics in the area and state. In general, as the clinical years progress, learning occurs more on the student's terms.

Concerning the match, roughly 30 to 40 percent of the students get their first choice and 70 to 80 percent get one of their top three choices. Faculty members are generally helpful with advice on programs and letters of recommendation.

Social Life

For fun outside class, MCW offers a wide variety of options, which run the gamut of intramural sports, a new exercise facility, and numerous student organizations based on everything from ethnicity, sexuality, and political interests to social concerns.

For students coming from larger, more glamorous cities, the best things about Milwaukee are that it has a medical school and it is only 90 miles from Chicago. Some of those naysayers, however, are won over in the end. Milwaukee has a variety of ethnic restaurants, numerous bars, baseball's Brewers in their brand-new stadium (scheduled for completion in 2), basketball's Bucks, one of the finest zoos in the country, a variety of fine arts, a natural history museum with an IMAX theater, annual ethnic festivals, and a giant ten-day music festival each summer. The Petit National Ice Center offers two indoor ice-hockey rinks. All of this lies on the shores of beautiful Lake Michigan. The lakefront area is made up of numerous beaches and harbors and is often the epicenter of activities.

One of the best aspects of Milwaukee is that even at rush hour, travel times from outlying areas to downtown are usually less than 30 minutes, even less if traveling the opposite way such as from an apartment downtown to school. Speaking of housing, rent is cheap. While students can spend more than $1,500 a month for a high-rise that overlooks the lake, many cheaper places are available in the hip downtown/East Side areas. Prices become even more reasonable the closer students get to school. One-bedroom places rent for about $400 to $600 per month, and three bedrooms run from $500 to $900 per month. These are for nice, safe neighborhoods within a few miles of school. A number of students actually buy homes.

The Bottom Line

MCW is the place for well-rounded and diverse students who want a medical education that offers a fair amount of hands-on experience. The setting is not necessarily high powered, but it does provide solid preparation for residency.

MEDICAL UNIVERSITY OF SOUTH CAROLINA COLLEGE OF MEDICINE

Charleston, South Carolina

Tuition 1996–97: $23,504 per year
Applications: 3,185
Size of Entering Class: 142
Total Number of Women Students: 223 (41%)
Total Number of Men Students: 326 (59%)

World Wide Web: www.musc.edu
Contact: Wanda Taylor, Director of Admissions
171 Ashley Avenue
Charleston, SC 29425-2
843-792-2055

Founded in 1824, the Medical University of South Carolina (MUSC) College of Medicine in Charleston was the first medical school in the southern United States. Students at MUSC will tell you that in addition to getting a top-notch education with one of the cheapest price tags in the nation, they have also been able, in fact encouraged by the University faculty members, to allow time for the humanities, to explore the phenomenal town of Charleston, and to develop their extra medical interests. The result? Year after year, MUSC places an overwhelming majority of the students in one of their top three choices for residency (including the big names) and graduates a group of tightly bound, highly satisfied students.

From an initial pool of 2,400 applicants, MUSC invites 600 to interview and admits about 135 students each year. The admission process, for many, is the clenching factor in choosing MUSC as their medical school. The interview day allows time for students to have lunch and provides a tour by current students who are not on the admissions committee. This allows applicants to gain an additional perspective without the worries of having to impress. Interviews are offered based on a formula that weighs GPA, MCAT scores, and a variety of other criteria. Once selected for an interview, students become equal once again. Selection is then based on a combination of their interviews and recommendation letters. The administration takes great pride in the fact that four students, one from each class, sit on the admissions committee as full voting members, with all rights and privileges. These students are involved in the interviewing process and play a role in selecting candidates. Students have two on-campus interviews: one with a committee member and one with a

member of the University faculty. Both carry equal weight, and if there is a large discrepancy between the two, the student is normally asked back for a third interview.

The average age of incoming student is in the mid-20s, although there is a handful of students from each class in their mid-30s. The overwhelming majority are South Carolina residents. However, understand that the University defines a resident as someone who has been living in the state for at least a year prior to the date of matriculation. Coincidentally, a number of first-year medical students have been South Carolina residents for only a year prior to their date of matriculation. The men-women ratio is approximately 60:40, and despite preconceived notions regarding the homogeneity of the Carolinas, each class has substantial ethnic diversity.

Preclinical Years

MUSC is currently in the process of revamping its medical curriculum. Up until now, there were two different ways a medical student could choose to attack the first two years: the traditional approach or the parallel approach. Of the 135 students in a particular class, about twenty can opt to participate in the Parallel Curriculum (PC) instead of the Traditional Curriculum (TC). The PC, established in 1994, is an alternative problem-based curricular track, in which students learn the same material that the TC students learn using a vastly different format. TC students learn through a combination of lectures, labs, small groups, and more lectures; the PC students learn from case studies and pseudo-lecture correlates. PC students work together on an ordered set of clinical cases (with faculty guidance) to develop learning issues and knowledge relevant to the basic sciences. An enormous benefit of the PC program is the fact that students begin learning to attack clinical problems from the first day of medical school. TC students, on the other hand, have two years of lecture about the very topics that the PC students are trying to solve on their own. It is sort of like the difference between being force-fed information and having to figure it out for yourself.

Advocates of the PC program say that students actually enjoy their medical education, and the students who participate in it admit that it mentally prepares them for the clinical years. Advocates of the TC program say that they need the structure that the lectures and exams provide. In addition, TC students seem to have an easier time adjusting socially than do the PC students, who are relatively sequestered in a small cohort of twenty students. The TC has an emphasis on small-group instruction, as does, although not to the same degree, the PC program. Both curricula address four major objectives during the first two years: provision of basic science concepts, acquisition of problem-solving strategies, development of skills that permit the performance of an adequate medical history and physical exam, and an introduction to the role of the physician in society.

The MUSC curriculum committee is currently attempting to take the best facets from each curriculum and combine them to maximize the students' learning, proficiency, and enjoyment. Similar to the parallel curriculum, more of the first two years of the traditional program are taught from an organ-system perspective instead of teaching each course separately. There is also a greater push for all courses to include as much problem- and case-based teaching as appropriate. Students also serve on the curriculum committee. They are encouraged to take an active role in shaping the direction of the various courses.

Microbiology and immunology is typically the most grueling course. Regardless, students are extremely well educated on the two subjects and perform above the national average on those sections of the USMLE Step I.

USMLE scores are typically at or above the national average, with only a few students from each class failing. This past year was the first year that the PC program had a 100 percent pass rate.

In conjunction with the College of Graduate Studies, MUSC offers the Medical Scientist Training Program, which leads to combined M.D.-Ph.D. degrees.

Clinical Years

Students perform their clinical years at a variety of facilities on the MUSC campus. The MUSC Medical Center is a comprehensive 600-bed facility composed of three separate hospitals (the University Hospital, the Institute of Psychiatry, and the Children's Hospital). The Medical Center includes centers for specialized care (Heart Center, Transplantation Center, Hollings Cancer Center, Digestive Diseases Center) and numerous outpatient facilities, including an extensive array of affiliated faculty practice association ambulatory-care centers. Students can also do a portion of their clinical years at the approximately 100-bed VA hospital on campus. Programs that have earned distinguished reputations at MUSC are neuroscience, substance abuse, cardiovascular medicine, drug sciences, perinatal medicine, burn care, ophthalmology, hearing loss, genetics, rheumatology, and cancer care.

The third year combines PC and TC students for the first significant period of time since their matriculation. Third year consists of eight weeks of internal medicine, pediatrics, surgery, obstetrics/gynecology, and psychiatry and four weeks each of neurology and family medicine. Students have the option to postpone their four weeks of neurology until fourth year so that they can do eight of family medicine at a rural location in South Carolina. Third year also has one week of intensive nutrition education.

Fourth year has limited requirements: four weeks of internal medicine, four weeks of surgery, and a four-week subinternship in pediatrics, medicine, or surgery. The remainder of the fourth year is filled with electives and has a large degree of flexibility with regard to what students do and where they go. In addition, students have up to twelve weeks of off time to interview, travel, get married, or take a vacation.

MUSC is like most medical schools: it has some amazing house officers and some house officers who are not that great. Generally speaking, though, the house staff is one of the School's best assets. No student leaves without having been permanently changed by his or her interaction with one of the attendings or residents. A formal student-initiated mentor program is currently being designed to assist with specific questions and guidance issues that concern students.

MUSC's strength is the clinical years. Students, having been exposed to a wide array of disease processes, therapeutic modalities, and diagnostic thought strategies, attend top-tier programs and are as clinically competent as anyone from any other school.

Social Life

Students fall in love with the city of Charleston. Attending medical school in a city like Charleston has inescapable implications for students' state of mental health during their four years here. It is not rare for students to go to medical school here, fall in love with Charleston, and then decide to train and eventually settle here. Granted, during the first couple of years of medical school, the degree of free time students have is limited. However, the free time they do get is spent doing some pretty memorable things.

Charleston is home to the Spoleto Festival, a 2½-week-long stretch where the city plays host to hundreds of artists, authors, and performance artists from around the nation and the world. The whole downtown area is permanently smothered in groovy little galleries and cultural happenings. A breath of beach air is the cure-all for a tough day at medical school, which is why the School hosts a Beach & Ocean program. Classmates teach each other how to sail and surf. They also water-ski together. Class parties and gatherings are held at the beach.

The city of Charleston is very old and has a unique history and feel. Bed and breakfasts abound, and the city is jam-packed with great restaurants.

All these elements about the city contribute to a general class cohesiveness that is not present in every medical school around the country. Students are amazed by the number of close friendships they derive from their experience. Classmates marry classmates, and students both study and socialize with each other. Some students are more competitive with each other than others are, but, overall, each class is a tight unit that it is fun to be a part of.

The Bottom Line

MUSC successfully combines an outstanding education, a low price, and an exceptional town to make the four years of medical school bearable and even enjoyable. MUSC does not offer the name recognition of some of the superhyped private universities; however, it does offer a rock-solid medical education that in no way limits career opportunities.

MEHARRY MEDICAL COLLEGE SCHOOL OF MEDICINE

Nashville, Tennessee

Tuition 1996–97: $20,785 per year
Applications: 4,908
Size of Entering Class: 80
Total Number of Women Students: 186 (48%)
Total Number of Men Students: 198 (52%)
World Wide Web: www.mmc.edu/sofm.htm

Contact: Allen D. Mosley, Director of Admissions and Records
1005 D B Todd Boulevard
Nashville, TN 37208-9989
615-327-6223

Meharry Medical College is the largest private, historically black institution exclusively dedicated to educating health-care professionals and biomedical scientists in the United States. The College's diverse student body represents a cross section of the United States and several other countries. The students and faculty have interesting backgrounds, and nearly everyone has undergone tremendous hardships, which they have surmounted. In January 1999, Meharry announced it is forming an alliance with Vanderbilt Medical School to enhance the educational, scientific, and clinical programs at and between both institutions; what this means for medical students and applicants, though, is still unclear.

Preclinical Years

Meharry follows a traditional preclinical program. The first semester consists of anatomy and biochemistry as the two heavy hitters. Unfortunately, the year also begins with Introduction to Clinical Medicine, quite possibly the worst-run class in the preclinical years; some students are lucky and begin interviewing patients the first week of school. If you survive the first semester, things do get a bit more interesting with physiology, neuroscience, and microanatomy. Because there is some overlap between the courses, students find that the second semester is less stressful than the first. The second year consists of a continuation of Introduction to Clinical Medicine as well as two semesters of pathology and behavioral sciences. Microbiology, easily the best-taught course in the preclinical years, is offered in the first semester of the second year. Pharmacology rounds out the second year in the second semester.

The grading system at Meharry is the traditional A-B-C-F. Luckily, this does not foster the cutthroat, take-no-prisoners competition that might be found in other schools that admit students with less-than-altruistic interests at heart. Working in groups and sharing ideas occurs very freely among classmates, because most students are generally willing to help each other.

Research opportunities are available. Some students tutor for extra money. If a student is lucky, a professor may ask him or her to go with him to another country to do research.

Clinical Years

Meharry students work in a number of hospitals in Nashville as well as throughout Tennessee and nearby Kentucky. Opportunities to perform procedures and to become involved with patients vary, depending on the rotation. As with most medical schools, surgery tends to be the most notorious for its long hours and highly demanding, difficult residents. Meharry's pride and joy, however, is its family practice curriculum, which tends to be a nurturing environment for learning. The fourth year includes electives and a primary-care clerkship, where students experience working in a rural portion of Tennessee. There tends to be a great deal of exposure to basic outpatient medicine as well as to managed care environments because the students work closely with private practitioners. There is, however, no pressure placed on the student to select one specialty over another. Students tend to be well prepared for the match process because they are given ample advice that begins early in their curriculum.

Social Life

Contrary to what many people think, Nashville does have roads, buildings, and indoor plumbing. And not everyone who lives there speaks with a drawl. One thing is for sure: if you like country music, you will have a great time at Meharry; if you don't, you will have a good excuse to study. The dance clubs tend to be pretty homogeneous if you are used to Los Angeles or New York. They don't all play country music, and students frequent them. Nearby Tennessee State University, Fisk, Vanderbilt, and Belmont allow some exposure to undergraduate activities in case anyone feels a bit nostalgic for collegiate life.

Housing is quite affordable. The closer to campus, the cheaper the rent. Average rent is about $700 per mont for a two- to three-bedroom condo. Living close to campus may have its price, though. Nashville is a relatively safe city, but Meharry has a reputation for being in a rough neighborhood. A few students have had their cars stolen when living close to campus.

The Bottom Line

If you want to attend an institution that consists predominantly of African Americans, with a rich heritage and culture founded on helping the underprivileged, this institution is for you.

MERCER UNIVERSITY SCHOOL OF MEDICINE

Macon, Georgia

Size of Entering Class: 56
World Wide Web: gain.mercer.edu/musm
Contact: Dr. Roger W. Comeau, Associate Dean
for Admissions

1400 Coleman Avenue
Macon, GA 31207-3
912-752-2524

Mercer University School of Medicine's mission is to train primary-care physicians to work in underserved areas of rural Georgia. Consequently, the School does not accept or even interview anyone who is not a resident of the state of Georgia. There are only seven medical specialties that are mission compliant: family practice, internal medicine, pediatrics, obstetrics-gynecology, general surgery, emergency medicine, and psychiatry. Applicants are screened closely for a commitment to pursuing one of the mission-compliant areas and for a desire to perform primary care in an underserved area of rural Georgia.

Admissions/Financial Aid

Mercer is the youngest and smallest medical school in the U.S. Founded in 1980, with its first class graduating in 1986, the School currently accepts fifty-six students in each class. Mercer accepts a number of nontraditional students, with most classes having 10 percent or more students over 30 and at least one student over 40. This demographic tends to make families and family concerns more of an issue than at traditional medical schools.

Preclinical Years

Mercer's basic science years are unique among U.S. medical schools. The entire basic science curriculum is organized upon Problem Based Learning (PBL). There are no lectures, only group meetings. The only scheduled sessions are on Monday, Wednesday, and Friday from 9 a.m. until noon. The first two years are divided into phases, which are case based and organ-system specific, and each session attempts to integrate the separate disciplines of medical science. The first consists of Phase A (Biochemistry and Cell Biology), Phase B (Genetics and Embryology), Host Defense (Immunology), Hematology, Neuroscience, Brain and

Behavior, and Musculoskeletal. The second year consists of Cardiology, Pulmonology, Gastrointestinal, Renal, Endocrinology, and Infectious Disease phases. Most of the phases are six weeks long and all culminate in a multidisciplinary exam (MDE) and oral exam on the last two days of the phase. The MDEs contain questions from each discipline studied in the phase for a total of about 200 questions. The orals are another unique aspect of the program at Mercer. Students are given a written case scenario with 30 minutes to read the case and prepare a presentation explaining the basic science of the case. Then, an additional 30 minutes are allotted for the student to give the presentation before two faculty members. Grading is a pass/fail system.

The Monday, Wednesday, and Friday group meetings consist of seven students and a faculty member (called a tutor) who read a case and then attempt to set issues relevant to the basic science foundation of the case. The issues are phrased as questions and are supposed to focus study for the next group session. The issues are then discussed among the group, with an attempt made to explain the basic science underlying the specifics of the case.

Though fine in theory, PBL at Mercer is little more than a semistructured environment for self-education. With rare exception, the basic science faculty members make no effort to interact with students. There is even a widespread perception among the students that most of the basic science faculty members actually avoid student contact. The majority of the group tutors are better described as nonparticipating monitors. This makes answering and explaining the case issues a disjointed discussion among students whose knowledge base is limited to a few random, self-acquired scientific facts. Unfortunately, Mercer produces students with an unstructured knowledge base, making it extremely difficult for them to incorporate clinical information in later years. The average USMLE Step I score is consistently several points below the national average.

The PBL system fosters neither competition nor cooperation, but isolation. The extreme demands of learning a complicated field exclusively by textbook, combined with the often-misleading student discussions during group, produce an environment in which students often try to remove themselves from contact with anything that might interfere with their unassisted self-acquisition of knowledge. No support system exists for those students who experience academic difficulty. The philosophy of the institution even leads to questioning the integrity and capability of those who seek help, because they are circumventing the system of adult self-directed learning by asking someone to directly teach them. An interaction called a resource session is allowed and usually consists of basic science faculty members answering specific questions submitted by the students. By School mandate, this session must be student initiated and student directed. The rare basic science faculty members who do teach are occasionally chastised by the more senior faculty, thus perpetuating an oppressive and ineffective system. Student input is rarely solicited and, when proffered, is routinely disregarded.

Two other programs are clinical skills and community science. Clinical skills and clinical experiences are introduced during the first year. The clinical skills program does a good job of teaching rudimentary skills, and the staff members genuinely try hard to implement useful training. Mercer uses actors as standardized patients, and sessions on performing a history and physical tend to overemphasize the psychology of physician-patient interactions over physical exam skills. Most students feel that they were not adequately prepared to perform a brief focused hhistory and physical, write a SOAP note, and make a patient presentation. The community science program is a combination of epidemiology, biostatistics, research design, and critical literature analysis. It also incorporates the idea of a physician with a social conscience and community orientation. The department administers visits to precepting physicians in rural communities in the first, second, and fourth years for two, four, and four weeks, respectively. Faculty members in the community science department are very helpful and try to accommodate most student concerns and considerations. Unfortunately, the time and work overload from the inefficient and inadequate PBL basic science curriculum causes students to view both clinical skills and community science as, at best, inconvenient distractions rather than distinctly interesting opportunities.

The medical library and Learning Resources Center are both outstanding resources staffed with the most professional and considerate people in the institution. The financial aid office is very helpful and works well with students to process financial aid forms. They also do an excellent job of being very clear and straightforward about the cost of medical education, particularly at this school.

Clinical Years

The third year is organized into two half-years: one consists of three 8-week rotations and the other of one 12-week plus two 6-week rotations. The eight-week rotations are family medicine, surgery, and pediatrics. Internal medicine is twelve weeks long and is held in conjunction with psychiatry and ob-gyn, which last six weeks each. All rotations in Macon are performed at the Medical Center of Central Georgia (MCCG, or The Med). Twenty students per class are given the opportunity to spend the third and fourth years at Memorial Medical Center in Savannah. Alternate sites are available for family medicine (Rome, Albany, Columbus, and Savannah) and ob-gyn (Savannah). Opinions on the rotations vary, depending on site location, residents, and attendings. In general, they are all viewed as at least adequate, with some even seen as excellent. Most sites contain a diverse enough population to provide exposure to a wide array of clinical pathology.

The youth, size, and geographic focus of the School contribute to obstacles some interviewing seniors must surmount. Most Mercer graduates go into either family medicine or internal medicine (more than 60 percent of each class) and do not go far outside the South for residency training. Consistent with the School's mission, most alumni return to Georgia for service after residency. With only fourteen graduating classes, there are less than 700 alumni. Outside Georgia and the South, interviewing seniors often must overcome the hurdles of simply identifying the School and attempting to explain its unique curriculum.

Social Life

Macon, Georgia, is a city that still views itself culturally as a very large Southern town rather than a city. Macon has the Georgia Music Hall of Fame, a Grand Opera House, the Tubman African American Museum, and a Museum of Arts and Sciences. Macon hosts two minor-league sports teams, the Macon Braves (baseball) and the Macon Whoopee (ice hockey). The city is replete with opportunities for dining out. It also has some excellent antebellum sites that were undamaged by the Civil War. Atlanta is a little more than an hour away and offers anything that Macon does not.

Mercer University has a well-developed intramural sports program, with very active participation by medical students. Organized social activities are a picnic during orientation, a Halloween Party for students' children, a family Thanksgiving dinner, a spring cookout, and a recently implemented Christmas formal. All are organized by students and/or their spouses, with attendance almost exclusively by students.

Before 1996, the medical school had few social activities and no support network for students, spouses, or families. That year, some of the student spouses formed a spouses' group separate from the medical school. The majority of married students, and especially most of those with children, feel that the School is, at best, unconcerned about their families.

The Bottom Line

The general consensus is that students believe they could have done better at a correspondence school. The ineffective educational philosophy and nonparticipatory basic science faculty members, coupled with the expensive tuition, motivated one student to sum his experiences at Mercer as *never have I paid so much to receive so little.* Mercer University School of Medicine is an institution where teaching is virtually nonexistent, assistance from basic science faculty is philosophically prohibited, students are ignored, and family members are viewed as nonentities.

MICHIGAN STATE UNIVERSITY COLLEGE OF HUMAN MEDICINE

East Lansing, Michigan

Tuition 1996–97: $22,531 per year
Total Number of Women Students: 270 (53%)
Total Number of Men Students: 240 (47%)
World Wide Web: www.chm.msu.edu/

Contact: Dr. Loran Bieber, Associate Dean for Graduate Studies and Research
East Lansing, MI 48824-1020
517-353-8858

Although Michigan State University (MSU) houses elite football, basketball, and hockey teams, there is much more to MSU than sporting events. MSU is the only University in the nation with an allopathic medical school, an osteopathic medical school, and a School of Veterinary Medicine on its campus. Founded in 1964 in response to the increasing need for primary-care physicians in the state of Michigan, MSU College of Human Medicine (CHM) has established itself as a front-runner in training primary-care physicians, who are nationally renowned for their skills and accomplishments. With a patient-centered philosophy, the College of Human Medicine emphasizes communication and patients' needs in addition to the science of medicine. Nestled in the college community of East Lansing, the College of Human Medicine prides itself on being a medical school that is cooperative, not competitive; diverse, rather than homogeneous; and fun, rather than dull and lusterless. *Consumer's Report* praised the College of Human Medicine in 1995 for the innovative and effective teaching methods incorporated into its preclinical and clinical curricula. *U.S. News & World Report*'s annual evaluation of graduate schools in the United States ranked the College of Human Medicine among the top quarter of medical schools in the nation for training primary-care physicians eight years in a row.

Admissions/Financial Aid

The College of Human Medicine accepts students with a myriad of interests that range from anesthesiology and orthopedic surgery to family practice and internal medicine from all over the United States. Of the 3,404 primary applicants in 1998, 421 were interviewed for a class of 106. Sixty-two percent were female students.

Although these numbers vary from year to year, the College of Human Medicine has been committed to diversity. Women outnumbered men for the first time in the last entering class, and the class includes young students with traditional academic backgrounds, older students entering a second career, and students from diverse cultural backgrounds. Since the College of Human Medicine is a publicly funded school, a majority of students are from the state of Michigan (approximately 80 percent in-state students and 20 percent out-of-state students). The in-state tuition and fees for the 1997–98 academic year averaged $11,951 (which varies from year one to year four), while the out-of-state tuition and fees for the 1997–98 academic year averaged $28,097. There are many opportunities for financial aid, including loans, grants, CHM-endowed scholarships, privately funded scholarships, and graduate assistantships.

Preclinical Years

In 1991, the College of Human Medicine introduced a new curriculum to its students. The goal of the curriculum is to provide a dynamic learning environment that enables students to master basic science concepts while developing the skills necessary to solve clinical problems. To foster additional cooperation, the first two years are graded using a pass/fail system. The first two years are separated into two blocks. Block I consists of three semesters (fall, winter, and summer). These courses focus on fundamental concepts (biochemistry, physiology, anatomy, physiology, histology, neuroscience, pharmacology, etc.) that serve as the foundation for the more advanced concepts encountered in Block II (year two). In addition, students are able to get their hands wet during the first year by going to the hospital and learning dynamics of the doctor/patient relationship, developing interactive skills with patients, and conducting general physical exams. Block II covers a thirty-three-week period of problem-based learning. Instead of taking traditional classes, such as pathology and microbiology, students take classes that are taught using a systems-based approach. For example, all students take a cardiology unit in which they learn the histology, pathology, microbiology, radiology, pharmacology, and physiology of the cardiovascular system. There is less lecture time than in Block I, as the students learn how to become independent, yet cooperative, thinkers in small-group settings. Advanced history taking and physical exam are also studied in Block II in preparation for the next two years in the hospital. Also packed into Block II are courses in medical ethics, epidemiology, and health policy.

Clinical Years

Block III, which extends through years three and four, comprises eighty weeks of required and elective clerkships. Clerkships are physician-supervised learning experiences in which students work with patients at clinical health-care sites. The required clerkships in family practice, internal medicine, pediatrics, obstetrics and gynecology, surgery, and psychiatry involve both hospital-based and ambulatory-care experiences. During the second half of Block III, students are allowed to take electives, which may include medical research or traveling to a hospital outside the state to enroll in a course. The College of Human Medicine is unique in that students have the opportunity to spend their third and fourth years in one of six available Michigan communities: the Upper Peninsula, Grand Rapids, Kalamazoo, Lansing, Flint, and Saginaw.

Social Life

East Lansing is a college community located just minutes from the state's capital. Most students are pleased to find comfortable and affordable housing that is less than 10 minutes from the medical school's campus. At the College of Human Medicine, medical education is more than books, classes, and exams; it is serving the community and learning to apply medical skills where they are needed the most. There are many student organizations and activities, including Friendship Clinic (a monthly clinic in which Block I and II medical students help physicians care for patients), Immunization Clinic (where medical students give free immunizations to children of the Lansing community), Students Teaching Aids to Students (STAT), Student Council, and many other interest groups (Family Practice Interest Group, Pediatric Interest Group, and Surgery Interest Group). The activities outside of school are endless; students may find a group of medical students at Beggar's Banquet for the ever-popular wine night or enjoy a production of Miss Saigon at Michigan State University's Wharton Center for Performing Arts. At MSU, the home of the Spartans, many students attend sporting events, where they can cheer on their favorite team.

The Bottom Line

It is the College of Human Medicine's mission to educate excellent, caring, compassionate, primary-care physicians who have respect for others who are different from themselves, are committed to a lifetime of ethical practices, and are committed to lifelong learning. The College offers students this opportunity as well as a chance to grow and mature.

MICHIGAN STATE UNIVERSITY COLLEGE OF OSTEOPATHIC MEDICINE

East Lansing, Michigan

Tuition 1996–97: $22,531 per year
Students Receiving Financial Aid: 89%
Total Number of Women Students: 226 (43%)
Total Number of Men Students: 300 (57%)
World Wide Web: www.chm.msu.edu/
CHM_HTML/CHM.Home.Page.html

Contact: Dr. Paulette Lovell, Director of
Admissions
East Lansing, MI 48824-1020
517-353-7740

Michigan is a D.O.-friendly state, where 20 percent of the physicians in the state are osteopathic physicians. Michigan State University (MSU) is the state-supported land -rant college. As such, the College of Osteopathic Medicine (COM) has a clear mission, which includes bettering the health and welfare of the people of the state. COM is not the only medical school at MSU. In addition to COM, there are the College of Human Medicine (CHM) and the College of Veterinary Medicine (CVM).

This environment makes for a fertile ground for both education and research. MSU-COM has an exceptional reputation for training osteopathic physicians, and this is confirmed by the growing ranks of past graduates who have become deans of other osteopathic medical schools and department heads at both osteopathic and allopathic hospitals throughout the country. The most recent rankings of exceptional graduate programs by *U.S. News & World Report* ranked MSU-COM tied with Mt. Sinai School of Medicine as the 31st best primary-care medical school in the nation.

Admissions/Financial Aid

Admission is competitive. Each year approximately 2,700 students apply and 250 are interviewed for 125 spots. Although the majority of students are Michigan residents (92 percent), applicants are encouraged to apply regardless of their state residency. The entering class of 1998 was a diverse group composed of students from a variety of ethnic and social backgrounds with a nearly equal percentage of men and women. This year, the average age of first-year students was 25 years, but ages range from 20 to 50

years. In fact, diversity is one of the defining features of the student body. Students seem to have something unique and special about them. This makes for interesting repartee during small-group discussions throughout the preclinical years.

Admission is on a rolling basis and early application is essential. The Admissions Committee interviews students who have the required academic numbers, but essays, interviews, and recommendations (especially from a D.O.) are considered important in the final decision. One aspect that seems to characterize the class is each student's overriding interest in the principles of osteopathic medicine. Students should come to the interview prepared to explain their interest and exposure to the osteopathic medical profession. Financial aid is available to students in the form of scholarships, grants, graduate assistantships, low-interest loan programs, and federal direct student loans. In-state tuition is reasonable, and additional aid is available for out-of-state students and those with exceptional need.

Preclinical Years

Currently, CHM and COM students at MSU take most of their first-year basic science courses together (the examination average scores for both schools are about the same). The two Schools' curriculums diverge during the second year.

COM students continue the lecture/lab/small-group format for their systems-based courses, while CHM students have a minimal lecture curriculum that emphasizes self-study. However, beginning with the entering class of 1999, COM and CHM students will take completely separate courses, with the COM curriculum going though a much anticipated overhaul. COM uses a pass/fail system that encourages cooperation among students. Fellow students are always willing to share notes, practice exams, and useful charts and mnemonics. There always seems to be a huge supply of study materials posted on the board in the Kobiljak Resource Center for students to share.

The pass level for most courses is 70 percent, but don't be fooled into thinking that no one will ever want to know your course performance. The academic affairs office maintains the percentage and class percentile ranks for most courses and this information is available to residency directors, but only with the students approval. Typically, the most difficult courses for students seem to be Gross Anatomy, Pharmacology, Cardiology, and GI. Also, former students note that Dr. Ralph Otten does a thorough job teaching the fine art of Electrocardiography.

The Department of Osteopathic Manipulative Medicine does a great job of teaching students the basic techniques and philosophy surrounding high velocity, muscle energy, myofascial, counterstrain, and craniosacral treatments. Overall, the exam schedule is rigorous from the beginning. You should be prepared to study weekends for exams almost every Monday. When it comes time for board exams, students run a free board review series where professors give two to three lectures intended to cull the massive amounts of information presented during the course down to the salient knowledge needed for the boards.

Clinical Years

Students begin their clinical education during their first year, with courses designed to develop basic skills in history and physical. Second-year students spend 80 or more hours doing a family practice preceptorship, which provides a prelude to the intensive clinical training that students gain as externs at one of thirteen hospitals located throughout the state. Currently, the extern rotations begin in August of the third year and graduation is in May, twenty months later.

At the end of the first year, students select a base hospital at which they will perform two thirds of their clinical rotations. The other one third of clinical rotations is made up of electives (unrestricted outtime) and selectives (out-time restricted to any MSU-COM affiliate) for students to explore their specialties of interest. Although the majority of affiliated

hospitals are located in major metropolitan areas such as Detroit, Lansing, Flint, and Grand Rapids, opportunities are available for rural medicine rotations. MSU-COM has a wide variety of affiliates, which includes top osteopathic teaching hospitals such as Botsford General, Pontiac Osteopathic Hospital, Mt. Clemens General, and Ingham Regional Medical Center.

Most affiliates are mixed staff hospitals (both D.O. and M.D.), which gives externs an opportunity to see a variety of different teaching styles. In addition, MSU-COM externs, through an affiliation with Horizon Health System and Henry Ford Health System, may choose to rotate at Henry Ford Hospital in Detroit. Generally speaking, Botsford General has the best teaching reputation, but students will end up doing more procedures at a place like Garden City Hospital.

MSU-COM has a primary-care–focused clinical curriculum. Externs are expected to spend six consecutive months in an outpatient rotation known as the Primary Care Ambulatory Clerkship. While this program gives student's a heads-up on the world of primary care, students have complained about the length and organization of this clerkship. The strength of specialty and primary-care clerkships tends to be very good; however, only a few of the primary affiliate hospitals have top Pediatrics or OB/GYN programs. Consistent with osteopathic principles, Botsford General has one of the best neurology departments in Michigan and Orthopaedics tends to be strong just about everywhere.

Through its COGMET Osteopathic Medical Education Consortium, MSU-COM supplies students with a pipeline to high-quality postgraduate medical education programs at its affiliate hospitals. One criticism some students have made is that the osteopathic philosophy expounded upon during their preclinical years never materializes into obvious differences between their D.O. and M.D. clinical instructors.

Social Life

The student population is diverse at MSU-COM. Many students are married or engaged and there is an active student auxiliary composed of spouses and significant others. Students are encouraged to participate in extracurricular activities.

The Emergency Medicine and Sports Medicine Clubs always seem to have an intriguing lecturer. The

Family Medicine club is sponsored by the Michigan Association for Osteopathic Family Physicians and tends to have the best free food for its meetings. It always seems as if there is something going on every lunch hour for students to get involved with during their preclinical years. Their are groups involved in exploring ethics issues, performing AIDS education, providing free public health screening and education, and going on medical missions to South America and Africa.

Whatever a student's area of interest, he or she will have no problem finding an established student organization to encourage those interests. Students still have time for social activities, and the prime-time bashes include Vegas Night, the annual Halloween party, and Fee Follies (a chance to parody professors and students alike). MSU has an excellent Division I athletic program, which makes for weekly social events at the local sports bars to watch football and basketball games. In 1999, the fan hype included a trip by the MSU basketball and hockey teams to the Men's NCAA Final Four tournaments and the annual Michigan State-Michigan football game, which is always a highly anticipated event. Most students live in reasonably priced off-campus housing. Although many students choose to live in Owen Hall, the graduate student dorm a short walk from Fee Hall (the main building for COM). Parking for off-campus students tends to be annoying but not a problem if you don't mind a 5 to 10 minute walk. Nightspots

around town include Crunchy's, Harper's, Landshark, and Rick's and Reno's just to name a few. A car is essential, especially during second year, when it is almost guaranteed that students will have to drive to get to their preceptors offices. Although the winter weather in mid-Michigan can be irritating, the spring and summer are excellent.

During the summer, food science runs a dairy with some of the best homemade ice cream you have ever tasted. Also, the horticultural gardens are a beautiful place for a walk. The University has several athletic buildings throughout campus for student recreation, and intramural sports are very popular, and owns a top-rated thirty-six–hole golf course. Everything changes at the end of second year, when 90 percent of the students leave East Lansing to move a short-distance (mostly 1 hour by car) away to their base hospital for third- and fourth-year clinical rotations.

The Bottom Line

In the end, MSU-COM churns out an excellent crop of well-trained physicians schooled in the osteopathic philosophy. Although most students seek careers in primary care, opportunities are limited only by the interests of the student. If applicants are looking for a first-class medical education with an emphasis in osteopathic principles and practice, Michigan State University College of Osteopathic Medicine may be the place for them.

MIDWESTERN UNIVERSITY ARIZONA COLLEGE OF OSTEOPATHIC MEDICINE

Downers Grove, Illinois

Size of Entering Class: 126
World Wide Web: www.midwestern.edu/Pages/ AZCOM.html

Contact: Office of Admissions
555 31st Street
Downers Grove, IL 60515-1235
888-247-9277

The Glendale, Arizona, campus of Midwestern University is a booming, bustling bastion of health education. The first program offered at the Glendale site, Arizona College of Osteopathic Medicine (AZCOM), first opened its doors to students in fall 1996 and will graduate its inaugural class in 2. AZCOM traces its roots back to Midwestern University (MWU) Chicago College of Osteopathic Medicine, which served as the model and springboard for the curriculum now used at AZCOM. The curriculum model was not the only item imported from Illinois—the sunny climes of Arizona were able to lure many of the best basic science faculty members from the bone-chilling winters of Chicago. What started as just one building has turned into an active campus, replete with a physician's assistant studies program, a pharmacy school, a physical therapy/occupational therapy school, and an osteopathic medicine clinic.

Admissions/Financial Aid

Although AZCOM is a relatively new school, gaining admission is a competitive process, as evidenced by the number of interested applicants. For the entering class of fall 1998, 3,295 students applied, 349 were interviewed, and 126 matriculated. During the interview process, applicants undergo a 30-minute panel interview, which is given by a basic science faculty member, a D.O., and a third-year medical student. Applicants also receive a tour of the campus and a financial aid presentation. Popular student opinion states that to be recognized as a strong applicant, one must have, in addition to the regular medical school requirements, a D.O. recommendation letter, an interest in primary care, and, above all, a strong understanding of osteopathic medicine.

Financial aid is relatively easy to obtain. It usually provides for tuition and some moderate living expenses. After that, it's (if students are lucky) either parents to the rescue or time to take out more loans.

Preclinical Years

During the first year of school, students spend many hours in anatomy lab soaking up plenty of juicy bits of anatomy. During one of the lab days that students rotate out out of the College, they shadow a physician for the afternoon. During both the first and second years, students work with a preceptor for an afternoon every other week. It is this preceptorship that truly teaches the students most of the clinical skills they need during their third and fourth years and provides a light at the end of the tunnel, something sorely needed after the weekly Monday morning tests. Other basic science classes studied during the first two years include histology, embryology, biochemistry, physiology, human behavior, immunology, microbiology, pharmacology, and pathology. Clinical courses, such as Introduction to Clinical Medicine and Clinical Correlates (ICM and CC), are taught in first and second years. First-year ICM and CC gently dips students' big toes into the water, while second-year ICM and CC dumps them in head first. Any student who can remember everything the professors teach shines on rotations. Every week, one professor hands out an unwieldy tome disguised as class notes, and when all notes for the quarter are assembled, they can easily rival Harrison's in information, if not girth alone, an intimidating sight to see, especially before the cumulative final. The other professor's handouts, on the other hand, are brief and succinct and concentrated with information.

Once a week, students attend a lecture and lab in osteopathic manipulative medicine (OMM). The OMM department is headed by the recipient of numerous teaching awards. It is a class enjoyed by all students, not only for different skills that are learned but also for the chance to lie supine in class.

The school's policy for passing any class or test is receiving at least a 75 percent, hence the slogan, "Seventy-five, stay alive," a phrase heard most often during the last couple days of finals week. There is hardly any competition among classmates, as class rank is generally kept confidential unless a student decides to make his or her rank known. Generally, a congenial attitude exists among fellow classmates.

Clinical Years

Rotations during third and fourth year are preceptor based, with a heavy emphasis on primary care. Students rotate through various hospitals and offices throughout the valley and, as a result, have a wide variety of experience. Since AZCOM is the first medical school in the valley, most of the doctors in Phoenix are eager to take on and teach students. Some allow students to take almost total control of patient care, while others do so under supervision. Four months of elective time is allowed, with one month of it occurring during third year. A month of vacation time is allotted each year, with two weeks usually scheduled around Christmas and the other two weeks scheduled by the student. Since the inaugural class is still in its third year, there is no data to report the school's percentages for interviewing and matching for residency.

Social Life

Nestled in a suburb of Phoenix, Glendale hasn't much to offer in terms of big-city life. However, plenty of opportunities to procrastinate before midterms abound in Glendale proper, but high culture is not what Phoenix is known for. Most students explore the outdoors with weekend trips to Sedona or Flagstaff and the occasional postfinals jaunt to Vegas. Common outdoor activities include hiking, mountain biking, and tubing down the Salt River, touted on billboards as Arizona's largest floating picnic.

During the first two years, most students live on or near campus. Housing is relatively affordable in Glendale, moreso if students have a roommate. By third year, most students migrate to the posh settings of Scottsdale. A car is a definite must during the last two years, since public transportation is virtually nonexistent in Phoenix and rotations take students all over the valley. Phoenix is a great city to live in and will be even better once they finish building it.

The Bottom Line

AZCOM is the school for the student dedicated to serving the needs of others. Community service is stressed highly, as evidenced by the University motto, "To teach, to heal, to serve." If practicing medicine is an applicant's ultimate goal, then he or she should consider AZCOM. The faculty is excellent, the clinical experiences enlightening, and the academic atmosphere rewarding.

MIDWESTERN UNIVERSITY CHICAGO COLLEGE OF OSTEOPATHIC MEDICINE

Downers Grove, Illinois

Size of Entering Class: 160
Total Number of Women Students: 253 (40%)
Total Number of Men Students: 377 (60%)
World Wide Web: www.midwestern.edu/Pages/
CCOM.html

Contact: Julie Rosenthall, Director of Admissions
555 31st Street
Downers Grove, IL 60515-1235
800-458-6253

The Chicago College of Osteopathic Medicine (CCOM), a college of Midwestern University, is rich in history and pride. Founded in 1900, CCOM has been part of an eventful century of growth and change within both the osteopathic profession and the world of medicine in general. The College has undergone some dramatic changes over the past decade, including the relocation of administrative and basic science facilities to a beautiful campus 25 miles west of Chicago in Downers Grove. The campus maintains a low profile, casually if not asynchronously interspersed between office buildings, private residences, and a forest preserve. In addition to the move, the Colleges of Pharmacy and Allied Health were created, thus forming Midwestern University.

Admission to CCOM is highly selective. For the class of 2002, almost 4,000 applications were received and only 434 interviews were granted. CCOM admits 150 to 160 students each year. The average age of incoming students is about 26. Anywhere from 37 to 45 percent of a given class is women, and members of minority groups account for 8 percent. By far, the majority of students are residents of Illinois and its surrounding states, although some hail from as far away as California and Hawaii (often necessitating a specialized orientation in the intricacies of Midwestern snowfalls and Chicago potholes). Some students are married with children, others are fresh out of undergraduate school, and still others have advanced degrees (M.P.H., M.B.A., and Ph.D.). The most unifying characteristic of each class, however, is solidarity in simply getting through the course work.

Preclinical Years

A common misconception seems to persist that osteopathic medicine is some form of alternative medicine. On the contrary, during the preclinical years, students are immersed in all of the basic medical sciences and begin to learn the art of osteopathic manipulation. According to the most recent school catalog, "CCOM strives to produce excellent osteopathic physicians, emphasizing primary care but including the traditional specialties and subspecialties." Beginning with the first week of school, students become acquainted with basic medical skills and techniques in the Introduction to Clinical Medicine course. First-year students develop interviewing and history-taking skills, and second-year students perform components of the physical exam (cardiac, neurological, pelvic) on professional patients as well as complete history and physical exams on hospitalized patients.

The first two years at CCOM can be summed up in one word: intense. The school follows a traditional format, with the first two years being primarily didactic in nature. CCOM operates on a quarter system, with three 10-week quarters per year. Typically, classes and labs are scheduled from 8 a.m. to 4 p.m. every day. Students endure one or two tests per week, peaking with a grueling finals week. The class schedule lightens somewhat during the second year, but overall, students are battered by an unwavering onslaught of information.

All courses are graded on a percentage scale, with a minimum passing score of 70. No grades are curved, and no honors are awarded, which provides an atmosphere basically free of competition. In fact, due to the intensity of the schedule, students in each class become remarkably close-knit, and students often rely on the help of their classmates. Between the department handouts and a class-run note service, many find it possible to skip class if they choose.

Following their first year, students take a long and well-deserved three-month summer break. Some take this time to pursue research fellowships offered by the school, others work, and still others travel abroad. For most, however, the last summer off is a time to kick back and relax, because come September, students cruise right through second year and begin clinical work with virtually no time off in between.

Clinical Years

Primary care lies at the core of the osteopathic profession. This is certainly true at CCOM and becomes evident during the clinical years. CCOM students are required to complete rotations in family, community, and emergency medicine as well as traditional core clerkships in pediatrics, general internal medicine, general surgery, psychiatry, and obstetrics/gynecology. As a result, students receive a tremendous amount of exposure to and experience in primary care. As expected, a large number of graduates become primary-care physicians, especially within the field of family medicine.

One of CCOM's main affiliate hospitals is Olympia Fields Osteopathic Medical Center, known simply as Oly to CCOM students. Located just southwest of Chicago, Oly is both a 213-bed community hospital and a level I trauma center. Students give general surgery, orthopedic surgery, and pediatrics rotations solid reviews. In addition, the hospital is the home of one of the largest emergency medicine (EM) residency programs in the nation. Fourth-year students are required to complete an EM rotation, and those who go to Oly assert that it is a great experience. However, one complaint occasionally heard is that some services may be unorganized and crowded with too many students and residents. The school maintains affiliations with many other top-tier hospitals throughout the Chicago area, including Cook County, Edgewater, Illinois Masonic, and Christ.

As mentioned, primary care is emphasized; however, this fact does not preclude students from pursuing any specialty they desire. During the clinical years, students are required to choose from numerous specialty clerkships in affiliated hospitals (cardiology, hematology/oncology, thoracic surgery, neurosurgery, etc.). In addition, several months of open electives can be completed anywhere in the city or throughout the nation. Some students even choose to set up international rotations. When it comes to these electives, Chicago is a medical student's playground. The variety and volume of pathology and clinical settings make the city one of the best places in the country to learn medicine.

Students generally feel that the clinical years are a blast. After two intense years at the Downers Grove campus, many students move downtown and experience life in the city while completing their rotations. At times, clinical life can be quite demanding, such as pulling a 36-hour shift while on the trauma service at Oly. Other times, especially on less intense rotations, students may find a lot of spare time to catch up on life. Regardless of the schedule, it's a time to experience real medicine.

Social Life

During the first two years, most students choose to live on campus or in the suburbs surrounding Downers Grove. Life in the Chicago area does not come cheap. One-bedroom apartments have a minimum monthly rent of $700, and the cost of living in a wealthy suburb adds up. Add room and board to private school tuition, and the price tag for medical education skyrockets to nearly $40,000 per year. Fortunately, the school offers financial assistance to any student who requires it, and many students seek alternative funding arrangements.

The Windy City provides plenty for all, including the Art Institute of Chicago, Field Museum, Adler Planetarium, an active theater district, numerous festivals throughout year, and, yes, Jerry Springer. The city hosts teams in all major-league sports along with numerous college athletics. Those who prefer the outdoors have Lake Michigan in their backyard and can find plenty to do outside of the city. Finally, no talk of Chicago would be complete without mentioning the incredible diversity of restaurants and nightlife. Whatever a student's preference, it's bound to be found in Chicago.

The Bottom Line

CCOM may not be a common household name, but the school has proudly, yet quietly, amassed 100 years of experience in training osteopathic physicians. If applicants are looking for a solid medical education against the backdrop of a great medical city like Chicago, they should consider CCOM.

MOREHOUSE SCHOOL OF MEDICINE

Atlanta, Georgia

Applications: 2,928
Total Number of Women Students: 86 (59%)
Total Number of Men Students: 59 (41%)
World Wide Web: www.msm.edu/
Contact: Karen Lewis, Assistant Director of
Admissions

720 Westview Drive, SW
Atlanta, GA 30310-1495
404-752-1650

The Morehouse School of Medicine (MSM) was founded in fall 1975 to train physicians for service in underserved areas. The School's mission continues to be the recruitment and education of students from minority and economically disadvantaged backgrounds for service as primary-care physicians. MSM graduates have, in fact, kept with this mission, with more than 85 percent entering and completing primary-care residencies. At the same time, the School has done a fine job training its students for the rigors of medicine; the School has a 97 percent first-time pass rate for USMLE I (June 1998) and a 96 percent first-time pass rate for USMLE II (August 1998). The School houses the nation's only Neuroscience Institute and the first NASA/Space Medicine and Life Science Research Center at a minority medical institution.

Admissions/Financial Aid

The admissions process at MSM is as competitive and intense as it is at other schools. The School receives more than 3,000 applications annually for only thirty-five seats. Applicants are microscopically analyzed for characteristics parallel to those of the School's mission. In short, if a student's career goal is plastic surgery in Hollywood, MSM is not the place for that student. MCAT scores and transcripts are also heavily considered.

The interview sessions are generally easygoing. In addition to your interview by a faculty member, you are served lunch/brunch with an MSM student who answers questions that you might have about the School. A word to the wise: be careful here, because this same student also sits on the admissions committee and has a deciding vote on who is accepted.

The entering class size is composed of thirty-five students. Seventy percent of the students are native Georgians. African Americans comprise 90

percent of the student population, with the remaining 10 percent white and/or international. Women students account for 55 percent of the population, and the ages range from the low 20s to mid-30s. All students are considered for financial aid, with more than 95 percent receiving some type of assistance.

Preclinical Years

The first two years include the traditional basic science courses in lecture format (7 to 8 hours per day, five days per week). The most challenging class of the first year is human morphology (HM), an amalgam of gross anatomy, histology, genetics, embryology, and cell biology. It is grueling and detail oriented and makes many students quite weary by the end. Neurobiology in the second semester is by far the best class of the first year. This course is taught by a group of seven professors who are committed to students' mental, physical, and spiritual well-being. In addition to regular office hours, students are welcome to meet with these professors at any time.

Students gain early exposure to clinical medicine and community advocacy through several courses. Monthly visits with local community doctors and rural clinics expose students to the team approach to health-care delivery (M.D., RN, social worker, and nutritionist). Students also participate in the legislative process of public health by researching major issues specific to underserved communities. In cooperation with local residents, students draft projects aimed at addressing community members' major health concerns. These programs are then presented before the State House of Representatives for consideration of funding and implementation.

The amount of reading picks up considerably in the second year. The best class is pathophysiology, taught by one of the School's most brilliant and dedicated professors, Dr. Janice Herbert-Carter. Although most students complain about the heavy reading and highly detailed exam questions, her class has been credited with preparing students extremely well for USMLE Step I and, even more important, for clinical rotations. In addition to her regular office hours, she makes herself available until midnight the night before exams for last-minute questions. On exam day, she can be found strolling the halls searching for students in need of assistance. Her grasp of the information and her ability to present it to students in concise, practical, and clinical terms makes pathophysiology the highlight of second year.

Clinical and laboratory research opportunities are available throughout the academic year, but most students prefer to take advantage of these during the summer months. Some favorite program sites include the National Institutes of Health, Centers for Disease Control, and NASA.

Students have two major concerns with the current curriculum. There is little time for electives during the first two years and the grading system is strictly A through F, with no curve (a grade of 69.5 percent equates to an F). Despite students' attempts to change the grading system, the administration has been quite resistant. Any change to pass/fail, the administration believes, would lower standards. Even though the grading system is harsh, students tend to work together closely. The School makes a powerful effort to emphasize teamwork rather than competition.

Clinical Years

Third- and fourth-year students receive clinical instruction at seven affiliate hospitals, but most of their clerkships occur at Grady Memorial Hospital, a 1,000-bed hospital for the city's indigent. This patient population provides a broad spectrum of clinical experience, including TB, HIV, hepatitis, alcoholism, injection drug use, gunshots, and burns.

In addition, students are delegated little real responsibility (they learn as much about dropping off lab requisitions as about delivering a baby). Despite its demanding schedule, surgery is known for its competent and dedicated residents and attendings, who also happen to be effective instructors. Many of the students and residents still recant the critical role they played during the 1996 bombing at Atlanta's Centennial Olympic Park, marked by several injuries and one fatality.

All third-year clerkships must be completed in Atlanta, but the fourth year provides opportunities for electives across the country as well as selected international sites. Overall, students are generally content with their clinical training. On average, 65 to 70 percent of the students match to their first- or second-choice residencies, with an average of 85 percent entering primary care (this percentage is among the highest in the country).

Social Life

With its growing population (in excess of 2 million), Atlanta is the ideal location for medical students infatuated with big-city living. Whatever a student's pleasure, this international metropolis has it, from salsa dancing to murder mystery dinner, from hiking at the nationally renowned Stone Mountain Park to in-line skating at Piedmont, from clubbing in Midtown to karaoke in Marrietta. Among the favorite relaxing activities is a trip to Virginia Highlands for a sidewalk massage or a foot massage session.

Housing prices vary, depending on students' proximity to the city (the closer they are to the action, the more they pay). In the city, one- and two-bedroom apartments range from $650 to $850 per month. Apartments located outside the city's perimeter range from $450 to $750 per month. However, what students save by living further out, they pay for in aggravation during their commute. The roads are congested and rife with accidents. If at all possible, students should avoid housing that requires a commute on the Interstate 75/85 connector, which is the accident hot spot of the southeast region.

As with any big city, Atlanta ranks among the highest in the country for crimes. Car-jackings, murders, and robbery exist throughout the city and its suburbs. The public school system in Georgia ranks among the lowest in the land, so those with children might want to consider private school.

The Bottom Line

MSM is the ideal place for those seeking training in preparation for service to the underserved. Tuition is considered affordable, with an average indebtedness of $65,000–$85,000. In addition to enhancing its dual programs (i.e., M.D./Ph.D., M.D./M.P.H.), MSM will double its class size by the year 2002. If applicants are interested in an intimate environment with great professor accessibility, MSM is the place for them.

MOUNT SINAI SCHOOL OF MEDICINE OF THE CITY UNIVERSITY OF NEW YORK

New York, New York

Applications: 5,273
Size of Entering Class: 105
Total Number of Women Students: 234 (49%)
Total Number of Men Students: 242 (51%)
World Wide Web: www.mssm.edu

Contact: Dr. Richard D. Kayne, Associate Dean for Admissions
1 Gustave L Levy Place
New York, NY 10029-6504
212-241-6696

Located at the edge of Manhattan's Upper East Side, Mount Sinai sits on the border that divides one of the city's wealthiest districts from one of its poorest. The location offers students the best of both worlds: a vibrant, though expensive, neighborhood for social activities and a diverse and underserved patient population. This contrast is best observed in the eclectic and challenging mix of patients on Mount Sinai's medical wards. A richly endowed school, Mount Sinai has undergone a lavish building boom in recent decades and offers lucrative financial aid packages. Women make up slightly more than 50 percent of recent classes, and a commitment to minority recruiting shows.

Preclinical Years

In the first year, gross anatomy and physiology are terrific. Biochemistry and histology have recently undergone some much-needed revamping and are now quite good. Microbiology and introductory pathology have been poorly organized in the past and continue to draw complaints. Across the first-year curriculum, the School has responded to students' requests for more small-group teaching sessions and seminars and pared back lectures.

The first year, however, is exceedingly long, and the School tries hard to ameliorate some of the resulting fatigue. Exams are blocked together and usually fall about once every month or two, so that students are not constantly in cram mode. The first two years are also conducted on an entirely anonymous pass/fail basis.

By the second year, students have already settled into the grind. The second-year curriculum generally receives higher marks from students than does the first year. Courses consist of monthlong modules based on individual disease systems and two longer, three-month classes—neuroanatomy and behavioral science and pharmacology. Joe Goldfarb's pharmacology course maintains its reputation as one of Mount Sinai's most difficult, but students routinely report that after the experience, they knew their drugs cold and did not have to review the subject for the Step I medical boards.

Among the shorter modules, which tend to be dynamic and easier, the cardiovascular medicine, gastroenterology, and bone and musculoskeletal sections are outstanding, owing in large measure to the dedication of the individual course directors. Asher Kornbluth, who teaches the gastroenterology segment, is well-known for offering a 4-hour review session the night before the exam, where he answers last-minute questions and doesn't keep you until all hours of the night. At the end of the second year, students are given a month off to study for the Step I board exams, a block of time everyone uses but few need.

One of the unique and widely regarded aspects of studying preclinical medicine at Mount Sinai is the School's organization around multidisciplinary labs. The first- and second-year classes are separated and given their own floors in Sinai's twenty-six-story Annenberg Building. Each student is assigned to an individualized lab space that includes a desk and chair, a table with a sink, a locked closet for books, and an Ethernet line. Students spend most of their study time in these open-hall labs and take most of their classes there as well.

In general, the administration, eager to buoy the School's reputation, responds quickly to student complaints. At the beginning of the first year, the School's Dean meets personally with each student and implores the students to tell the Dean what they don't like. Students lamented a lack of common meeting space, and the administration responded by building a multimillion-dollar student center, complete with three large-screen televisions and high-speed computers. In response to student complaints that there were not enough conference rooms for studying in groups, the medical school built a half dozen.

Clinical Years

Emphasis on grades does not begin until third year, when clerkships are conducted on a pass/fail/honors basis. Students rotate through clinical clerkships in groups of about fifteen to twenty. In some rotations, competition for grades can be fierce, especially in groups dominated by students pursuing competitive specialties. For everyone else, it's not high pressure but remains demanding. Clinical years are spent mostly at Mount Sinai's tertiary-care hospital or at one of its main teaching facilities (the Bronx Veterans Administration Hospital or Elmhurst, a city hospital in Queens that is among the best run of New York City's public hospitals). Students generally welcome the opportunity to go to Elmhurst, where the patient population, which consists of immigrants from Asia, Africa, and South America, often presents the student with rare diseases.

Most of the third year is spent at Mount Sinai Hospital, the flagship institution. In addition, in recent years, the medical center has been adding far-off hospitals to its network. Among these sites are two in New Jersey (Newark Beth Israel and Saint Barnabas in Livingston, where a few unlucky students can be shipped for a month to rotate through surgery, obstetrics and gynecology, or both). Although housing is provided at these sites and a daily shuttle bus runs to and from Mount Sinai, few students enjoy the 45-minute commute.

Among the clerkships, medicine is consistently outstanding. Students meet weekly with the department chair for a didactic session on a topic of their choosing. Pediatrics is also very good. Surgery can be grueling, depending on the site and the team to which students are assigned. The clerkship hasn't received the department's full attention, and, at times, it shows. Surgeons come late or skip lectures, and some residents tend to ignore medical students. Obstetrics and gynecology is good and has a new, dedicated course director. Psychiatry at Mount Sinai is housed in the medical center's posh new East Building and is considered fun and easy. Neurology lasts three weeks, anesthesiology lasts one, and each is relatively easy after some of the core blocks.

Fourth year is largely composed of elective time. Students must complete twenty-one elective weeks in

all, with some students using the time to audition at programs to which they would like to match and others using it to craft thinly disguised vacations (e.g., research time, clerkships in exotic locations). There are also required rotations in emergency medicine, geriatrics, a four- to six-week subinternship in either medicine or pediatrics, and a block of primary care, instituted in response to a new California law that requires primary-care training to qualify for a California state license. In addition, owing to a recent merger between Mount Sinai and New York University Medical Center, students can take classes at any of the NYU graduate schools and receive elective credit.

Social Life

Attending medical school is difficult enough, and life in the Big Apple can get expensive, which doesn't make circumstances easier. To help, the medical center provides subsidized housing located across from the hospital. Apartments range in price from $535 to $550 per person, in arrangements of four to six single bedrooms. More expensive housing for couples is also available. The School also provides deeply discounted tickets to Broadway events and the New York Philharmonic. The best sections of Manhattan's Upper East Side are a few short blocks away, although entertainment here can stretch a student's budget.

Extracurricular activities at the school range from standard fare, such as journal clubs and research tutorials, to the Mount Sinai Student Chamber Orchestra and a student-run theatrical group. Community service has been a big draw as well, and various health education programs in nearby Harlem are constantly springing up.

Winters can be dreary for those not from the Northeast. Mount Sinai is located right off New York's Central Park, where, during the summer, most students bike, jog, and in-line skate. Student housing offers three basketball courts, an outdoor racquetball facility, and a well-equipped gym. The majority of students hail from the tristate area of New York, New Jersey, and Connecticut, although most states are represented. A Northeastern energy and an unusual social and intellectual activism mark the student body.

The Bottom Line

Mount Sinai ameliorates many of the time-honored hardships of learning medicine and fosters an environment that accepts life outside medical school and promotes extracurricular and elective learning within.

NEW YORK INSTITUTE OF TECHNOLOGY, NEW YORK COLLEGE OF OSTEOPATHIC MEDICINE

Old Westbury, New York

Tuition 1996–97: $22,000 per year
Applications: 4,400
Total Number of Women Students: 428 (45%)
Total Number of Men Students: 531 (55%)
World Wide Web: sunp.nyit.edu/NYCOM

Contact: Michael J. Schaefer, Director of
Admissions
PO Box 8
Old Westbury, NY 11568
516-626-6947

Part of New York Institute of Technology, the New York College of Osteopathic Medicine (NYCOM) focuses on educating primary-care physicians, with an emphasis on osteopathic manipulation and philosophy. More than 60 percent of graduates choose residencies in family practice, internal medicine, pediatrics, and obstetrics/gynecology. For those who enter specialties, the most popular are emergency medicine, radiology, anesthesiology, surgery, physical medicine, and the NYCOM-sponsored neurosurgery residency, the only such program at an osteopathic school. NYCOM is not considered a major research institution but does some notable research, especially in Parkinson's disease, anatomy, and osteopathic manipulation medicine.

The 750-acre campus of the New York Institute of Technology is 25 miles east of New York City on the north shore of Long Island. However, few would ever know that one of the biggest cities is so close; the campus and surrounding residential community is wooded and secluded. The College's first building, the Nelson Rockefeller Academic Center, was established on campus in 1977 and was named for the former U.S. vice president, who was instrumental in founding the School. This building houses the Office of Admissions, the library, and study rooms. Another building houses the clinic, lecture halls, and labs. NYCOM is currently constructing a third building, planned to open fall 1999.

In 1998, 4,700 students applied for 220 seats. About 12 percent of applicants are invited to interview. At least one letter of recommendation from a D.O. is helpful but not essential. The interview begins with a short secondary essay followed by the interview and a tour that ends with lunch and a question-and-answer session. The interviews are conducted by faculty members (D.O., M.D., or Ph.D.) and may also include a student or intern. In addition to the usual factors, interviewers also seek to gauge interest in osteopathic medicine.

The average age for the entering class is 24. Some students come from careers in pharmacy, allied health, or engineering. Admissions prefers students from New York and New Jersey, with up to 80 percent of the class from these two states alone. About 50 percent of NYCOM students are women; African Americans and Hispanics comprise 12 percent.

Several special programs are available. The College has an accelerated program to educate émigré physicians in osteopathic medicine (APEP). APEP students follow a three-year program composed of two years of didactics and one year of clerkships, which is designed to reeducate émigré physicians for practice in the United States. Concurrent degree programs include D.O./M.B.A. and D.O./M.S. in clinical nutrition. There are also fellowships available in the anatomy and osteopathic manipulation medicine (OMM) departments for students interested in teaching and research. The office of minority affairs sponsors several programs for education of underrepresented minorities, including a basic science summer program for prematriculated students.

Preclinical Years

The curriculum at NYCOM incorporates OMM into the conventional medical curriculum. The OMM course is the only course that requires the full two years and part of the third. Teaching of osteopathic theory and practices is restricted to the OMM lab and lecture, while the osteopathic philosophy in the approach to a patient is part of virtually all courses, especially second year.

The College's content and delivery systems of courses are examined and revised on an ongoing basis. Some of the recent modifications include instituting problem-based learning to correlate basic science and clinical subject matter in the first two years. All lecture halls are now fitted with the latest equipment for computer-aided instruction. Small-group instruction is an essential part of basic science labs and the OMM and family practice courses. The departments vary in teaching quality, but physiology, anatomy, pharmacology, pathology, cardiology, nephrology, and OMM stand out as being consistently strong. Notes put together by the professors supplement each lecture and are available online. Classes are typically scheduled daily from 9 a.m. to 4 p.m. Grades are recorded as honors/pass/fail, with a minimum requirement of 70 percent to pass.

The first-year curriculum consists of fourteen courses from late August to early June. In general, the courses emphasize the basic sciences and include a balance of clinically relevant information. The first block is relatively easy, with histology, biochemistry, physiology, and OMM. A heavier volume starts in mid-October with anatomy. Students usually find that they are always trying to play catch-up for the rest of the first year. Three-hour exams come virtually every Monday, and, as expected, most students start to feel some burn out by February. Unfortunately, this coincides with the start of the most difficult part of the year, when neuroscience, general pathology, and pharmacology run concurrently. At least a refreshing, and somewhat easier, family practice course accompanies these.

Students can apply for a scholarship award to participate in research during the first summer in the labs of anatomy, neuroscience, physiology, and biomechanics. The hottest clinically oriented research at NYCOM is on Parkinson's disease.

During the second year, didactics are more intense and clinically based than first year. Courses overlap according to system. For instance, the cardiology course runs concurrently with cardiovascular pathology, cardiovascular pharmacology, and sections on the cardiovascular patient in the OMM and family practice courses. Relentless weekly tests continue in the second year.

If this is not enough, some choose to take elective courses, such as medical Spanish, advanced cardiac life support, or sports medicine. Students can also apply for teaching fellowships in anatomy or OMM that require delaying graduation for one year to combine research, teaching, and clinical clerkships in three years. There is more than a month to study for COMLEX (osteopathic licensing exam) Step I in June. All students take this test, and some also choose to take the USMLE (allopathic licensing exam). More than 95 percent pass the COMLEX on their first try.

Clinical Years

Students choose clinical rotations from more than fifteen local clinical affiliates in urban, suburban, and rural areas, including St. Barnabas, Good Samaritan Medical Center, the North Shore Hospitals, Long Island Jewish Hospital, and several rural affiliates in upstate New York. The affiliated hospitals range in size from 160 to 705 beds and allow the opportunity for a diverse clinical experience. Third- and fourth-year students may also choose to see their own patients on an outpatient basis during a primary-care rotation at the NYCOM Health Care Center. Since there are many hospitals to choose from, students must do some homework to find out which will best suit their needs and interests. Students rank their desired rotation slots, and a computer program sifts through them to make the assignments. This lottery system has not caused any problems, since most get their first or second choice. One complaint about the rotations is that some clerkship slots don't coincide with those of the hospital faculty. This causes a problem because faculty may have only half of the clerkship to get to know a student's ability, therefore affecting the value of a recommendation letter.

All graduates are accepted into postgraduate internship or residency programs. Seventy percent pursue a one-year osteopathic rotating internship, with 64 percent in the NYCOM educational consortium of affiliate programs. After internship, most choose to continue with an osteopathic residency, while up to 40 percent enter an allopathic residency. Approximately 60 percent of graduates enter primary care.

Social Life

Living on Long Island lends the opportunity to travel an hour west to experience the excitement and culture of Manhattan or drive east to some of the more rural areas and state wildlife preserves. The College is 10 minutes from the north shore beaches of Long Island Sound, where some students make time to windsurf, water ski, or fish. Also, there are plenty of good restaurants and shopping and in the area, but most students head west toward New York City to nightclubs or jazz bars.

On campus, many clubs and chapters of national organizations offer a chance to become involved in community service as well as to learn more about a specific medical specialty. There are also exercise and wellness organizations, intramural soccer and football, and even the School's own NFL (NYCOM Foosball League).

There is no campus housing. Most students live in the quiet residential communities that surround the School, although many do make the commute from NYC. Rent ranges from $300 per person for a house shared to more than $700 a month for a studio. Total living costs (rent, food, utilities, transportation) are estimated at $17,500 for twelve months. Most students find that borrowing the maximum subsidized and unsubsidized Stafford loans (currently $38,500) is sufficient to cover the $22,000 tuition (both in- and out-of-state) and living expenses. The financial aid office is very good at helping students through the process.

The Bottom Line

NYCOM is the school for students interested in learning and applying the osteopathic principles and practice in primary-care medicine. Medical research and subspecialty medicine are not emphasized.

NEW YORK MEDICAL COLLEGE

Valhalla, New York

Tuition 1996–97: $28,835 per year
Students Receiving Financial Aid: 17%
Applications: 10,985
Size of Entering Class: 190
Total Number of Women Students: 313 (40%)

Total Number of Men Students: 467 (60%)
World Wide Web: www.nymc.edu/
Contact: Dr. Fern Juster, Admissions Office
Valhalla, NY 10595-1691
914-594-4507

New York Medical College (NYMC), founded in New York City in 1860 by a group of civic leaders led by the noted poet William Cullen Bryant, is located in the bucolic hamlet of Valhalla in suburban Westchester County, New York. Today, the College's affiliation with St. Vincent's Hospital and Medical Center, Metropolitan Hospital, and Our lady of Mercy Medical Center continues a long relationship with New York City hospitals. The large network of affiliated hospitals allows students to train at clinically and demographically diverse settings. Westchester Medical Center, a tertiary-care referral center, is located on campus in Valhalla.

The school graduated the first female physician in the country in 1867 and three years later graduated the first African-American female physician in New York. Students from all parts of the United States make up the typical entering class of 190. However, California represented about 40 percent of one recent class.

Preclinical Years

Students spend the first two years at the main campus in Valhalla studying the basic sciences. The traditional lecture-oriented basic science curriculum has recently been revised to place more emphasis on clinical medicine and problem solving, as evidenced by direct patient contact beginning in the first year. Students work one-on-one in the office of a primary-care physician, fostering a personal mentor relationship. This experience can be continued into the second year to fulfill the clinical skills/physical diagnosis requirement.

Each student is assigned to a module and given a desk with a locked cabinet for personal use throughout the year. Gross anatomy and cell biology take up the first three months, followed by biochemistry and physiology. Neuroscience and behavioral medicine courses complete the first-year curriculum.

The anatomy department is outstanding and offers the standout class of the year. The lectures are well structured, and faculty members are invested in helping students learn. A student-run transcript service is well worth the money. The neuroscience course is usually very good. Behavioral medicine, the easiest class of the year, offers good lectures, although many students rely on transcripts. The year is rounded out by small-group seminars on the principles of primary care and lectures in epidemiology and biostatistics.

The second year is more difficult and reflects a redesign of the first- and second-year curriculum, which encourages early mastery of clinical skills fostered by exposure to patients. The clinical skills/physical diagnosis training continues throughout the second year in preparation for the third-year clinical clerkships. Students spend less time in the large lecture hall and more time in small study groups.

Pathology/pathophysiology is a yearlong class that is divided into two parts, the first of which students must pass to advance. Infrequently, a student is asked to decelerate and repeat this course. Microbiology and pharmacology, two well-taught classes, are offered concurrently with pathology part I and part II, respectively. Tests occur together in two 3-hour periods and can be exhausting. Generously, the week before each test day—there are three test days per class—no classes are scheduled.

The faculty is generally quite accessible. Transcripts can be quite a crutch during second year. Although the pharmacology department does not allow students to use the system to tape lectures, students use their own tape recorders to prepare transcripts.

Clinical Years

The clinical experience at the school is excellent. As a result of its continued success, NYMC was one of sixteen schools recognized by the Robert Wood Johnson Foundation for its dedication to educating primary-care physicians.

Students perform required third-year clerkships at hospitals in New York, New Jersey, and Connecticut, placements at which are determined by a lottery. Students are well integrated into treatment teams at the large hospitals. St. Vincent's Hospital in Manhattan and Westchester Medical Center are usual favorites among students.

Surgery is outstanding at all the university hospitals. As a tertiary care center, Westchester Medical Center offers exposure to all surgical subspecialties, including cardiothoracic surgery and neurosurgery. The medicine clerkship has also been an excellent experience at most hospitals. The psychiatry clerkship is terrific, especially at St. Vincent's Hospital and Medical Center, which offers students exposure to a large volume of patients with varying psychopathology. Obstetrics and gynecology and pediatrics can be hit-and-miss at Westchester Medical Center.

When students have poor experiences at affiliates, the school is receptive to complaints and often discontinues its affiliation with the offending hospitals. Because of its affiliation with the archdiocese, the College has been seeking affiliations with Catholic hospitals in the tristate area. St. Agnes Hospital is a recent addition.

Fourth-year electives are diverse and flexible. The fourth year lasts eleven months that consist of sixteen weeks of required clinical experience and eighteen weeks of electives and culminate in a grand graduation ceremony at Carnegie Hall in Manhattan.

Social Life

A university housing complex located in Valhalla to accommodate 300 first- and second-year students was built in 1993. Rent for first-year students is $530 per month. Alternately, neighboring communities provide good opportunities for students to rent apartments or houses. Nearby Tarrytown, about 5 minutes from Valhalla, has been a favorite of many students. To serve those students who spend their clinical years in New York City, the College recently bought an eighteen-story luxury apartment building on the Upper East Side of Manhattan that offers East River views, recreation facilities, and 24-hour security. The building offers furnished suites of one to four bedrooms, and the cost depends on how many students share each apartment. The average price per student (utilities included) for a five-bedroom apartment is $535 per month; for a three-bedroom apartment, $603 per month; and for a two-bedroom apartment, $645 per month. A limited number of studio ($985 per month) and one bedroom ($1,235 per month) apartments are available; gas is included, but the student pays the electric bill.

For those who live in Manhattan, the cultural and entertainment opportunities rival the best cities in the world. However, the Valhalla campus, located 30 minutes away, offers a wide range of nonacademic activities as well. Numerous sites for outdoor activities are close by, including the Rockefeller estate in Tarrytown, and provide lots of open farmland and forest to find your way through. Of local interest is the town of Sleepy Hollow (a.k.a. North Tarrytown), which inspired Washington Irving's *Legend of Sleepy Hollow*.

Academic, social, and athletic clubs are active, and the student senate plays an important role in the College community. One tradition is the rugby club, which plays rival medical and graduate schools at weekend tournaments. The rivalry with Columbia is particularly intense. If bloodletting isn't a student's favorite sport, facilities for basketball, softball, golf, tennis, and winter sports are all available.

The Bottom Line

NYMC is an excellent school with opportunities that afford students enough flexibility to achieve both personal and academic goals.

NEW YORK UNIVERSITY SCHOOL OF MEDICINE

New York, New York

Tuition 1996–97: $26,800 per year
Size of Entering Class: 150
Total Number of Women Students: 364 (39%)
Total Number of Men Students: 564 (61%)
World Wide Web: www.nyu.edu/homepage.html

Contact: Raymond Brienza, Assistant Dean,
Admissions
70 Washington Square South
New York, NY 10012-1019
212-263-5290

New York University (NYU) usually conjures up images of heady days in Greenwich Village, appearing as an extra in a Woody Allen film shot on campus, or, at the very least, the shot of Sally dropping Harry at the Washington Square Arch.

Unfortunately for NYU's medical students, however, the medical center is not in Manhattan's perennially hip Village. The NYU School of Medicine, which was established in 1841, is just one component of the largest private university in the U.S. and is still located in the most exciting city in the world, in that city's most vibrant borough: Manhattan.

Preclinical Years

Living in New York and attending medical school at the same time can make it seem as though medical school is just a time- and money-consuming obstacle between a student and all those things a student would enjoy. That probably explains why the faculty has seen fit to jam-pack first-year schedules with more hours of class (usually 9 a.m. to 4 or 5 p.m., four days a week, and a day of 9 a.m. to 1 p.m.) per week than they attended in all four years of college. After a week of orientation—being introduced to the city they'll be calling home for the next four years—it's suit up for your first anatomy lab on the first afternoon of classes.

Things get better. By December, students will have decided which classes to attend, which classes to sleep through, and how great a bargain (at $60 per year) the student-run transcript service is. It doesn't hurt that once anatomy is over, first year is a breeze. NYU is in the process of reorganizing the curriculum into modules of linked subjects, so things are constantly changing. At the same time, NYU is at the forefront of integrating computer-based learning into the basic sciences curriculum through its well-funded Hippocrates Project. In general, most professors who teach the basic sciences are accessible, care a

tremendous amount about the students, and keep their ears to the ground for student grumblings. One perennial complaint is the size of the library, which is among the smallest of medical school facilities in the country. Study space was formerly a problem near exam time, but a recent major renovation of two areas of campus has alleviated the space crunch.

Exams are scheduled, for the most part, two or three at a time, spread out over a week. Two very important words become a mantra: pass/fail. The first two years are completely pass/fail, which takes away all that competitive pressure that was supposed to be left at undergrad classes. About once a week, first-year students are introduced to clinical medicine through interviewing patients. This experience is the prelude to psychiatry interviews and physical diagnosis, which take place during second year.

The first summer can be a lot of fun. For those who couldn't get enough anatomy, NYU is home to the Anatomy Fellows Program, which trains about a dozen students each year to teach visiting anatomy students and, later, to tutor first-year students—a free service to those students having trouble. The Bellevue Emergency Department also sponsors about a dozen summer students, who spend several 12-hour shifts per week learning everything from physical exams to suturing. Other students opt for lab research or travel opportunities.

The second year is much like the first, although pathology, pharmacology, and introduction to clinical medicine are all more or less integrated into one class. At its conclusion, students are given a month off to study for the USMLE Step I, and they consistently score above the national average on the exam, with few or no failures.

Clinical Years

Because of NYU's strong tradition of providing health care for Bellevue Hospital, New York City's flagship public hospital, students receive an unparalleled hands-on approach to medicine. Interns who attended NYU typically are among the best in their classes at drawing blood, starting IVs, and performing other common procedures. The overwhelming amount of work to do sometimes leaves teaching behind and makes some rotations somewhat disorganized, but self-starters do extremely well. Although NYU for several years had adopted a flexible block curriculum, allowing students to schedule rotations at any time in the third and fourth years and giving them more flexibility, the administration has recently modified the curriculum to require the majority of rotations to be completed by November of the fourth year.

Unfortunately, a larger-than-average class size (more than 160 in the past few years) and the pressures of the New York metropolitan area health-care market, squeezed by managed care, have made it necessary for NYU to increasingly farm out students to many outlying hospitals. These include Lenox Hill, a posh private hospital on the Upper East Side; North Shore University Hospital, a first-rate community hospital in Manhassett, Long Island; and NYU Downtown Hospital. Some of these do not have the same commitment to teaching shared by the home institutions of Bellevue (on First Avenue and 26th Street), the Manhattan Veteran's Administration Medical Center (First and 23rd Street), and NYU's own Tisch (University) Hospital (First and 33rd St.). NYU also staffs the Hospital for Joint Diseases, about fifteen blocks from the main medical center. Shuttles to the various centers are available, but traveling remains inconvenient.

A standout rotation is psychiatry, which is well organized and provides good hands-on, as well as, didactic experience. Other rotations receive mixed marks, depending on where they were completed; overall, teaching tends to be better at NYU's private institutions, while hands-on experience is better at Bellevue. NYU is also trying, although somewhat reluctantly, to ride the crest of the primary-care wave by incorporating a four-week ambulatory care rotation. The culmination of the fourth year, the required subinternship in medicine, is tremendous experience, and is longer (six weeks) than at most schools.

Electives are plentiful and range from studying literature and humanities at the main campus (or at the medical center) to working one-on-one with Dr. Benjamin Sadock, coeditor of the *Comprehensive Textbook of Psychiatry* to working at the New York City Medical Examiner's Office (located on the NYU campus) to more traditional electives such as diagnostic radiology subspecialty rotations and months on intensive care units.

One caveat: The effect on the merger between NYU's hospitals and Mount Sinai's hospitals has yet to be seen. Some observers say it's only a matter of time before the two medical schools merge, although for now the Schools remain separate, with separate applications.

Social Life

Situated in New York, NYU has about a thousand more opportunities for meeting people, experiencing culture, and staying out all night to get into trouble than any medical student could possibly enjoy. There's plenty of socializing among students. A recent graduating class included about a dozen interclass couples who were married, engaged, or close.

Many of NYU's students tend to be from the New York metropolitan area (including New York, New Jersey, and Connecticut), but most of the fifty states are represented because NYU is a private institution with no particular obligation to residents of the state. The average age in the class tends to be on the young side, with a few students over 30 years old in each class. NYU is loyal to its alumni and faculty; chances are that 10 percent or more of an incoming class will have parents who attended or teach at the School.

On-campus housing isn't terrific, but considering the current real estate market in Manhattan, it is quite reasonable. In the neighborhood that surrounds the campus, for example, studios can go for $1,100 a month, with one-bedrooms starting at $1,200. Cheaper housing can be found in other areas of Manhattan, but cheap is a relative term. The majority of students start off in Rubin Hall (about $500 per month), which is more dormlike than any college dormitory, with single rooms off a hallway featuring a common bathroom and kitchen), or Greenberg Hall (about $700 per person, per month), which consists mostly of two-bedroom apartments and a converted living room/third bedroom, plus a kitchen and a bathroom. A third option is Skirball Residential Tower (about $750 per person, per month), which is a luxury building that features one-bedroom apartments that are usually shared by two students.

The Bottom Line

NYU gives students a great hands-on chance to become doctors at one of the top twenty-five medical schools in one of the greatest cities in the world.

NORTHEASTERN OHIO UNIVERSITIES COLLEGE OF MEDICINE

Rootstown, Ohio

Applications: 1,183
Size of Entering Class: 105
Total Number of Women Students: 185 (44%)
Total Number of Men Students: 237 (56%)
World Wide Web: www.neoucom.edu/

Contact: Karen Berger, Associate Director of
Admissions
PO Box 95
Rootstown, OH 44272-0095
330-325-6270

Northeastern Ohio Universities College of Medicine (NEOUCOM) was founded in 1975, with the intention of increasing the number of primary-care physicians in northeastern Ohio. The school is one of the ten or so six-year B.S./M.D. programs in the country. One of the best features of this program is that students are accepted to medical school straight out of high school. What makes it even better is that there is almost no competition. In phase I, students are not competing against anyone but themselves. The lack of competition continues through medical school because students have spent their undergraduate years together forming strong friendships that strongly discourage competition.

Admissions/Financial Aid

Each year approximately 1,000 high school students apply to the six-year B.S./M.D. program. About 300 are interviewed and, ultimately, 100–105 are accepted. The bulk of the students accepted are from within the state of Ohio, as the school gives preference to Ohio residents. However, the school has a policy to accept 3 to 5 percent of the students each year from out of state.

Students apply to the program in their senior year of high school. Interviews are held at each of the undergraduate universities. Students rank order their preference of which of the three universities they would like to attend, and through a match-like system, approximately thirty students are accepted into each undergraduate university. The interviews seem to focus around assessing the student's level of maturity, often asking ethical and current event questions. The average SAT and ACT scores and high school GPAs of accepted students change from year to

year but remain competitive. Ideally, SAT scores of more than 1250 and high school class rank in the top 10 to 15 percent makes students competitive enough to obtain an interview.

The second type of admission is the direct entry. These are students who already have done their undergraduate work elsewhere and are applying to medical school via the traditional route. Approximately ten direct entries are accepted into NEOUCOM each year. Since there are only ten slots, these students tend to have a very competitive resume, exceeding the B.S./M.D. requirements for promotion from phase I to phase II.

The average cost of tuition is $10,000 for the first, second, and fourth years, and third-year tuition is $14,000. The staff members in the student services office are very knowledgeable about all the different kinds of loans, scholarships, and grants. Also, for students who are horrible with finances and with making sure their loan checks last through the whole term, NEOUCOM offers school-based emergency loans.

Preclinical Years

The first year is very rigorous. It is divided into three terms, and students cover as many as six different basic sciences in one term. Classes run from 8 a.m. to 5 p.m. daily. Life tends to become monotonous, and students get those med school blues. To make it worse, at the end of the term is exam week. A single exam determines your grade for the past ten to fifteen weeks of work. Although this sounds bad, it can be advantageous because this grade is purely objective. If you study hard, you will do well on the exam; it does not matter what the instructor thinks of you. No one else has a say in a grade except for a student.

The second year of medical school is not quite as rigorous, but it is pretty rough. It is better than the first year because students gain some clinical experience through the Introduction to Clinical Medicine class. It is in this class that students learn physical diagnostic techniques and procedures. Students have interviews with standardized patients to help build a foundation of interviewing skills. However, the curriculum is still geared more toward basic sciences in the second year.

Each student receives a grade of honors if he or she does well, satisfactory for passing, and either a conditional unsatisfactory (which is erased if the student passes the remediation exam) or an unsatisfactory (which stays on a student's transcript even after passing the remediation exam) if the student fails. The majority of the students earn a satisfactory in each subject, five to ten will receive honors, and usually two to three will fail.

There is plenty of vacation during the first two years: two weeks of Christmas vacation, one week for spring break, and about three months of summer vacation after the first year.

Clinical Years

Students can choose from doing their clinical years at Akron, Youngstown, or Canton. Each has its advantages and disadvantages, depending on the student and what field he or she wants to enter. The third year offers the core clinical clerkships in internal medicine, surgery, psychiatry, pediatrics, and obstetrics/gynecology. In addition, NEOUCOM offers a clerkship in family practice. This is unique because few medical schools offer family practice clerkships. This clerkship is viewed as a hassle to some medical students, but others find it an interesting one for many reasons. It gives the student a relaxed environment in which to not only learn the medicine associated with being a physician, but also to learn the communication skills needed to establish a physician-patient relationship. The internal medicine clerkship allows the students to see and manage patients while under the supervision of a resident. Students can take as much responsibility for the patients as they feel comfortable handling. There are a large number of patients and diseases, as well as a very friendly and helpful residency program staff. The surgery clerkship at Canton is unique because there is no residency program. The students work in the operating room one-on-one with the attending. Some students in Canton get the opportunity to assist or even do whole operations with their attending, which is more than a third-year surgical resident could hope for. Pediatrics is a popular rotation due to Akron Children's Hospital, and ob/gyn is well liked by most students.

Call nights are rough at times and sometimes permit students to get only 1 hour of sleep. Most attendings are well liked, and students are given ample chances for procedures such as delivering babies. Students more hesitantly recommend psychiatry, although one does see quite a variation of psychotic individuals and procedures such as electroconvulsive shock therapy.

Social Life

NEOUCOM is located in the small rural town of Rootstown. There is little social activity there, but bigger towns with more social life are just minutes away. There are no dorms provided by the school, so most students live in apartments in the surrounding towns. Only 15 minutes away is downtown Kent. Kent State University is one of the largest colleges in Ohio, and there are many bars, dance clubs, and restaurants to choose from in this college town. On weekends, it is always a good time to go to downtown Cleveland (only 45 minutes), where there are hundreds of clubs and bars.

The Bottom Line

NEOUCOM is a great medical school for enthusiastic high school students who know that they want to enter medicine. It provides a guaranteed admission to medical school right out of high school. Students do not have to worry about the pressures of doing well in college, taking the MCAT, and applying to medical school. Plus, they graduate two years ahead of their peers.

NORTHWESTERN UNIVERSITY MEDICAL SCHOOL

Evanston, Illinois

Applications: 9,522
Size of Entering Class: 171
Total Number of Women Students: 355 (50%)
Total Number of Men Students: 351 (50%)
World Wide Web: www.nums.nwu.edu/

Contact: Charles A. Berry, Associate Dean for
Admissions
Evanston, IL 60208
312-908-8206

Between the stretches of Lake Michigan's shoreline and Chicago's Magnificent Mile lies Northwestern University Medical School. Northwestern's solid academics and enviable location make the School an appealing choice for students undeterred by private school tuition. The Medical School's philosophy of self-directed learning encourages students to assume an active role in shaping their professional growth. Furthermore, the proximity of several other Northwestern professional schools lends diversity to the Medical School experience. Dual-degree M.D./M. B.A., M.D./M.P.H., and M.D./Ph.D. programs are among the options that students with special interests may pursue.

Preclinical Years

Students are introduced to the Medical School and the many attractions of Chicago during orientation week. Soon thereafter, students begin MDM-I, the first of three short courses on medical decision making. Subsequent morning lectures build upon basic science principles, whereas the afternoon curriculum focuses on the physician-patient relationship, the physician's role in society, and medical ethics. Depending on students' personal comfort level with biochemistry and cell biology, the early weeks in Medical School may be a time for the beach, the nightlife, or long stressful nights bent over textbooks.

The playing field is soon leveled, however. About the time when the first frost hits, the curriculum kicks into high gear, with anatomy lab and problem-based learning, which together emphasize independent responsibility, maturity, and teamwork. These early experiences fuel the annual humorous student production. The well-equipped Learning Resources Center, part of the newly constructed Galter Health Sciences Library, offers more avenues for learning than most busy medical students find time to fully explore. Those students who can't seem to get enough

note with mild discontent that the library closes at midnight and somewhat earlier on weekends.

Lecturers are attentive to students' needs and take pains to make lectures interesting and useful. For the rare professor who is a bit too eager to share her personal research exploits (rather than the scheduled topic), there is a lecture evaluation system through which students can voice grievances. An active student government works closely with the Medical School's curriculum review committees.

First-year basic science lectures are integrated into a single yearlong course called Structure-Function, which is broken up into three to six week blocks, with most blocks organized by organ system. These blocks are generally arranged to coincide with the corresponding topic in histology and anatomy labs. For example, dissection of the limb musculature in anatomy lab takes place during the musculoskeletal block of Structure-Function. Students find the cardiovascular, renal, and respiratory physiology lectures particularly strong, whereas they are more likely to appeal to their textbooks for endocrinology because these lectures can sometimes be overly academic.

Exams are given roughly once a month and are graded on a pass/fail system, which relieves much of the competitive edge. Most students supplement their class lectures with extensive reading, although some swear by Mednotes, the student-run lecture transcript service. During the summer following first year, many students take advantage of research grants offered through the Medical School. Others undertake clinically oriented projects, participate in extramural programs, or travel.

Second year is similar to the first, although the emphasis changes from basic science to pathology, pharmacology, and microbiology. Students get clinical exposure through training in physical exam skills, medical diagnosis, and patient interviews and physicals. Sessions geared toward the USMLE are offered, and students are allotted a few weeks off prior to the exam.

Clinical Years

Students attest that Northwestern's clinical curriculum is among the School's greatest strengths. Because of the diverse settings in which they train, Northwestern medical students develop expert technical skills and see a mixture of rare and common diseases. Recently, Northwestern implemented a system that ensures students enter each clerkship with comparable experience.

The McGaw Medical Center of Northwestern University includes Northwestern Memorial Hospital (Wesley, Passavant, and Olson Pavilions; Prentice Women's Hospital Maternity Center; and the Institute of Psychiatry), the Rehabilitation Institute of Chicago, and the Veterans Administration Lakeside Medical Center. In addition, Northwestern is affiliated with excellent community hospitals, most of which require commutes of varying length.

Northwestern's unusually high faculty-student ratio of 1:2 gives students many opportunities to work closely with the clinical faculty members. The third-year clerkships include surgery, medicine, obstetrics and gynecology, pediatrics, neurology, psychiatry, and primary care. Most Northwestern students regard medicine and surgery as their core clinical experiences during the third year, but the pediatrics and obstetrics/gynecology departments are also notable for their academic strengths. Students interested in specialties such as otolaryngology, plastic surgery, or orthopedic surgery find the strength of these programs an added asset when it comes time to apply for residencies in their fourth year.

Northwestern has not traditionally been at the forefront of national trends in primary care, but in the past few years, the School has made efforts to encourage student interest in such disciplines. For example, a required four-week primary-care clerkship was recently added to the third year. A six-week multispecialty surgical clerkship, which emphasizes what the primary-care physician should know about surgical specialties, now supplements the surgery rotation. On a restructured pediatrics clerkship, students split time evenly between inpatient and ambulatory care settings. Almost all students have looked upon these curricular changes favorably. At the same time,

students considering specialties are grateful for the School's commitment to supporting students' interests in specialty as well as primary-care fields.

Northwestern prides itself in success in residency placement, with more than 75 percent of students matching in their first-, second-, or third-choice programs. About half of the students stay at Northwestern for their residency training.

Social Life

Chicago has been described as a city with the personality of a small town. Probably most famous for its night life—blues, jazz, dance and comedy clubs, and festivals—Chicago is also justly proud of its beaches, bike paths, lakefront attractions, and Navy Pier. Shared experience brings classmates together, while the nearness of Northwestern's other graduate schools exposes students to a diverse group of individuals during their schooling.

On-campus housing is terrific, as long as students don't mind eating out. The most common reason students opt out of University housing is the dormitory food plan. Abbott Hall and Lake Shore Center, the two student dorms, offer mostly single rooms, some with lake views, in prices that range from $450 to $750 per person per month. Lake Shore Center features a well-equipped weight room, pool, gym, and bar and grill. Abbott Hall houses the cafeteria, the bookstore, and several administrative offices. After their first year, most students move into university apartment/studio complexes, which are only slightly more expensive than the dorms. Others move to Lincoln Park, a scenic area a few miles north of campus.

Many of Northwestern's students are from the Midwest, but most of the fifty states are represented. One third of Northwestern's classes of 175 is part of the Honors Program in Medical Education, a seven-year combined B.A. or B.S./M.D. program. As a result, about 120 slots are available for new applicants, and the average age tends to be in the early twenties, with a few students in their thirties or older.

The Bottom Line

Northwestern offers students the autonomy to shape their own development into physicians at one of the nation's finest Medical Schools, while sampling the delights of the ritziest part of Chicago.

OHIO STATE UNIVERSITY COLLEGE OF MEDICINE AND PUBLIC HEALTH

Columbus, Ohio

Tuition 1996–97: $31,650 per year
Students Receiving Financial Aid: 63%
Applications: 4,413
Size of Entering Class: 210
Total Number of Women Students: 499 (44%)
Total Number of Men Students: 648 (56%)

World Wide Web: www.med.ohio-state.edu/
Contact: Dr. Mark A. Notestine, Assistant Dean of Admissions and Student Affairs
Columbus, OH 43210
614-292-7137

As the fourth-largest medical school in the nation, the Ohio State University College of Medicine (OSU-COM) is a premier place to become a physician. Since 1914, the school has been known for producing outstanding clinicians and researchres. Thanks to the Dean (who is a former Director of the National Institutes of Health), the school has recruited several top-name researchers in the past several years, guaranteeing that students are exposed to the cutting edge in medicine.

Admissions/Financial Aid

OSU-COM is one of the largest medical schools in the country, with an average class size between 210 to 220. Though the majority of students are straight out of college, a large number have other professional degrees or nonscience hobbies. On average, students have at least a 3.5 GPA and a MCAT score of 31 or greater. By state mandate, 80 percent of the entering class is Ohio residents, 20 percent nonresidents. The class is usually 35–40 percent women.

Tuition is the lowest of all medical schools in Ohio, though it is still substantial. Summer and yearlong research scholarships exist and are relatively easy to secure. Upon graduation, the school offers several more scholarships (some up to $10,000) awarded for a job well done.

Preclinical Years

Students begin the year with gross anatomy. Teams are assigned alphabetically at the beginning of the year, and students spend every third day in dissection. The two days off of dissection are spent studying

cross-sectional anatomy and imaging technology or working with multimedia computer programs. The Anatomy instructors are excellent and readily available to answer questions during dissections.

During this first semester, students spend one day per week in medical humanities and behavioral sciences (MHBS). Patient interviews, tutorials, small-group discussions, and hands-on experiences deal with subjects such as bioethics, death and dying, human growth and development, alternative medicine, and community medicine. Many graduates credit MHBS with making them better communicators and helping them to better understand their patients' experiences.

After the first twelve weeks of class, the class is split up into three different educational tracks. Students must decide early on which track they wish to pursue—didactic, problem-based, or independent study. Most choose the didactic pathway. Classes are arranged according to system and are taught primarily via lectures, labs, and tutorials.

Lectures typically run from 8 a.m. or 9 a.m. until noon, Monday through Friday. Afternoons are either spent in labs (histology slide review, small group tutorials, etc.) or are free for studying. There is a student run note taking service.

A very popular alternative is the problem-based learning (PBL) pathway. Students are assigned to groups in which they review cases under the supervision of an attending physician. This pathway is limited to a certain number of students and, thus, usually the best applicants are chosen. Since this is a relatively new program (begun in 1991), the students going through the PBL pathway have been tracked closely.

They tend to score somewhat above the rest of the class and far above the national average on the USMLE. Perhaps this is because the strongest students are selected, or perhaps it is because this way of learning medicine works better.

The third educational track is independent study. Students who choose independent study are usually those with children who need a flexible schedule, those who learn better on their own or from books, those in the M.D./Ph.D. program who want time for research, and those motivated to finish school in less than four years. This track provides set goals and excellent study resources, including preassigned study areas. Tests are shelf board exams.

Regardless of what track a student chooses, the school stresses cooperation over competition. Grading is honors/pass/fail. Casual study groups are formed, and there are tutors available (usually high-performing students) to assist those in need.

Clinical Years

The clinical years begin with a four-week Introduction to Clinical Medicine (ICM) class. The class covers history and physical skills and interpretation of lab results. The last week of ICM is spent rounding with a ward team, learning to gather and present data. The final consists of examinations on volunteer patients and interpretation of X-rays, EKGs, and labs. The class is not particularly difficult and gives students a good introduction to the third year.

Third year consists of six 8-week blocks. Rotation choices include Internal Medicine (four weeks each of two different medicine specialties), Primary Care Medicine (four weeks of general internal medicine, four weeks of family medicine), ob/gyn, Pediatrics, Surgery, and Psychiatry. Students take in-house call every fourth night with their team during these rotations except for Psychiatry and Family Medicine. There is no elective time allotted for third year, but for those seeking to enter a particular specialty, it is possible to push a third-year rotation (e.g., psychiatry) into the fourth year in exchange for a specialty rotation.

Fourth year is much less structured. Every student completes four weeks of neurology, and four rotations in the Differentiation of Care (DOC) curriculum. The DOC sequence consists of clinical experiences in different realms of patient care that include the undifferentiated patient (emergency care),

ambulatory patient, chronic care patient, and acutely ill patient (ICU). The remaining time is twelve weeks of electives and four weeks of vacation.

All third-year rotations, neurology, and the DOCs have to be completed in the Columbus hospitals or the Cleveland Clinic. Overall, the clinical experience is superb. The main hospitals are the Ohio State University Hospital, the James Cancer Institute, and Columbus Children's Hospital. There are several excellent community hospitals affiliated with the medical school where many students rotate: Riverside Hospital, Mount Caramel Hospitals, and St. Ann's Hospital. These hospitals are all located within the Columbus area and do not require long commutes. In addition, Ohio State has an affiliation with the Cleveland Clinic Foundation. Since 1992, students have been able to do one or more of their rotations at the Cleveland Clinic.

Attendings are of extremely high caliber and committed to teaching. Many take students out to dinner at the end of rotations. Medical students are active in patient care. Every patient on a team is assigned to a medical student, and students are expected to know their patients well. Students deliver lots of babies on obstetrics and can occasionally first assist in surgery.

Students do quite well in the residency match. Sixty percent receive their first choice in residency selection, and 85 percent get one of their top three choices.

Social Life

Ohio State is located in Columbus, the state capital. The city is the sixteenth-largest city in the U.S. Columbus offers a great diversity. From the artsy Short North area to the hip Brewery district and the quaint Victorian village, there is something for everyone. The quality of life is good, and the cost of living is relatively low. Surrounding suburbs are growing rapidly, and some married students can afford to buy homes in the suburbs.

The medical school is located on the edge of the undergraduate campus, which is one of the largest universities in the country. More than 55,000 undergraduates make the campus a little city within the city. The Ohio State University is well known for its sports teams, and there are many events to keep students from the medical school library on a nightly basis.

Since there is a strong undergraduate population, the music scene in Columbus is great. From small venues to large outdoor amphitheaters, local bands and national acts are easy to find. Cultural activities include the Ballet Met, Opera Columbus, Columbus Museum of Art, and the Columbus Symphony. Outdoor activities are plentiful. From golf at the famous Muirfield course to rowing on the Olentangy River to biking or boating, there is something for just about everyone—except the downhill skier, who will need to get a fix in the yearly student ski trip scheduled for the Martin Luther King, Jr. holiday weekend.

The Bottom Line

Ohio State offers students a diverse educational experience, including three preclinical tracks and several teaching hospitals in Columbus and Cleveland. Students take an active part in all phases of their education and receive solid instruction from physicians who care about teaching.

OHIO UNIVERSITY COLLEGE OF OSTEOPATHIC MEDICINE

Athens, Ohio

Tuition 1996–97: $16,035 per year
Students Receiving Financial Aid: 93%
Applications: 3,127
Total Number of Women Students: 181 (43%)
Total Number of Men Students: 239 (57%)

World Wide Web: www.oucom.ohiou.edu
Contact: Dr. James Artis, Director of Admissions
Athens, OH 45701-2979
740-593-4313

Ohio University College of Osteopathic Medicine (OU-COM) offers students a strong comprehensive curriculum in a student-friendly environment. Located in Athens, a rural town in the southeastern corner of Ohio, the school was established in 1975 to increase the number of family physicians in the underserved areas of the state such as southeast Ohio. A large percentage of the school's graduates pursue careers in primary care, the majority of whom practice family medicine.

Admissions/Financial Aid

Last year there were 2,875 applicants, 185 of whom were interviewed and 98 of whom matriculated. Applicants need to have good grades in their science courses, solid MCAT scores (average MCAT 25), and diverse extracurricular experiences. Interview days consist of an information session with the Director of Admissions, a tour, lunch with currently enrolled students, and three interviews. A typical interview team consists of a D.O., a basic science professor, and an administrator. Every applicant meets one-on-one with each of the team members for about 30 minutes each.

The admissions staff is helpful in making the process as painless as possible. The Assistant Dean of Admissions is particularly helpful with counseling prospective students. In the past, the Assistant Dean of Admissions joined up with members of the Student National Medical Association to help minority applicants through the admissions process. The school notifies all students of the status of their application within one week after their interview.

Students tend to come from many different paths. Each class has a large number of people who are pursuing their second career or who are also raising families. In 1998, 27 percent of the entering class

was underrepresented minorities, and 50 percent of the class was women. Students who apply to OU-COM must commit themselves to serving in the state of Ohio. Out-of-state applicants are required to sign a contract with the state to practice in Ohio for five years after graduation (residency training in Ohio counts for five years of practice). Approximately 90 percent of the students at OU-COM receive some type of financial aid. The average indebtedness for graduates in 1998 was approximately $86,000.

Preclinical Years

There are two separate curricula students can pursue: System-Based (SB) and the Primary Care Continuum (PCC). All students participate in the osteopathic manipulative medicine labs together. Both curricula have simulated patient labs as well as gross anatomy and microanatomy labs. Each track, however, approaches the basic sciences differently.

The Systems-Based curriculum is a traditional lecture-driven approach to the basic sciences. Some classes are well-known for their devoted teachers. The anatomy instructor is well liked for her mnemonics, charts, and charming personality. Pathology and microanatomy are highly detail oriented, but their instructors are well-known for helping out students whether it is early morning or on the weekend. The systems-based approach begins in the second year and covers the relevant material in an organized fashion. Students also participate in Early Clinical Contact (ECC) sessions, in which they follow a physician in his office. After the first part of the national board exam, students must take a host of clinically oriented classes. Most students feel this is the most challenging quarter, particularly because the weather is warm and they are looking forward to their clerkships. The SB curriculum is being revised to emphasize clinical case presentations and more active learning.

The Primary Care Continuum was established in 1994. It is a problem-based learning format that incorporates extensive ECC experience and focuses on topics common to primary-care medicine. The program introduces more clinical cases and topics at an earlier stage than the SB curricula. A group of twenty students are divided into three small groups. The groups meet several times a week to discuss case studies. The students are required to identify clinical problems, outline learning objectives, and determine which objectives need to be investigated. Students are evaluated once a quarter. These assessments are based on a content exam that includes the learning objectives covered during the quarter, participation, and group dynamics. This curriculum requires many hours of independent studying and is ideal for self-motivated students. Along with case discussions, the PCC students also spend 4 hours a week in a physician's office getting early patient exposure. After boards, PCC students return for a summer session. This session integrates the basic science principles with clinical workup and management of patient cases.

Clinical Years

Students rotate through a group of hospitals known as the Centers for Osteopathic Regional Education (CORE). The CORE hospitals are located in various cities throughout the state (Athens, Dayton, Columbus, Toledo, and Cleveland) and offer clinical clerkships for osteopathic students from four different schools. Students' experiences are highly varied, depending on the location they choose. Some learn rural medicine at seventy-five–bed hospitals, while others experience the diversity of big city medical centers. All hospitals, however, are linked by videoconferencing for weekly didactics sessions. Each hospital also has its own set of morning and noon lectures. Students, in general, are quite satisfied with their clinical experience, though the amount of hands-on training varies between settings.

Since OU-COM is committed to producing family physicians, students are required to do a minimum of fourteen weeks of family practice. All students are given sixteen weeks of elective time and approximately nine to twelve weeks of vacation (for third and fourth year combined).

Social Life

Athens is a quaint and quiet college town with 20,000 permanent residents. It's known for its famous Halloween party, which allows the town to show off its vibrant fall colors. Most people cherish the outdoors and spend time cycling the many trails, hiking at Old Man's Cave, and touring the weekly Farmer's Market. Most students spend their free time participating in various medical school organizations. Intramural sports are particularly competitive.

The cost of living in Athens is relatively cheap, with apartments that rent from $200 to $700 per month. Many students with families buy homes when they first arrive and have little problem selling them when they move away for their clinical rotations. Families also appreciate the good schools and low crime rate. The best shopping, however, is found in other towns, including Columbus (70 miles away) or Parkersburg, West Virginia (40 miles away).

The Bottom Line

OU-COM is a great choice for those interested in practicing primary care in the state of Ohio. The school offers students a unique choice of learning environments in both the preclinical and clinical years.

OKLAHOMA STATE UNIVERSITY COLLEGE OF OSTEOPATHIC MEDICINE

Tulsa, Oklahoma

Applications: 2,107
Size of Entering Class: 87
Total Number of Women Students: 117 (34%)
Total Number of Men Students: 231 (66%)
World Wide Web: osu.okstate.edu/osucom.html

Contact: Dr. Daniel Overack, Assistant Dean for Admissions
1111 West 17th Street
Tulsa, OK 74107
918-582-1972

Oklahoma State University College of Osteopathic Medicine (OSU-COM) is one of nineteen osteopathic medical colleges. Since its inception in 1972, OSU-COM has trained more than 1,500 physicians, with representatives in all fields of medicine.

Graduates of OSU-COM earn a D.O. (Doctor of Osteopathic Medicine) degree. A D.O. is a fully licensed physician who chooses to specialize in any field of medicine, from anesthesiology to family medicine to surgery, depending on what postgraduate residency training is pursued. In addition to traditional medical training, D.O.'s are trained in the art of osteopathic manipulative therapy (OMT), a unique hands-on approach to diagnosis and treatment. They use skilled palpation with modern laboratory tests, diagnostic imaging, and complete history and physical exams when arriving at a diagnosis.

OSU-COM also offers a Ph.D. in biomedical sciences and a combined D.O./Ph.D. program.

Admissions/Financial Aid

OSU-COM is a state-supported school, with 84 percent of its students from Oklahoma. With a smaller class size (only eighty-eight students per year), the application process is competitive, especially for out-of-state students. The school processes 1,500 to 2,000 applications per year, with 325 to 375 of those applications from Oklahoma residents. The 1998–99 average MCAT score is 8.8, with an average GPA of 3.54, which are well above the basic requirements. Of the 348 students, 66 percent are men and 34 percent are women. Minority students represent about 20 percent of the total enrollment. The interview process itself is a relaxed and comfortable experience. Prospective students are made to feel welcome during the half-day event. Applicants interview with a faculty member and a community D.O., as well as tour the

facilities and meet various medical students. Tuition is approximately $9,000 for Oklahoma residents and $22,000 for out-of-state students. This is a relatively inexpensive education, especially considering the low cost of living in the Tulsa area. Financial aid through government grants and loans is readily available and easily accessible through the financial aid office.

Preclinical Years

From anatomy to histology to biochemistry, first-year students are inundated with the foundations of medicine. Most classes are held in the mornings, which leaves the afternoons for anatomy, histology, microbiology, and osteopathic clinical skills labs. Teams of three students each work 6 hours per week with a cadaver in the anatomy lab. Actually, most students spend extra hours at night and on weekends in the labs to keep up with assignments.

Students also find that OSU-COM faculty members are willing to spend many extra hours with them in the learning process, most without appointment. For those who just can't wait to get their hands on live patients, a preclinical educational experience is offered. Students are placed with preceptors at the school's teaching hospital and with doctors in the Tulsa community for hands-on training in both the first and second year. In the summer between first and second years, the dean encourages students to take a relaxing break. However, there are many opportunities for work-study, research with faculty, and rural externships.

Faculty members, students, and residents are currently involved in biomedical research on artificial vision, arthritis, reproductive endocrinology, and kidney physiology, as well as studying the efficacy of new drugs for treatment of HIV/AIDS, cardiovascular diseases, and asthma. There is also a summer class in radiology offered. Second year brings even more challenges to the lowly medical student. Pathology, the cornerstone class, nudges students to the next level of learning—integration. In preparation for the clinical years, the curriculum is oriented around problem-solving skills, represented by the 9-hour clinical problem-solving class. Pathology, pharmacology, and clinical skills training are interlaced in a small-group setting. Each group is facilitated by a practicing D.O. Several 1- to 2-hour classes are also required, including health promotion/disease prevention, multicultural health, and medical information sciences. The grading system is A–F for required courses.

OSU-COM students are expected to assist and support each other in learning, which is one of the best aspects of the school. Study groups of two to three students begin to form after the first few weeks of class. Unlike many schools, class attendance is expected and professors hand out detailed class notes. No note groups are needed.

Clinical Years

There are two main clinical options for OSU students: there is training available at Hillcrest Hospital in Oklahoma City or at Tulsa Regional Medical Center in Tulsa. Students may opt to move to the Oklahoma City area for the final two years, except for two months of required training at the school's health care center in Tulsa in the fourth year. Five months of core training are required at either hospital, which consist of two internal medicine rotations, one month of surgery, one month of obstetrics and gynecology, and one month of emergency medicine. Other required rotations reveal the primary-care emphasis of the school and consist of rural family medicine and rural hospital training.

There are eight months of elective rotations, with opportunities in all areas of the United States and beyond. During the core hospital months, students see large volumes of patients, perform and dictate extensive numbers of histories and physical exams, and study for case presentations. Internal medicine at Tulsa Regional provides excellent training and is one of the best osteopathic medicine programs in the nation. Students attend daily morning reports and noon lectures and are given an opportunity to present cases with backup from residents and attendings. Other good training programs include general and thoracic cardiovascular surgery and emergency medicine. The obstetric and pediatric departments are smaller, but experience is also available at other Tulsa hospitals. Most students train with private pediatricians around the Tulsa area.

The American Osteopathic Association (AOA) requires osteopathic physicians to complete one year of general internship training (or the equivalent) following medical school for licensure. After that year, residents may continue on in specialty programs, either osteopathic or allopathic. Osteopathic students have more than twice the opportunities for postgraduate training (allopathic and osteopathic), though there is a different matching process for D.O. and M.D. programs. OSU-COM students are accepted into a wide variety of programs that are generally their first or second choice.

Social Life

Life in Tulsa is fairly low key. A city of 400,000, Tulsa has a wide variety of cultural events, including the symphony, the ballet, and various seasonal and ethnic festivals. Many concerts are held on the banks of the Arkansas River, just a short walk from the school. Students are often seen walking, running, biking, and inline skating on the 5-mile path around the river park. Oklahoma's weather includes all four seasons and is known to change without warning. As the native Will Rogers stated, "If you don't like the weather, just wait a few minutes."

Though many students are nontraditional, students form close social bonds, with various club and class parties. Each August's orientation cookout and December's holiday ball bring all students together for fun. Each spring the faculty members challenge the first- and second-year classes to a game of softball on Lesion Field. Tulsa and the surrounding communities offer excellent schools and programs for children. The cost of living and crime rate are quite low compared to the rest of the country, making Tulsa an ideal place to raise a family. The school does not provide housing, but there are affordable apartments within walking distance.

The Bottom Line

OSU-COM offers a quality education at a reasonable price. Older or nontraditional students need not fear applying. Students who function best in a friendly atmosphere, with supportive faculty members and small class size, will reap the benefits of this medical education. Students considering primary care find that this is the school's greatest strength. As a doctor of osteopathic medicine, students will be members of a select and growing group of physicians dedicated to holistic patient care.

OREGON HEALTH SCIENCES UNIVERSITY SCHOOL OF MEDICINE

Portland, Oregon

Size of Entering Class: 98
Total Number of Women Students: 278 (48%)
Total Number of Men Students: 306 (52%)
World Wide Web: www.ohsu.edu/som

Contact: Dr. Joseph Bloom, Dean
3181 SW Sam Jackson Park Road
Portland, OR 97201-3098

Ask ten people about Portland, Oregon, and you will hear ten radically different answers. Some might mention 11,235-foot Mount Hood, Mount St. Helen's, and Mount Adams, all ever visible on the horizon. Others describe a relaxed quirkiness. Portlanders can ski in the Cascades, windsurf in the Columbia River Gorge, and visit the Pacific Ocean all in the same day. Overlooking the city and the Cascade Mountains is the Oregon Health Sciences University (OHSU).

OHSU, which is ranked second among comprehensive medical schools by *U.S. News & World Report,* is widely honored for its commitment to primary care. Moreover, OHSU's Top-50 research status attracts national and international dollars.

Admissions/Financial Aid

OHSU's student body, which historically consists of more than 90 percent Oregon residents, is slowly changing, with nonresident matriculation rates up to 25 percent. Tuition can't be the draw, as the in-state tuition of $16,800 almost doubles to $32,760 for out-of-state students. Thankfully, the financial aid office placates everyone with loans and scholarships. As Oregon's only medical school, OHSU's selection process is very competitive. More than 2,100 applicants are pared to 400 interviewees, ultimately reaching a 7 percent acceptance rate. Several applicants thus choose to augment their chances through application to the M.D./Ph.D. and M.D./M.P.H. programs. Although active recruitment occurs, cultural diversity remains a weak point at less than 1 percent.

OHSU students are inquisitive, energetic, and people oriented. Currently, the group includes teachers, writers, lawyers, a sailor, and a cabinetmaker. Although mean class age is 25 to 26, more than a handful of students are in their 30s and 40s, leading to a friendly and well-seasoned atmosphere. Students, as a rule, teach, advise, and support each other here.

Preclinical Years

The OHSU theme-based system operates upon an objective-driven curriculum. Professors must give students a list of learning concepts for each lecture. The official party line is that if students master the objectives, they will score at least an 85 percent on the multiple-choice exams. This is probably not true, but using objectives does help focus cram sessions before bimonthly tests. The first and second years consist of lectures, small group discussions, and labs from 8 a.m. until 12 p.m., Monday through Friday, which leaves three afternoons per week free for self-study and other pursuits.

OHSU has an integrated block system through which all students move simultaneously. For example, Gross Anatomy, Imaging and Embryology, winner of Most Outstanding Preclinical Course in the past four to five years, synthesizes anatomy, embryology, radiology, and some physiology. As always, professors determine the class quality, but occasional stand-up comedy and ER clips provide needed relief. Due to the thinly veiled grading system (honors/near honors/satisfactory) and information overload, students also band together for notetaking supergroups.

OHSU's crown jewel is the two-year Principles of Clinical Medicine course (PCM). Each week, it consists of an afternoon of clinical community preceptorships and an afternoon of physical exam education and small-group discussions. Thus, almost from day one, OHSU students are immersed in providing real clinical care. Group topics range from physician-assisted suicide and cultural diversity to managed care. Despite isolated grumbles, students applaud the early clinical exposure. On the other hand, the experience in the small groups depends upon luck, facilitator skill, and group dynamics.

Popular preclinical electives include Literature in Medicine, Reproductive Health, and International Health. The three months that follow the first year are open to pursue research, travel, or relax. At the end of second year, more than 20 percent of students score in the top quartile nationally for USMLE Step I.

Clinical Years

Rubbing elbows with internationally known faculty can be a humbling experience. Luckily, the faculty and housestaff collectively believe in education, scholarship, and most important, student respect. Barring the occasional drill sergeant, scut work is rare. Students write orders, see the gamut of diseases, deliver babies, and debate clinical minutia with staff. Because of large Russian, Southeast Asian, and Latino populations, students discover more cultural diversity among patients than they might otherwise expect.

Following a Transition to Clerkship course, the third year is chock-full of six-week clerkships in internal medicine (six weeks at OHSU or VAMC and six at Providence, Emanuel, or Good Samaritan); Surgery; Ob/Gyn (OHSU or Emanuel); pediatrics (OHSU or Emanuel); psychiatry (OHSU or VAMC); family medicine; and primary care. The primary care clerkship allows students to choose from a plethora of rural Oregon sites and is hailed as a fantastic experience. However, since electives must wait until fourth year, some feel primary-care-overloaded and delayed in exploring specialty careers. Ultimately, clerkship experiences depend upon who is teaching rather than where. OHSU rotations are highly ranked by students for the teaching quality and hands-on patient care. Pediatrics, surgery, and obstetrics/gynecology, though, are more dependent on housestaff attitudes. With characteristic humanity, OHSU frowns upon such unsavory activities as squashing your classmates during rounds.

Neurology, advanced surgery, outpatient pediatrics, a choice of subinternship (surgery, medicine, or pediatrics), subspeciality electives, and a Transition to Residency course flesh out the fourth year. Most students have at least ten weeks for interviewing and personal downtime. In recent years, students have worked around the globe, clerked at other medical schools, and enjoyed a wealth of clinical electives.

Ultimately, medical school should lead to the right residency. More than 85 percent of OHSU students match at one of their top three residency choices.

Social Life

Portland has an average of 37 inches rain per year (usually November to March), but the climate is mild. Mount Hood, with year-round world-class skiing, is within an hour, as are the Oregon Coast's treasures. Portlanders enjoy hiking, cycling, jogging, and boating year-round. The arts scene includes the Oregon Symphony, "First Thursday" art gallery open houses, and musicals at the Civic. Students also frequent the dizzying array of coffeehouses, microbreweries, and bars in the area. Blazers' NBA basketball, minor-league ice hockey, and soccer satisfy sports fans. Popular OHSU events include the Holiday Party, all-Hill ski trip and the Follies, a hilarious show staged by the second-year class that pokes fun at the realities of medical student life.

OHSU's beauty comes at a price. With land at a premium, parking is a true commodity. Since students cannot buy parking permits, the school distributes free TriMet bus/train passes to ease the crunch. But the most preferred solution has been renting among the student slums located on the Hill. The apartments are old, but rents are reasonable. Tolerable-to-very nice one-bedroom apartments rent from $460 to $750 per month, and two-bedroom apartments are available from $500 to $900 per month; be forewarned, however, that with a 10-minute drive to groceries and entertainment, a car is almost a necessity. OHSU's surrounding neighborhoods are idyllic, with negligible crime. Additional housing options are the artsy Southeast neighborhoods, lower income Northeast, yuppie Northwest, and the relative comfort of suburbia in Hillsdale and Beaverton.

OHSU also operates a dormitory on the Hill. The environment would rate an AAA 1 (bare bones yet comfortable). Pin-drop silence typically enshrouds the dorm, but it is a good option for singles. Rent runs around $400.

The Bottom Line

OHSU is a school for those with energy, enthusiasm, and an interest in primary care. Budding cardiologists and surgeons do have a place here, but those with no desire to discuss the subtleties of community medicine and managed care should probably go elsewhere.

PENNSYLVANIA STATE UNIVERSITY MILTON S. HERSHEY MEDICAL CENTER COLLEGE OF MEDICINE

Hershey, Pennsylvania

Tuition 1996–97: $24,550 per year
Size of Entering Class: 110
Total Number of Women Students: 194 (45%)
Total Number of Men Students: 241 (55%)
World Wide Web: www.hmc.psu.edu

Contact: Dr. C. McCollister Evarts, Senior Vice President and Dean
500 University Drive
Hershey, PA 17033-2360

The Pennsylvania State University College of Medicine (PSCOM) is located in Hershey, Pennsylvania, also known as Chocolatetown USA. With the world-famous chocolate factory located only a couple miles away, the smell of sweet chocolate is truly in the air. The Hershey Medical Center is situated in the rolling hills of central Pennsylvania and affords students a uniquely relaxed atmosphere in which to study medicine. With the establishment of the first department of humanities in a college of medicine in 1967, PSCOM emphasizes a humanistic approach to medicine. PSCOM is consistently one of the top primary-care schools in the country. Although the school has a primary-care focus, Hershey Medical Center is the premier trauma center in central Pennsylvania and recently performed the first robotically assisted heart bypass surgery in the U.S. The students are generally easy going and the air of pretentiousness and competition of some private schools is absent at this state institution. Graduates note the friendly and personable atmosphere as one of PSCOM's greatest assets.

Admissions/Financial Aid

Last year 6,894 students applied to PSCOM, 280 of whom were granted interviews, and 110 of whom matriculated. A Second Look program in the spring gives accepted students a chance to revisit PSCOM to help them clarify their decision. Forty-five percent are women and 25 percent are members of minority groups. One of the most attractive aspects of the school is the price. In-state tuition last year was only $17,000, and total expenses were under $30,000. Out-of-state costs begin to approach private school prices, yet 45 percent of students were non-Pennsylvania residents, which is relatively high for a state school. During the admission process, it is claimed that

preference is given to in-state residents but out-of-state residents are also encouraged to apply. On interview day, a prospective student has two to three short individual interviews with faculty members. Free Hershey chocolate is given to everyone, and escorts take students from one interview to another. Pressure interviews are not conducted but interviewers may ask about current topics in medicine, such as managed care, since Hershey Medical Center has recently affiliated with Geisinger HMO. Ninety-one percent of the students receive financial aid. Merit scholarships and grants are not readily offered, but student loans are available to cover the entire cost of school.

Preclinical Years

PSCOM adopted a new integrated curriculum two years ago, which combines the traditional lecture track with the case-based learning track. The option to choose one format upon matriculation is no longer available, and all students participate in the same program. The first year is split into three blocks or trimesters. The first block is anatomy, which is taught by the most dynamic and entertaining lecturer of the first year, who treats everyone like they were his own children and makes the transition to medical school enjoyable. Another bonus is that class doesn't begin until 1 p.m. so the night owls can maintain their routine. The second and third blocks deal with other basic sciences such as physiology, biochemistry, genetics, pharmacology, microbiology, etc. The first year is more lecture based than case based. Tests are all multiple choice, with some additional essays in anatomy. The grading system is pass, high pass, and honors, with the top 20 to 30 percent of the class receiving the higher distinctions. The battle cry for the majority of the class is "P=MD," which dissipates much of the competition among students. The learning atmosphere is very friendly and group oriented. Of the two-week spring break during the first year, one week is spent on a primary-care preceptorship, which is a more "hands-on" shadowing program that integrates everything learned during the first year. After the first year, most of the students begin work on their Medical Student Research (MSR) projects because this is the only free summer in medical school. The MSR is a requirement at PSCOM and gives students an opportunity to pursue research in any field of interest and to interact one-on-one with faculty. Compared to the first year, the second year is a rude awakening into the world of hard work. The second year consists of more case-based learning and less lecture. The biggest complaint of the second year is the lack of formal pharmacology lectures. Neuroanatomy is not taught until the spring of second year. A physician, patient, and society (PP&S) course is taught during both preclinical years and exposes students to nonscience issues of humanities, behavioral science, and similar courses. This course also teaches clinical interviewing and examination skills, which are sharpened during the second year. With the volume of scientific knowledge that is expected of students, the PP&S material is not greeted with open arms.

Clinical Years

The clinical years begin nearly a month after national boards and mark the first opportunity to travel to other hospitals in the Northeast. PSCOM is affiliated with the well-known Cleveland Clinic and provides students with a chance to study in a major urban medical center. Rotations are also possible at York, Reading, and Lehigh, which is popular for its burn unit. The medicine subspecialties, such as dermatology and cardiology, are generally considered some of the strongest at PSCOM. Cardiothoracic surgery is another well-respected field since the first artificial heart and robotic CT surgeries were developed here. Pediatrics is one of the best-organized rotations while ob/gyn is not as popular due to the limited number of deliveries at Hershey and friction between residents and students in the past. Student responsibility is considered adequate and the amount of exposure a student receives is neither exceptional nor disappointing. Third-year rotations can be taken in any order, and two electives are offered, which is helpful. Electives are quite easy to schedule, even at other hospitals. During the fourth year, two months are afforded for personal activities, and another two months are given to conduct research. Match counseling is considered satisfactory and about 85 percent of

students receive one of their top three choices and 91 percent are placed in one of their top four. Future Shock is a residency financial planning seminar that helps graduates ensure that they pay their student loans. Unlike most of medical schools where no one holds your hand to do anything, this program goes out of its way to make sure that graduates have completed all of the necessary forms and are aware of their financial future.

Social Life

Contrary to a recent medical school review, students at PSCOM are very close and socialize a great deal with each other. This is fostered by the rural location of the campus and the proximity of student housing. More than half of the students live on campus, which is 3 minutes from the hospital and classes. Campus housing is not brand new but spacious living rooms and free electricity and water make this an attractive option. Housing is very affordable and parking is cheap since space is easy to find in central Pennsylvania. A car is helpful because public transportation is nonexistent in Hershey. Crime is not an issue. There is a greater chance of injury from a barnyard animal than there is from a mugger. This makes schoolwork the only daily stress and provides a great atmosphere for studying, relaxing, or raising children. The campus Fitness Center is new and is free to all students and provides free weights, Cybex machines, and a full assortment of cardiovascular equipment. On-campus programs include a Halloween party, a Christmas semiformal, and the semiannual CoffeeHouse talent show. The serene setting also has its downsides. Downtown Harrisburg is 20 minutes away and is the only source of nightly entertainment. The bars and clubs of Harrisburg leave a little to be desired for the single thrill seeker. Harrisburg has its share of minor-league sports teams as well as cultural experiences such as museums and theaters. For the true urbanite, a 90-minute trip to Philadelphia, Baltimore, or Washington, D.C., will better satisfy the hunger for entertainment.

The Bottom Line

PSCOM is tough to beat when it comes to getting the most for the money. The educational dollar goes a long way at Hershey and not often will you find a major medical center in such a beautiful and safe area. At the expense of heart-pounding entertainment, PSCOM prepares students to practice medicine anywhere in the world and does it with a smile along the way.

PHILADELPHIA COLLEGE OF OSTEOPATHIC MEDICINE

Philadelphia, Pennsylvania

Total Number of Women Students: 387 (39%)
Total Number of Men Students: 595 (61%)
World Wide Web: www.pcom.edu
Contact: Carol A. Fox, Associate Dean for
Admission and Enrollment Manage

4170 City Avenue
Philadelphia, PA 19131-1694
215-871-6700

The Philadelphia College of Osteopathic Medicine (PCOM) was founded in 1899 in a two-room suite of a downtown office building and has evolved throughout the last 100 years to now occupy a 17-acre state-of-the-art campus on City Avenue in Philadelphia. Students find comfort in the sense of community that exists at PCOM. Even on an applicant's interview day, it is not unusual to meet students who gladly answer questions or provide tips on the best places to live.

PCOM receives more than 5,000 applications per year for 250 spots. Last year, 590 students were interviewed and 249 matriculated. Applicants range in age from 21 to 42 with the majority being 22–25. The class of 2002 is 41 percent female and 20 percent minority. The PCOM family includes single and married students and even students with families. Many have come directly from college, although some are pursuing medicine as a second career.

Preclinical Years

The first two years at PCOM are spent in the classroom, based on an intense trimester system. An optional five-week summer start program to introduce students to some of the core subjects, such as anatomy and biochemistry, is available. The first year begins with anatomy and continues with histology, biochemistry, pathology, pharmacology, and immunology and microbiology. After the first two trimesters, most courses are taught as systems. For example, in the obstetrics/gynecology course, students cover all the relevant physiology, pathology, and pharmacology. This style is a hit with students, many of whom state that it is easier to learn and comprehend subjects when the whole picture is presented at one time. It also agrees with the basic osteopathic tenet to view the body as a whole.

During the first two years, tests are given about every three weeks in each class. Most tests are multiple choice. Throughout the years, the question format has become more case based in an effort to better prepare students for osteopathic board exams (COMLEX) and real-life clinical scenarios. A visit to the Student Council back test file is a good idea before all tests. Back tests are usually photocopied and distributed with scribe notes. The student-run scribe service provides students with a hard copy of scribed lectures from all classes during the first two years. These notes allow students to skip classes such as physiology, a weak class that most students prefer to learn on their own. Classes that students cannot afford to skip include pathology and pulmonary medicine.

During the preclinical years, students gain clinical exposure through Primary Care Skills, a course that teaches basic physical exam techniques and helps students overcome anxieties about examining patients. This class also provides students with a simulated patient session once a term to practice their history and physical exam skills. Osteopathic Principles and Practice is another course that provides hands-on learning and sets PCOM apart from allopathic medical schools. In this class, students learn the basic tenets of osteopathic medicine and principles of osteopathic manipulative medicine, which provide students with another tool to assist patients in returning to and maintaining health.

The two months between the first and second years provide a much-needed break. Some students do clinical externships in rural areas through the National Health Service Corp. Others participate in Bridging the Gaps, a community health internship that offers a stipend for seven weeks of work. This program allows students to serve the Philadelphia community through projects that assist people with AIDS, educate women about breast cancer, or encourage inner city kids to avoid drugs and violence. Other students decide to skip work and spend the summer at the New Jersey shore enjoying some much-needed rest and relaxation.

Clinical Years

Students rotate (in groups selected by lottery) through rural and urban sites in Pennsylvania, New Jersey, and New York. Hospitals include Mercy Fitzgerald, City Ave Hospital, Geisinger Medical Center, St. Francis Hospital, St. Luke's Hospital, Einstein Hospital, and Clarion Osteopathic Hospital. The third year consists of two electives and core rotations in family medicine, osteopathic manipulative medicine, pediatrics, surgery, internal medicine, radiology, and cardiology. Radiology is a favorite; the professor uses high-tech equipment and puppets and sings to illuminate and animate the world of films.

The fourth year includes more time for electives, along with rotations in internal medicine, surgery, ambulatory surgery, emergency medicine, community medicine, urban medicine, and rural medicine. In the urban health-care centers, fourth-year students run the show (with supervision from attendings), seeing patients on their own and getting a feel for what it will be like in just a few short months when they will be interns.

Clinical experiences vary based on a student's motivation and the interns and residents with whom he or she ends up working. For example, doing a July rotation in obstetrics with a first-year resident affords fewer chances to catch babies than later in the year. PCOM's Student Council publishes current third- and fourth-year students' opinions on the various clinical sites in the Rotation Evaluation Guide to help students pick sites that best suit their needs and interests.

Two weeks of vacation are worked into clerkships at the end of December during the third and fourth years. Also, fourth-year students have some time off to study for COMLEX Part II.

Social Life

PCOM has many clubs and sports teams to join during the limited and valuable free time. Clubs include those affiliated with professional organizations, such as the Student Osteopathic Medical Association, Undergraduate American Academy of Osteopathy,

American Medical Student Association, and American Medical Association Medical Student Section. PCOM has clubs that represent many different faiths, including the Christian Medical and Dental Society, the Jewish Physicians' Network, and the Islamic Medical Society. Other clubs include the Science in Medicine, Computers in Medicine, Public Health Club, Sigma Sigma Phi (National Honor and Service Fraternity), and Ballroom Dance. The Student Council is active and well respected by the administration and faculty, with representation on every major committee in the school and on the Board of Trustees. The Student Council sponsors events such as the annual spring dinner dance and the student and faculty performance known as Follies that parody the lives of medical students.

Philadelphia offers a world of entertainment. Students can obtain discounted tickets to many theaters downtown for shows and musicals. The Franklin Institute with the Fels Planetarium, the Art Museum, and the Convention Center are all within a 20-minute drive of City Ave. The night life and restaurant scene provide any cuisine imaginable, from the posh and expensive Bookbinders to Manayunk, an artsy twenty-to-thirty-something hangout. Don't forget the Flyers, Eagles, Phillies, and 76ers. The new Student Activity Center will serve as the new practice site for the 76ers as well as a place for frustrated medical students to sweat their frustration and stress away.

No on-campus housing is available for students. However, the surrounding city and suburbs offer many reasonable options, from rooms to apartments to duplexes. Prices range from $575 to $825 a month. Student Affairs compiles a book with rental options and a list of students who are looking for roommates. Student support systems include tutoring from upperclass students, accessible faculty and administrators, and a psychiatrist.

The Bottom Line

PCOM offers a collegial environment, a diverse student body, and an opportunity to learn osteopathic medicine. This is the place for students interested in primary care or those who have a desire to integrate primary care into specialty medicine. The tuition is competitive for a Philadelphia medical school, and the area offers big-city entertainment options.

PIKEVILLE COLLEGE SCHOOL OF OSTEOPATHIC MEDICINE

Pikeville, Kentucky

Students Receiving Financial Aid: 90%
Applications: 450
Size of Entering Class: 120
Total Number of Women Students: 14 (23%)
Total Number of Men Students: 46 (77%)
World Wide Web: pcsom.pc.edu/

Contact: Stephen M. Payson, Associate Dean for Student Affairs
Sycamore Street
Pikeville, KY 41501
606-432-9640

The country's newest medical school is located in Pikeville, a small town nestled in the Appalachian Mountains of eastern Kentucky. The mission of the Pikeville College School of Osteopathic Medicine (PCSOM), founded in 1997, is to provide medical education that emphasizes primary care and to produce physicians who are committed to serving the patients of the Appalachians. Students are typically from Kentucky and the surrounding states, but there are also several students from the Northeast and Northwest. Most students have had extensive medical work experience and are familiar with osteopathic medicine.

Preclinical Years

PCSOM's student-oriented approach is evident from the first day of classes. Included in the cost of tuition are all required textbooks, memberships to several important professional organizations, a stethoscope, an otoscope, a lab coat, an osteopathic manipulation table, and a new laptop computer.

Passing in all classes is 70 percent, so there is a spirit of completion instead of competition. This is encouraged by a network onto which teachers and students place lecture presentations, notes, study guides, and practice exam questions that may be helpful in learning the material. The network and the Internet can be accessed through plug-ins in classrooms, labs, and the library. A dial-up server is available for off-campus access.

Clinical medicine is emphasized from the start. A bright point in the weekly grind is guest lecturers who present current topics in medicine. A clinical skills class prepares students before biweekly clinical

rotations begin in October of the first year. First-year students perform these rotations in local hospitals and clinics, which emphasize primary care, while second-year students perform clinical rotations with specialists. All classes incorporate case studies and clinical concepts with the applicable didactic material to prepare students for medical practice and the national board exams that are now clinically oriented.

In addition to a traditional first- and second-year curriculum, PCSOM students have an added bonus: Osteopathic Manipulative Medicine. The course director, a highly acclaimed manual medicine practitioner, has arranged the class according to the following osteopathic techniques: muscle energy, functional, strain-counter strain, myofacial, and high velocity, all of which are strategies used to treat musculoskeletal problems. The class helps students remember gross anatomy because it is taught as a clinically oriented functional anatomy course. At first, most students are a bit skeptical, but the results of this kind of treatment can be amazing.

A number of recent construction projects have provided additional facilities. The Armington Science Center's new floor, which features a state-of-the-art lecture hall and laboratory, is dedicated to the medical school's use. Allara Library, Pikeville's college library, was recently renovated and has a growing medical section. The Telemedicine Center and medical library building will soon be completed, which should allow virtual rounds.

Clinical Years

Because PCSOM is new, students have yet to experience the clinical aspects of the curriculum. Students may choose their clinical rotations within one of seven mandatory hub sites: Ashland, Corbin, Hazard, London, and Pikeville/Prestonburg, Kentucky; Norton, Virginia; and Williamson/South Williamson, West Virginia. The rotations are preceptor based and students are assigned to an area physician for the entire one- to three-month rotation. Four months of elective rotations are available and may be performed at areas other than the seven hub sites. The months before both national board examinations are left free for study or participation in preparatory classes.

The Telemedicine Center will be used for real-time videoconferencing with physicians and students on distant rotations. PCSOM students join medical students from the University of Kentucky, who are already participating in this venture.

Social Life

Although Pikeville is a small city, Pike County, in which it is located, is one of the largest counties in Kentucky. The result is that there are a number of restaurants and shopping centers within a 20-minute drive of Pikeville's quiet downtown. The local YMCA is an excellent facility, and medical students receive a discount. Groups of students usually play tennis, basketball, and racquetball or hit the weights at the YMCA. Buying or renting a home is also feasible, and Pikeville is a great community in which to raise a family. Dormitories and apartments are available at reasonable rates ($200–$700 per month).

Coal mining is a major economic factor in the area; as a result, the socioeconomic spectrum is heavy on both ends and somewhat light in the middle. The Cut-Through Project was completed in 1988 and solved a flooding problem in downtown Pikeville by moving the Big Sandy River through a mountain. Now, Pikeville is one of the fastest growing cities in Kentucky. One of the latest developments is a technical school that is under construction just two blocks from PCSOM. Pikeville Methodist Hospital (currently 221 beds) is undertaking the area's largest ever construction project, a new ten-story tower for patient services that will more than double the size of the facility.

The Bottom Line

PCSOM students are groomed for primary care in the rural Appalachian region. Graduates have clinical experience and a strong background in osteopathic principles.

RUSH UNIVERSITY RUSH MEDICAL COLLEGE

Chicago, Illinois

Applications: 5,216
Size of Entering Class: 120
Total Number of Women Students: 215 (44%)
Total Number of Men Students: 279 (56%)
World Wide Web: www.rushu.rush.edu/medcol/

Contact: Jan L. Schmidt, Director of Admissions
600 South Paulina
Chicago, IL 60612-3832
312-942-6913

Named for Benjamin Rush, the father of modern psychiatry and the only physician to sign the Declaration of Independence, Rush Medical College at Rush University is best characterized by it students and graduates, who are extremely interested in clinical medicine. This interest includes but is not limited to primary care. The Rush Medical Center is an 872-bed hospital with 29,000 admissions and 21,000 surgeries performed every year. The type of research carried out at Rush is almost exclusively clinical in nature. For those whose interests lie in finding the biochemical marker for an obscure disease, Rush is probably not the best place. For those who hope to become well-trained clinicians, however, it's a perfect fit.

Preclinical Years

Chicago is a terrific city in which to be a medical student, but the challenge is finding the time to enjoy it. Orientation is a good start. There are enough structured events to get to know your classmates and second-year students and also enough free time to be able to explore the city.

The academic years are divided into quarters. Fall quarter runs from September to Christmas (sixteen weeks). Winter quarter is short and runs from January to mid-March (ten weeks). Spring quarter starts after a week of spring break and runs from the third week of March until the third week of June (fourteen weeks). July and August make up the summer quarter. Lectures and labs generally run from 8 a.m. until 5 p.m. four days per week, and from 8 a.m. until noon one day per week. The transcript service is a big help.

Most official school literature describes a choice between two curriculum tracks (traditional lecture/lab) and alternative (problem based/case based). As of fall 1999, however, the alternative curriculum will no longer be offered. Administrators say the traditional-only curriculum will be modified to incorporate more case-based learning strategies.

The curriculum follows a traditional pattern with anatomy, histology, physiology, biochemistry, immunology, and microbiology in the first year and pathology, pharmacology, and pathophysiology in the second year. Short courses in epidemiology, behavior, and ethics tend to be shuffled back and forth between the first and second years. Historically, students rate gross anatomy and pathology as very strong courses and biochemistry as very weak.

Midterm and final exams come in groups of three or four and are spread out over a week. The exams are almost exclusively multiple choice, with a smattering of extended match questions similar to those being phased out of the USMLE. Grades are honors, pass, and fail, which results in some competition among students striving for honors. Rush students generally perform well above average on the USMLE Step I.

Exposure to clinical medicine is significant in the first two years. Each student is assigned to a primary-care physician in the community and is expected to spend one afternoon a month in that physician's office. Students are free in July and August between first and second year. There are numerous opportunities for funding of health-related projects in the U.S. and abroad. Students who are considering competitive specialties are welcomed by faculty members as student researchers.

One of the school's greatest strengths is its flexibility for students who are experiencing unfortunate academic or personal problems. Students struggling in their first year can choose to split the year, making medical school a five-year process, and those needing time off for health reasons or for maternity/paternity leave are given many flexible options. Those who fail a course are always given a chance to retake exams.

Clinical Years

Students perform clerkships at four different hospitals. Rush Medical Center is the large tertiary-care center where most training takes place. Rush North Shore and Illinois Masonic are smaller community-based hospitals where more primary care takes place. Cook County Hospital (CCH or County), a public hospital, is a jewel of a resource for the Rush medical student. It's not uncommon to be assigned a child with malaria, another with lead poisoning, and several with asthma. The learning curve is steep, and students are given a large degree of responsibility for case management as well as for hands-on procedures such as blood draws and catheter placement (IV and urinary).

Strong rotations include general surgery, internal medicine, psychiatry, and family practice. Obstetrics and gynecology and pediatrics have scored weaker on student evaluations. The trauma elective at Cook County is one that students may never forget, for mostly positive reasons.

The administration encourages students to defer all electives until the fourth year. However, the schedule can be quite flexible, and the administration is usually amenable to making necessary changes. The administration is also quite flexible with vacation and interview time, with the exception of core clerkships.

Formal and informal advising is quite good, and Rush students seem to match well, with the bulk of students matching at one of their top five choices.

Social Life

Homogeneity rules over diversity, with respect to student backgrounds. Ninety-five percent of students are from the Chicago suburbs and have attended either a Big Ten school or a Midwestern liberal arts college. A dozen or so out-of-state students (almost exclusively California and Washington) round out the class. There are, however, a significant number of older students.

Housing is available on campus, and in the safe neighborhood around Rush, two-bedroom apartments usually rent for $800–$900 per month. Rush offers tremendous, well-organized community volunteer projects through the Rush Community Services Initiatives Program, in which a majority of Rush medical students participate. One downside to life at Rush is that there are no sports or workout facilities and students are left to join private gyms in the city, which can be expensive. The only intramural sport at Rush is flag football.

The Bottom Line

Rush is a great opportunity for students who wish to train to become clinical practitioners in a flexible and compassionate environment.

SAINT LOUIS UNIVERSITY SCHOOL OF MEDICINE

St. Louis, Missouri

Tuition 1996–97: $28,500 per year
Students Receiving Financial Aid: 85%
Applications: 4,912
Size of Entering Class: 150
Total Number of Women Students: 274 (40%)
Total Number of Men Students: 408 (60%)

World Wide Web: medschool.slu.edu
Contact: Dr. William C. Mootz, Acting Dean of
Admissions
221 North Grand Boulevard
St. Louis, MO 63103-2097
314-577-8205

St. Louis University (SLU) School of Medicine is the oldest medical school west of the Mississippi and has provided quality medical education for 160 years. The University is affiliated with the Society of Jesus (the Jesuits), a Roman Catholic religious order. This affiliation is evident in SLU's commitment to training physicians who know more than just medical facts and their application and who are also competent in the ethical and psychosocial aspects of the profession. As a result, the School attracts many mature students with varied backgrounds, which often include prior careers. This adds a breadth helpful to those students who came to medical school directly from college.

Preclinical Years

The four-year curriculum has been recently restructured to decrease the amount of time spent in the lecture hall and to provide more problem-based learning. The administration wanted to find a compromise between programs that are entirely problem based and those that are entirely didactic. The curriculum in now divided into three phases. Phase one comprises the first year, phase two consists of the second year, and phase three comprises both the third and fourth years.

Phase one, thirty-seven weeks in length, consists primarily of a series of courses entitled the Fundamentals of Biochemical Sciences. These include human anatomy, cell biology, metabolism, molecular biology and genetics, microbes and host responses, and principles of pharmacology. In addition, there are several smaller courses that cover issues such as ethics, communication skills, biostatistics, health information resources, and electives. Courses are graded honors/pass/fail, but near-honors and weak-pass categories are used for internal purposes (e.g., to enhance letters of recommendation and to identify students in need of

assistance). After the first year, students have a fourteen-week summer break. Some stay at SLU to continue research that was started in elective blocks.

Phase two, which is also thirty-seven weeks in length, is divided into eight organ-based modules. Each module covers normal anatomy and physiology, pathophysiology, disease prevention, and treatment modalities. The eight organ systems include nervous, cardiovascular, respiratory, hematopoietic and lymphoreticular, renal and urinary, endocrine and reproductive, gastrointestinal, and, finally, skin, connective tissue, and musculoskeletal. At the end of the year, an Introduction to Clinical Medicine course provides a symptom-based approach to diagnosis and treatment and a smooth transition into the clinical years.

Thus far, the two classes that have gone through this new curriculum are pleased. The first two years offer a significant amount of free time for self-study, and self-motivated students use this time most effectively. After year two, students have seven weeks before phase three starts. Most choose to take four weeks to study for Step I of the USMLE examination and then three weeks of vacation before beginning the clinical years.

Clinical Years

Phase three consists of eighty-four weeks of clinical training, which are performed over the final two years. The third year is forty-eight weeks long and includes rotations in internal medicine (twelve weeks), surgery (eight weeks), pediatrics (eight weeks), obstetrics and gynecology (six weeks), and psychiatry (six weeks). The remaining eight weeks comprised two of the following four-week rotations: neurology, family medicine, or electives. This allows a student with a strong interest in a particular field to begin to explore that area while still in the third year. Neurology or family medicine is then completed during the fourth year. Again, courses are graded honors/pass/fail.

Additional fourth-year requirements include a subinternship (four weeks) and surgical subspecialties (four weeks). The remaining twenty-eight weeks are comprised of electives, much of which can be taken at other institutions to help with residency selection. There are four weeks of vacation in the third year and twelve in the fourth year.

Some unique and attractive features of the curriculum include a Basic Science Correlation course that runs throughout the third and fourth years and emphasizes recent developments in basic science and application to clinical medicine. In addition, an increasing amount of the clinical training is performed in the outpatient setting and now comprises thirteen of the required forty-eight weeks of the third year. This provides students with close access to attending physicians in both general and subspecialty fields.

Clinical rotations are performed primarily at Saint Louis University Hospital, a tertiary-care hospital that was recently purchased by Tenet Healthcare Corporation. The hospital will continue to be the primary teaching hospital for SLU students and residents, and the impact of the purchase has been minimal, with no major changes planned. Pediatric rotations are located at the connecting Cardinal Glennon Children's Hospital, an incredible learning environment and enjoyable place to work. Inpatient and outpatient psychiatric care is provided at Wohl Memorial Institute, also connected to the hospital. Medicine, surgery, and obstetrics and gynecology rotations are also taken at the nearby (within 2 miles) John Cochran Veterans Affairs Medical Center, St. Mary's Health Center, and Deaconess Hospital.

Occasional rotations are also provided through the Jefferson Barracks Veterans Affairs Hospital, St. John's Mercy Medical Center, and St. Joseph Health Center, which are all within a 20-minute drive of campus. Ambulatory rotations are taken at these various health centers and at numerous private physicians' offices throughout the greater St. Louis area.

Students tend to enjoy pediatrics at Cardinal Glennon Children's Hospital, and pediatrics is one of the stronger residency programs at SLU. In medicine, SLU Hospital offers more rigorous but rewarding rotations. St. Mary's offers obstetrics and gynecology rotators the opportunity to work in the high-risk birthing center for St. Louis, and while all students take some calls there, St. Mary's is a good choice for those interested in obstetrics and gynecology as a career. Future surgeons should note that there is lots of hands-on experience to be had at the Veterans Affairs Hospital and in the trauma portion of the surgery rotation. Anesthesia and otolaryngology are highly ranked by students.

Social Life

St. Louis, a moderately large midwestern city, is a friendly, comfortable, and affordable place to live. A large number of students live in apartment complexes within a 5- to 10-minute drive of the health center. One-bedroom apartments start at $500 per month, and two-bedroom apartments start at $600 per month. Suburban areas 20 to 30 minutes south of the city offer one-bedroom apartments from $350 per month and two-bedroom apartments from $400 per month.

School social events regularly dot the calendar, and St. Louis offers bars and restaurants of all varieties. The city also offers numerous attractions, including the Gateway Arch, St. Louis Zoo, St. Louis Art Museum, Muny Opera House, St. Louis Science Center, St. Louis Forest Park, and Missouri Botanical Garden. Sports enthusiasts enjoy various professional and amateur sporting activities. The St. Louis Cardinals are regular pennant contenders, and the addition of home-run slugger Mark McGwire has increased the level of excitement in St. Louis. Hockey fans attend Blues games, while football fans can trek to Rams games.

Public service opportunities abound. The volunteer student–run health clinic is held each Saturday throughout the year and serves one of the poorest communities in St. Louis. Students take the histories and perform the exams, all under the guidance of an attending physician. Many students are also involved in education of local elementary students through the AIDS Awareness Task Force and the Child Abuse Prevention Programs.

The Bottom Line

SLU provides a balance of excellent practical clinical training and a strong research presence. It is an ideal school for those who want to live in a comfortable midwestern city and learn from dedicated teachers.

SOUTHERN ILLINOIS UNIVERSITY AT CARBONDALE SCHOOL OF MEDICINE

Carbondale, Illinois

Tuition 1996–97: $27,348 per year
Size of Entering Class: 72
World Wide Web: www.siumed.edu/

Contact: Dr. Carl J. Getto, Dean and Provost
Carbondale, IL 62901-6806

Southern Illinois University's small class size and commitment to education make it one of the Midwest's best kept secrets. If students want to be treated as adult learners with an emphasis on effective teaching techniques instead of obscure research lectures, then this is the school for them.

Admissions/Financial Aid

Like many state schools, SIU gives preference to in-state students with the hope that they will eventually practice in the area. This fits well with the School's mission to provide primary care to central and southern Illinois. In fact, the Chicago area is almost considered out of state, although many up-staters have somehow managed to squeeze by the downstate Illinois border patrol. There are even rumors of out-of-state students being accepted by applying early admission.

Preclinical Years

During the first two years students choose between two tracks, the Problem Based Learning Curriculum (PBLC) and the Sequence (lecture-based) Curriculum. Both tracks are pass/fail and structured around organ systems. Recently, the School has created a task force to develop a single curriculum that incorporates aspects of each track. The School is especially known for the PBLC, one of the first in the country. In fact, SIU develops and sells patient cases for PBL programs nationwide. Problem Based Learning students meet in small groups with tutors and work through carefully designed patient problems that permit free inquiry, as in a real clinical situation. Sometimes the patient problem may be presented via actors who have been known to do everything from vomit and collapse to pace the room repeating auditory hallucinations in response to your questions. Many students in the PBLC love being directed by patient problems in their search for information while avoiding a traditional lecture and test schedule.

Sequence students, however, often claim they like the security of being told what they need to know and the motivation that the tests provide. The Sequence lectures are usually well developed, thanks to the School's Department of Medical Education, whose job description is to avoid wasting students' time with useless information. Influenced by large volumes of student feedback, the department strives to design an educational program that teaches what is important in an effective manner. It has not reached perfection yet, but at least it cares.

Both tracks are committed to providing early clinical experiences as much as a half day each week starting from the first day of school. This keeps many students going when the basic science stuff starts taking over their lives and they wonder why they came to medical school in the first place. In addition, clinical reasoning is often taught and evaluated in the form of computerized clinical cases, thanks to a faculty member who is also responsible for putting Netter's Anatomy atlas on CD-ROM. First-year students are often seen listening to heart tones through a stethoscope connected to a computer.

Clinical Years

Both curricula come together for the clinical years, which mimic most other medical schools. Rotations are performed at two large hospitals, just far enough apart that it is almost worth using your car and enduring the 2-minute drive and 20-minute walk to and from the distant student parking lots. Memorial Hospital, which is attached to the medical school, is a newer facility with bright, sunny rooms and halls. The main building of St. John's Hospital is lacking in sunshine, but there are some brand-new additions, including beautiful pediatrics and obstetrics floors where all students do their third-year rotations.

Students have very limited choice in when and where they do their rotations third year. But everyone soon realizes that the order does not make much difference and at least third-year students are guaranteed to have most of their rotations close to home. This is much appreciated for those who do not want to lose nearby support systems during their most difficult year. The exceptions to this rule are family practice, which is done in a rural setting outside of Springfield, and occasionally psychiatry, in which a small number of students are sent to Carbondale for their rotation.

Students take on increasing responsibility as they go through their third-year rotations. Most clerkships are well organized and students like or dislike them based on the students' interest, not on the clerkship design or the way they are treated. In fact, even in surgery, students are usually respected and time is spent learning not doing scut work. Usually there is always one fearfully dreaded elective at every school, and at SIU, obstetrics takes the prize. Perhaps this fear comes from the tales heard about rounding on thirty patients in one hour or the fact that a student call room is missing from the obstetrics floor.

Throughout the third year there is a significant amount of outpatient time, especially during internal medicine, psychiatry, pediatrics, and family practice. Students are assigned mentors in almost all clerkships and usually work with them one day in clinic. As a regional health center, Springfield draws from many neighboring rural towns and farming communities, which influences the specialist patient population.

During the fourth year, there are three 2-week-long required clerkships: neurology, medical humanities, and anesthesia. Aside from those six weeks, the senior year is amazingly flexible. There is plenty of time to escape to distant U.S. sites and Third World countries if a student's heart desires. SIU also has an established relationship with a Chinese medical school and students may spend elective time in China studying acupuncture. Fourth years get 10½ weeks for vacation and residency interviews. While primary care is emphasized, SIU also has strong surgery departments that have been known to convince students to choose specialty careers. Students interested in more competitive residencies have no trouble getting matches if they have the grades and board scores to back them up. In 1998, 60 percent of students received their first choice in the match and 14 percent received their second choice. On average, 26 percent of students choose family practice, 16 percent internal medicine, 9 percent pediatrics, and 12 percent surgery.

Social Life

While SIU seems like a perfect school to many, the location is definitely not for city lovers. The first year is spent in Carbondale at the main SIU undergraduate campus. Although Carbondale has a reputation for out-of-control Halloween parties, many medical students do not have time for such follies. They prefer to spend their free time rock climbing and hiking in the surrounding Shawnee National Forest and other beautiful lakes and parks that surround the campus.

Students who enjoy the beautiful hills of southern Illinois sometimes dread the move to Springfield, which occurs between the first and second years. Altough Springfield is the capital, it is a rural farming town with a landscape more typical of the Midwest—flat farmland. Students still seem to find things to do, including hanging out at pubs, visiting the well-known Thai restaurant on the outskirts of town, playing basketball, singing with the Illinois Symphony Choir, and continuing the tradition of the medical school band. Many students also spend some of their free time volunteering for local shelters.

SIU has a good mix of traditional and nontraditional students with a variety of backgrounds. There are a small number of students in each class who participate in the M.D./J.D. program. Half of the students are married or partnered. Some have families. Housing is about the cheapest anywhere and most students with families choose to buy homes, especially when moving to Springfield. Renting students pay between $250 and $550 for a single apartment, while others live in group houses for $150 to $250 per person.

The Bottom Line

SIU is a small, student-friendly medical school with innovative education techniques and an excellent program in primary care. If students are lucky enough to be from Illinois and enjoy the small-town atmosphere, then this is the school for them.

STANFORD UNIVERSITY SCHOOL OF MEDICINE

Stanford, California

Tuition 1996–97: $27,381 per year
Applications: 7,075
Size of Entering Class: 86
Total Number of Women Students: 373 (45%)
Total Number of Men Students: 449 (55%)

World Wide Web: www.med.stanford.edu/school/
Contact: Admissions Office
Stanford, CA 94305-9991
650-723-6861

Stanford University School of Medicine is a unique school with outstanding opportunities. Stanford adopts a mission common to many of its peer institutions, namely to train leaders in medicine. A flexible curriculum, an entirely pass/fail grading system, the abundance of research opportunities, and support for numerous extracurricular activities combine to encourage, and even compel, the Stanford medical student to seek much more from a medical education than what is learned in the classroom and clinic.

Graduates rarely seek to just practice medicine, but rather are committed to leadership careers in research, policy, or community service.

The heart of Stanford's unique approach to medical education is its flexible curriculum, designed to allow students every opportunity to expand their experiences. While there are requirements for completion of the preclinical and clinical years, students are able to complete these requirements in any order and in any amount of time they choose (within reason). Most students take advantage of this flexibility through the five-year plan, usually by spreading the preclinical requirements over three years, thus making available substantial time to pursue other interests. Other options include spending an extra year during the clinical curriculum, taking a year off, or even spending an extra two or three years pursuing additional degrees.

Research opportunities abound in the medical school and in the main university, in fields from molecular biology to clinical medicine to sociology. The medical center in particular is clearly one of the top few research institutions in the world. Many students serve as teaching assistants for medical school and undergraduate courses. Some pursue experiences in public health, international medicine, or public policy.

Additional course work at the business school, law school, or undergraduate campus is readily avail-

able, and some students obtain second degrees in public health, public policy, or health services research. The chances are that appropriate resources are available for students to explore almost any interest they may develop.

What makes the five-year plan possible is the tuition policy; after paying for the equivalent of four years of full tuition, the fifth year is charged at a nominal rate. In fact, spending five years can often be more economical than spending four years, as many research and teaching positions come with substantial stipends and, more important, up to 50 percent tuition remission. Other key elements of the flexible curriculum include an entirely pass/fail grading system (which allows students to study appropriately but not excessively for classwork), options to place out of preclinical courses by passing a final exam equivalent before the course, and a relatively modest number of total preclinical and clinical requirements. While the majority of students do choose the five-year plan, it is not necessary to enjoy the benefits of the flexible curriculum; many students complete the requirements in the traditional four years but are still able to enjoy significant outside experiences.

Preclinical Years

The preclinical curriculum is a mixed blessing. The courses are generally well structured, well developed, and led by outstanding and often internationally famous professors and certainly provide students with a solid base of fundamental knowledge as they enter the clinics; however, there is no denying that students spend their share of long hours in dark lecture halls at early hours of the morning. Stanford has made significant progress in recent years in complementing its reasonably traditional preclinical structure with different types of educational experiences, most important, by introducing clinical medicine and patient interactions from day one of medical school.

The first year can be difficult at times, with daily course work, such as histology, biochemistry, neuroanatomy, statistics, and immunology, designed to test students' ability to remain awake. Then again, general anatomy, completed in the first quarter, with more than 20 hours of laboratory time per week, will be students' most intensive and rewarding academic experience to date. The second and third years become substantially more interesting, built around yearlong courses in physiology, pathology, and pharmacology, filled in by quick little electives such as emergency room procedures, rural medicine, and medical Spanish (and, for many, golf). By the time boards part I and clinical rotations roll around, students are well prepared.

Clinical Years

Clinical clerkships are centered on four hospitals: Stanford Hospital and Lucille Packard Hospital for Children are the main academic teaching tertiary/quaternary centers adjacent to the medical school, Santa Clara Valley Medical Center is the nearby county hospital for the majority of Silicon Valley, and the Palo Alto Veterans Administration (V.A.) Hospital. Kaiser Permanente is also an affiliated teaching institution. Stanford and Packard are beautiful, well-staffed, and well-supported institutions that provide cutting-edge care to the local communities as well as VIPs flown in from around the world.

The Santa Clara Valley Medical Center is considered to be a model for county hospitals in the quality and depth of care. Both the county and V.A. hospitals within the past one to two years have had brand-new main buildings built, significantly improving the resources available at both institutions (not to mention making them much nicer places to work).

If there is a common criticism of Stanford medical school, it is that the clinical experiences for students are not as intensive as they are in many other medical schools with city and county hospitals, although graduates of Stanford who are in various residency programs consistently report that their clinical training is on par or superior to that of their colleagues from other schools.

The clinical requirements are reasonable and leave plenty of time for away clerkships, clinical research, or even international experiences. Electives are available in any field imaginable and allow

students close contact with world-famous attendings who quickly become mentors and advisers. The required clerkships can be taken in any order and at any time students wish, allowing them, for example, to defer required clerkships in fields in which they are not interested to their last year, leaving them more time for electives in their first clinical year.

For the most part, the environment is supportive and friendly—and students find that most house staff members and attendings want students to learn. While some rotations have written exams, they are for a student's benefit only and cannot be used in evaluations.

Students need to do well in their clerkships, however, as the pass/fail system and the lack of exam scores make written evaluations from rotations a very large part of their residency application.

Social Life

Students' daily lives are centered in Palo Alto, perhaps the model of American suburbia, and the surrounding Silicon Valley, a relatively affluent area with many restaurants, bars, and cultural attractions to keep students busy. Weather permits outdoor recreation year-round.

San Francisco is 45 minutes to the north. Napa Valley, Monterey, and Carmel are all within a 2-hour drive. Lake Tahoe is 4 hours away and offers skiing comparable to Colorado and Utah as well as recreational activities that are particular to Nevada. Tahoe is a frequent weekend destination. Los Angeles and Los Vegas are easily reached by quick and reasonably priced flights.

The Bay Area is one of the most popular areas to live in the country and offers the combination of a comfortable, relaxed, and enjoyable daily life, with an endless list of spectacular diversions for day or weekend trips. With this, however, comes a price; the cost of living is high, rents are comparable to San Francisco or Boston, and a car is a necessity.

The Bottom Line

Students receive an outstanding medical education from a top-ten school and enjoy life tremendously while they are learning. Stanford is the ideal school for students who want to take advantage of the flexible curriculum and the vast resources to make themselves into leaders of medicine.

STATE UNIVERSITY OF NEW YORK AT BUFFALO SCHOOL OF MEDICINE AND BIOMEDICAL SCIENCES

Buffalo, New York

Tuition 1996–97: $22,905 per year
Size of Entering Class: 139
Total Number of Women Students: 357 (47%)
Total Number of Men Students: 409 (53%)
World Wide Web: www.buffalo.edu/

Contact: Dr. John R. Wright, Dean
Capen Hall
Buffalo, NY 14260
716-829-2775

The State University of New York (SUNY) at Buffalo School of Medicine and Biomedical Sciences is unique as a state school with low tuition and excellent resources because its roots are as a private school with a long history, traditions, and strong alumni ties. The original University of Buffalo (UB) was founded as a medical school in 1846 and was incorporated into the SUNY system in the 1960s. It is now part of a large two-campus university of undergraduate, pharmacy, dentistry, law, and many other graduate programs. UB attracts chiefly New York State residents, with perhaps a larger variety of backgrounds than would be found at more financially demanding schools. Admissions preference is given to in-state residents, and, of 3,000 applicants, about 450 are invited for interviews for a first-year class of 135. Tuition is $10,840 for in-state residents and $21,940 for out-of-state residents per year. About 90 percent of students receive some form of financial aid.

The School offers a primary-care focus, but with ample subspecialty and research opportunities. Students definitely feel a primary-care push. Funded partly by a Robert Wood Johnson primary-care initiative grant, the Primary Care Resource Center links students to primary-care experiences. These include summer externships with urban, suburban, or rural physicians. Some lasting bonds between students and preceptors have formed through these programs. Whatever the impetus, slightly more than half of the graduates enter primary-care residencies.

Students interested in subspecialties need to make a greater effort to find similar experiences. The teaching hospitals include mostly tertiary-care experience. Opportunities exist to pursue basic science and laboratory or clinically based investigations, with an annual student research competition. Interested students can apply to the combined accelerated M.D.-Ph.D. program or M.D.-M.P.H. and M.D.-M.B.A. programs.

Preclinical Years

The first year operates on a block system, with each semester divided into three segments, followed by a week of exams. Students like this approach, which starts on a clean template of new material each block. The first semester fires an unimaginable number of facts at students, but this is made more pleasant by a solid, dedicated faculty—one anatomist recently went to medical school to make his classes more clinically relevant. First-year students are introduced to insulin superstar and other superstars of biochemistry by an energetic paradigm-blasting professor. Faculty members are available for one-on-one instruction either in labs or after lecture. Second semester maintains the block system but has less time spent in lecture. Neuroscience in the second semester has excellent integration across anatomy, physiology, and clinical neurology. Clinical exposure begins in the first year, with a Clinical Practice of Medicine course that extends into the second year. Small-group problem-based learning also spans two years and has resulted in decreased lecture time. The library system quickly becomes indispensable, with a large campus library linked by computer and fax to smaller in-hospital libraries. This allows quick access to virtually any journal from any hospital.

The summer between first and second years offers opportunities to do primary-care externships, do research, or travel and play. Second year abandons the block system and offers excellent pharmacology, pathology, and microbiology instructors. More time is spent in the clinical setting as well. The curriculum seems to be in a constant state of evolution, but the good news is that the administration is fairly responsive to student feedback. It may take time, but groans about a course will benefit someone down the line.

The diverse student body is remarkably cohesive. Free time is filled with hanging out in the large modern student lounge, playing on medical school sports teams, and joining a variety of student organizations. The camaraderie formed during the preclinical years carries over to the clinical years, with acquaintances becoming friendships as students take on rotations together.

Clinical Years

One of the School's strengths is its affiliation with eight teaching hospitals. Buffalo General Hospital, Millard Fillmore Hospital, and Children's Hospital of Buffalo have recently merged financially, but current students say this has not impacted their experiences. Erie County Medical Center (ECMC), the Veterans Administration hospital, Roswell Park Cancer Institute, Sisters of Charity, and Mercy Hospital complete a consortium that provides exposure to a broad range of patient groups. Students are educated about managed care, which has a strong presence, while its impact on clerkships is minimized. Resident and attending teaching is generally strong and parallels the quality of each residency. Pediatrics is an especially well-liked third-year clerkship, thanks to excellent generalist and subspecialist teaching staff members. Surgical experiences vary among hospitals, with trauma at ECMC being a particularly sought-after rotation. Family medicine was added in the mid-1990s and is perhaps the most varied experience. Most of the rotation is spent one-on-one in a precepting physician's practice. Experiences are variable in family medicine—it can offer the most individual student responsibility or merely a call-free oasis during third year.

While experiences do vary from hospital to hospital, they are more the same than different. Students are brought together for weekly group

classes. One-week electives, vacations, and an ongoing ethics course are integrated into the third year. The fourth-year emergency medicine elective is a great chance to work on a plethora of patients and learn to suture anything and everything. Fourth year includes time for subinternships, away electives, School-organized trips to China or Hungary, and ample time to schedule residency interviews. When match day finally arrives, students traditionally do well, with 80–90 percent getting one of their top three choices, and two thirds getting their top choice.

Social Life

Buffalo offers four seasons in a moderate-sized affordable city. The metropolitan population is slightly more than a million. Lake Erie, an extensive park system, Niagara Falls, and Canada all offer plenty to do year-round. Winters are cold and there is plenty of snow, but roads are usually in good shape and there are numerous winter activities. Students choose a variety of housing—Victorian apartments in the city, college neighborhoods within walking distance of the campus, or newer condos in the suburbs. Housing is affordable for those looking to buy as well. Those living in the city ought to lock their cars to keep their radios, and the buddy system is a good idea in some areas, but security is available at both the campus and hospitals. Alternatively, nearby suburban Amherst is the safest town in the area, with a population of more than 100,000. Food abounds, with plenty of standard and ethnic restaurants, the real chicken wings, and Wegmans, which is grocery store nirvana. A large student population energizes nightlife that includes jazz, alternative, and college-type bars and coffee shops. The die-hard urbanite would need to drive 2 hours to Toronto to find true urban chic, but others will do just fine. Major-league hockey and football teams and a fun minor-league baseball team are also easily accessible.

The Bottom Line

The School offers private school roots with state school prices in a moderate-size city. It is a great choice for any New York State resident seeking a primary-care emphasis without closing the doors to other opportunities.

STATE UNIVERSITY OF NEW YORK AT STONY BROOK SCHOOL OF MEDICINE, HEALTH SCIENCES CENTER

Stony Brook, New York

Applications: 3,568
Size of Entering Class: 100
Total Number of Women Students: 229 (43%)
Total Number of Men Students: 304 (57%)

World Wide Web: www.uhmc.sunysb.edu/som/
Contact: Norman H. Edelman, Dean
Stony Brook, NY 11794

The State University of New York (SUNY) at Stony Brook is a major academic and tertiary-care center located less than 60 miles from New York City on the beautiful suburban north shore of Long Island. Its focus on academics, research, and patient care provides the perfect environment for a medical education. As part of the University's Health Sciences Center, established in 1972, the School of Medicine is a young, yet evolving, institution that strives to meet the changing needs of the health-care system while providing the best education for its students.

Preclinical Years

The curriculum is a systems-based approach to medicine that allows students to learn the basic sciences in an integrated format. Subjects such as biochemistry, physiology, and histology are organized into single-topic areas or organ systems. By eliminating much of the repetition involved in the individual course format, students learn the material more efficiently. Clinical lectures that build on the basic sciences are also integrated into the lecture series and provide students with an early understanding of the relationship between the basic sciences and clinical medicine.

Since the systems approach presents the basic science information in a more comprehensive fashion, it minimizes the amount of time students must spend in lectures. For instance, during the fall of the first year, most lectures do not start until 10, a.m. and some days, students are done by 2 p.m. Three afternoons a week are spent in anatomy lab, which is certainly one of the best classes at Stony Brook. Like the rest of the faculty, the excellent professors take the extra time needed to ensure that the students keep up with the work. In addition to the traditional medical

curriculum, students take a variety of other courses such as nutrition and Introduction to Human Behavior. Introduction to Clinical Medicine, in which students learn basic interviewing skills and practice physical exam techniques on real patients, also begins during the first year.

The School strives to create a supportive environment, with the emphasis on learning and not grades. A Big-Sib/Little-Sib program pairs all incoming students with second-year students. The second years hand down all their old exams and transcripts, and, most important, words of advice and encouragement to help make the transition to medical school a little easier. A student-run note service transcribes all lectures. The grading system is honors/pass/fail. Nearly all exams are scheduled on Mondays, which leaves students with fewer free weekends. For students in academic difficulty, there are tutors available and professors who offer extra help to ensure that everyone learns the basics.

Students have the summer between the first and second years off. For most, this is the perfect time to relax. For others, there are opportunities to do research, work in physicians' offices, or spend time doing community service.

Clinical Years

In the 1998–99 academic year, Stony Brook made major revisions to the third- and fourth-year schedule. Although some details are still being finalized, the revisions have in general been well received. The new schedule is designed to better prepare students for the evolving demands of today's health-care market, including increased exposure to primary-care and community-based medicine. The required clerkships during the third year are twelve weeks of medicine, eight weeks of surgery, eight weeks of pediatrics, six weeks of family medicine, six weeks of obstetrics and gynecology, four weeks of psychiatry, two weeks of radiology, and two weeks of emergency medicine.

University Hospital and Medical Center is the only tertiary health-care center that serves the 1.3 million residents of Suffolk County. As a result, it offers a diverse patient base, and students are exposed to a wide variety of clinical conditions and experiences. In addition to University Hospital, four affiliates serve as major resources: Winthrop-University Hospital, Nassau County Medical Center, Veterans Affairs Medical Center at Northport, and Brookhaven National Laboratory Clinical Research Center, Medical Department. Students at these far-flung affiliates can often feel isolated from the rest of the class.

At Winthrop-University Hospital, there is more emphasis on learning the basics of managing different medical conditions and less on actually managing individual patients. Nassau County Medical Center provides students with much more hands-on experience, especially in obstetrics and gynecology, with less emphasis on structured learning. At the Veterans Affairs Hospital at Northport, students have many opportunities to practice basic procedures, such as venipuncture, and are given a fair amount of responsibility for patient management. Brookhaven National Laboratory sponsors basic and applied research in which many students, including the M.D./Ph.D.'s, participate.

The fourth year includes a one-month subinternship in medicine, family medicine, pediatrics, or surgery; one month of neurology; one month of a surgery selective; one month of didactic experience in emergency medicine, laboratory medicine, therapeutics, or surgical anatomy; and a two-week outpatient psychiatry experience. Students can spend up to four months of their fourth year off-site doing various electives, and many take the opportunity to work at other institutions or to go abroad. Finally, all students must successfully complete an exercise with standardized patients, designed to evaluate clinical competency at some time during their fourth year. Students have two free months during their fourth year to take time off or to interview for residency programs.

Social Life

SUNY at Stony Brook is perfectly situated in a beautiful area just minutes from Long Island beaches and is still less than an hour from New York City. The University is also home to the Staller Center, Long Island's only arts facility to offer professional music, dance, theater, fine art, and film. For many, Stony Brook offers the best of both worlds.

Because Stony Brook is still a young institution, the administration is receptive to students' ideas and supportive of new student initiatives. These include a wide range of student organizations. The Family Medicine Interest Group organizes National Primary Care Day, a full day of events, which includes hands-on workshops in suturing, splinting, and casting as well as the basics of a pediatrics exam or female annual visit. SUNY at Stony Brook also has active AMA and AMSA chapters, and students frequently travel to national conferences to express the views of their classmates through resolution writing and policy formation. Unfortunately, because Stony Brook is a state-funded school, students must often seek their own sources of funding for such conferences.

The School also sponsors social events for students, including an annual Potluck Dinner and Talent Show and An Evening of Art, when students and faculty can display their creative talents. Panacea, the School's very own a cappella singing group, performs several times a year, with the highlight performances during the holiday season. Intramural sports are also a popular activity, with medical students fielding teams in sports such as soccer, flag football, and basketball.

A wide variety of housing options are available, with most students choosing to live off campus. One-bedroom apartments range from $600 to $900 per month. Those who share an apartment or house may pay between $400 and $600 per month per person. Most students live within a 15-minute drive of the School, while others may choose to live within a 45-minute drive. Public transportation is limited, so access to an automobile is a consideration. At the same time, parking is limited.

The Bottom Line

SUNY at Stony Brook offers an excellent medical education at a very affordable price to New York State residents.

STATE UNIVERSITY OF NEW YORK HEALTH SCIENCE CENTER AT BROOKLYN COLLEGE OF MEDICINE

Brooklyn, New York

Tuition 1996–97: $21,940 per year
Applications: 4,070
Size of Entering Class: 180
Total Number of Women Students: 329 (43%)
Total Number of Men Students: 442 (57%)

World Wide Web: www.hscbklyn.edu/
Contact: Liliana Montano, Director of Admissions
450 Clarkson Avenue
Brooklyn, NY 11203-2098
718-270-2446

The State University of New York Health Science Center at Brooklyn (SUNY HCSB) College of Medicine, formerly known as Downstate, is located in the heart of one of New York City's most multicultural boroughs. As the only academic medical center in Brooklyn and the only public medical school in New York City, the school offers its students the benefits of a well-rounded education, diverse patient population, rich cultural environment, and tuition that is half of most private medical schools.

Preclinical Years

After orientation week, which includes a white coat ceremony and a boat cruise around Manhattan, medical school begins. An exciting new curriculum was initiated with the incoming class of 1998. Prior to that, there were two different tracks—the Problem Based Learning (PBL) Track, consisting of group sessions for eight to ten students, and the Traditional Track, which consisted mainly of lectures and labs. Some of the lectures were excellent and some were worth skipping (thanks to the affordable student-run transcript service). The new curriculum incorporates both tracks, which translates into less emphasis on didactic lectures and formal lab hours and more emphasis on practical applications and small-group learning via case studies. Some students do not like small-group learning and are unhappy with the sessions, but most students enjoy the experience.

The transcript service is still available, as are transcripts from previous years. The first-year schedule is now organized in system-based blocks. A new course, Doctoring Experience, consists of a series of lectures on clinical practice and an afternoon per week with a local physician and allows students hands-on

experience starting the first week of medical school. If students can't get enough classwork, electives are also available. The most popular are Introduction to Emergency Medicine (one afternoon a week at the King's County emergency department, a Level I trauma center) and Introduction to Laboratory Medicine (a weekly lunch hour).

SUNY HSCB's grading system is honors/high pass/pass/fail. Exams consist of multiple-choice and short answers, along with practical exams. The Office of Academic Advancement offers plenty of group and private tutorials for students experiencing academic difficulties.

In the two months between first and second year, the school offers various opportunities, including clinical or basic science research and shadowing a preceptor. Other students choose wisely and take vacations.

The second-year schedule is organized into organ-based blocks that concentrate on the pathology and pathophysiology of a disease. Introduction to Clinical Medicine is also incorporated into each block. The year ends about five weeks before USMLE Step I, which allows plenty of time to prepare. Most students take a board review course that is offered on campus, and most do well, with a more than 90 percent pass rate for the past few years.

Clinical Years

SUNY HCSB is affiliated with several hospitals of all types: county, university-based, and community hospitals. Most affiliates are located all over Brooklyn, with a few in Staten Island and one in Manhattan (Lenox Hill Hospital). In general, students prefer to stay at the home sites—King's County and University

Hospital—where students receive excellent teaching and opportunities for hands-on procedures. By the end of third year, students are experts at blood drawing, IVs, and simple suturing and have been exposed to a wide variety of pathology. The affiliates, on the other hand, tend to emphasize teaching less (with the exception of Staten Island University Hospital) but leave students with more free time and less work. Students from international medical schools and osteopathic schools also rotate in the affiliate sites, occasionally creating competition for procedures.

On top of the clinical work, most rotations require write-ups and presentations as well as end-rotation exams. With the exception of neurology and obstetrics and gynecology, rotations end with multiple-choice USMLE Step II shelf exams. Oral exams are administered in every rotation except pediatrics.

The fourth year is payback for the hard work. Only two rotations are required: a month of subinternship (in medicine, pediatrics, obstetrics and gynecology, psychiatry, surgery, or neurology) and a six-week block of ambulatory care (most sites are in one of the five boroughs, but two lucky students from each block go to Miami). The rest of the year only requires twenty weeks of electives, which leaves about two months of vacation time.

Students tend to match with good residency programs, with about 70 percent getting their top three choices and most staying in the New York City area. Passing the USMLE Step II is not a requirement to graduate, but it is highly recommended.

Social Life

Opportunities abound in the New York City area. Most students travel the 30 minutes by car or subway to Manhattan for the nightlife, since there is not much to do in the neighborhood. Student housing is available, from studios to two-bedroom apartments, with prices ranging from $3,000 to $5,000 per semester. A good number of students opt to live in the beautiful neighborhood of Park Slope (about 15 minutes by car or subway), although rent is much higher.

A number of student organizations offer social events on campus, and there are weekly happy hours every Thursday, monthly coffee houses, an annual semiformal, ski trips, an annual faculty-student softball game, and more. The Student Center offers a well-equipped gym, pool, sauna, hot tub, and ticket office that offers good discounts on plays and Broadway shows. The University is also home to students from other health-related schools, such as nursing, occupational therapy, and physical therapy, as well as other graduate programs.

The Bottom Line

Students at SUNY HCSB obtain a well-rounded education and become well prepared for internship and residency while enjoying all New York City has to offer—all at a tuition half that of most private medical schools.

STATE UNIVERSITY OF NEW YORK HEALTH SCIENCE CENTER AT SYRACUSE COLLEGE OF MEDICINE

Syracuse, New York

Tuition 1996–97: $21,940 per year
Students Receiving Financial Aid: 87%
Applications: 3,222
Size of Entering Class: 150
Total Number of Women Students: 283 (45%)
Total Number of Men Students: 339 (55%)

World Wide Web: www2.ec.hscsyr.edu/
Contact: Ronald W. Wolk, Associate Dean
750 East Adams Street
Syracuse, NY 13210-2334
315-464-4570

State University of New York Health Science Center at Syracuse College of Medicine is known as SUNY HSC at Syracuse for short, and locals are used to calling it simply Upstate Medical Center. SUNY HSC is a state school located in Syracuse, New York. On the upside, this means cheap tuition ($10,840 a year for in-state tuition—almost double that for out-of-state students) and a great value for medical education. On the downside, this means lots of red tape.

Admissions/Financial Aid

Chances for admission to the school are greatly enhanced for state residents. In the class of 2002, 97 percent are state residents and 46 percent are women. There were 2,918 applicants, with 626 being granted interviews and 153 students matriculating. Besides a solid academic background, strong interpersonal and communications skills are important criteria for admission. Students hold degrees ranging from engineering to math to anthropology to history. The average GPA is 3.52, and the average MCAT score is 29 for matriculated students. Students who belong to underrepresented minorities undergo a special admissions process, and they have the option of starting medical school early by taking gross anatomy in the summer.

Financial aid is available for almost anyone who wants it (more than 95 percent of students receive financial aid annually), and students' needs and expectations are generally met.

Preclinical Years

The first semester of first year is rough. Gross anatomy and biochemistry are the two main courses in the first four months. These are complemented by courses in embryology and cell and molecular biology—a course so hated that less than 20 percent of the students attend its lectures. The four courses are jam-packed with thirteen exams in a fifteen-week period. The rest of the year gets better with histology, neuroscience, physiology, genetics, and nutrition. Classes don't end until the first week of June.

Gross anatomy and histology faculty members are the nicest in the school and come in on weekends and invite students to their homes for holiday dinners. Besides courses, the clinical faculty run small demos on how to use the diagnostic equipment (stethoscope, oto-ophthalmoscope, and sphygmomanometer) that each student purchases during the first month on campus.

Between the first and second years, students do all sorts of things. Many students travel around the country or world and just have fun; others pick up a work-study research job on campus. Still others participate in an internal medicine four-week elective designed to give first-year students early exposure to what clinical medicine is all about (and rack up four weeks of elective credits in the process).

Second year starts with what is probably the longest pathology course in the country (September to March, four days a week, 2–4 hours a day). Pathology is taught in such minute detail, as if the students are pathologists in training. Microbiology and immunology and an Introduction to Clinical Medicine course are taught side by side with pathology for the first five months. Students are also given exposure to an actual autopsy and spend one week (1 hour each day) drawing the morning labs with a registered phlebotomist.

The roughest time in medical school comes when pharmacology and pathology overlap for a four- to five-week period. The second year ends with courses in behavioral science and epidemiology. Pharmacology is extremely well taught, with the most up-to-date information and an excellent set of notes. Students survive second year by talking with third-year students and realizing that the grass is much greener on the other side.

A student-run note service system works effectively here and gives absolute transcription of the lecture, usually within three to four days of when the lecture was given. That process can be sped up if an exam is upcoming. Many students also listen to the lecture tapes, which are available for all lectures in the Health Science Center Library.

The grading is done in a fairly new honors/high pass/pass/fail system that is still in the feeling-out phase. Students work together in an attempt to learn the great volume of material being presented. The overall attitude is definitely more cooperation than competition. More than 97 percent of the students pass the USMLE Step I the first time around, and all students must pass Step I by January of their third year.

One additional program for students is the Medical Student Research Program. This program allows students to spend thirty-six weeks in a research setting while in medical school. They spend twelve weeks in between years one and two, twelve weeks at the beginning of third year, and twelve weeks at the end of fourth year working on a research project with a faculty member of their choice (some students have also done research projects at other institutions).

Clinical Years

For the third and fourth years, students are divided among the school's two clinical campuses. About two thirds of the students stay in Syracuse, while the other third go to the Binghamton (New York) Clinical Campus. For the most part, the clerkships are essentially the same. There is also the opportunity to do a Rural Medical Rotation for a total of nine months, during which a student is assigned to a rural site and rotates through a variety of different clerkships/departments in a hospital and outpatient setting. This program is for students interested in rural medicine or for individuals who like to work independently and be challenged in doing so. In addi-

tion, students can also go abroad for parts of their clinical education.

The third-year clerkship schedule is determined by a random lottery system. The core required clerkships are internal medicine (eight weeks inpatient, four weeks outpatient), pediatrics (three weeks inpatient, three weeks outpatient), surgery (six weeks total, three of general surgery), obstetrics/gynecology (two weeks gynecologic surgery, two weeks outpatient, two weeks labor and delivery), family medicine (four weeks), and psychiatry (six weeks). Shorter clerkships are required in radiology, neurosurgery/neurology, ophthalmology, urology, orthopedic surgery, otolaryngology, and anesthesia. The students at the Binghamton Campus spend time throughout the year with a family doctor instead of in the core family medicine clerkship and are also required to complete a geriatric rotation.

The family medicine rotation is commonly known as Family Vacation, and for radiology, all students need is a big mug of coffee to stay awake in those dark rooms. Psychiatry is also one of the easier rotations during the third year. An informal survey revealed that in 1998, the most disliked clerkship of the third year was obstetrics/gynecology. Even residents in the program who were former students say that the third-year rotation was not that great when they were students.

Pediatrics is on the opposite end of the spectrum and is one of the best clerkships. There are many opportunities to learn, and most of the residents let third-year medical students act as interns by taking care of patients, helping write orders, and discussing the patients with the attending.

Fourth-year electives are chosen by a very complicated random lottery system. Some common fourth-year electives include acting internships, EKG reading, dermatology, and emergency medicine. As the only Level 1 trauma center in the region, the University Hospital Emergency Room sees all sorts of interesting cases.

Guidance meetings about residency and match placement start in March of the third year. The deans are always available for consultations and truly do help guide students through this difficult process. In the 1999 graduating class, 55 percent entered a primary-care residency (pediatrics, internal medicine, or family medicine).

Social Life

Syracuse is not a large city and lacks the clubs and nightspots of New York City or Los Angeles. However, Syracuse also lacks the crime and violence of a big city. Medical students often get together with law students from Syracuse University (at least as students they are friends) and sponsor joint functions at a local bar. The students often go to Syracuse University sporting events, take an evening to see a play or drama, go to a concert, or catch a recently released movie on campus for only $2.

A car is usually not needed for transportation until the third year. The train/bus station is less than a 5-minute cab ride, and the airport is only 10 miles away. For those who like to shop, Carousel Mall has more than 125 shops (plans are under way to double its size) and is located only 4 miles from campus.

The four seasons are well represented here. People who don't like snow should consider schools south of here. In the winter, students ski at one of the nearby peaks or travel to Lake Placid, which is only 3½ hours away. In the summer, students jog or in-line skate along Onondaga Lake and enjoy the sun and warm temperatures.

Many students live in on-campus dorm-style apartments for the first year and then move to apartment complexes within a 10-minute walk of the hospital. Rent at these nearby apartments ranges from about $550 per month for a one bedroom to $750 to $850 per month for a two-bedroom apartment. Ample parking is available regardless of where one lives downtown.

The Bottom Line

SUNY Health Science Center at Syracuse is a top-forty hospital in a nice upstate New York setting that has the right balance of city amenities and rural experiences. Students learn to be great doctors and do not go broke in the process—the school offers all of the education at only a fraction of the cost.

TEMPLE UNIVERSITY SCHOOL OF MEDICINE

Philadelphia, Pennsylvania

Size of Entering Class: 189
Total Number of Women Students: 327 (39%)
Total Number of Men Students: 508 (61%)
World Wide Web: www.temple.edu/medschool/
admission.html

Contact: Dr. Audrey Uknis, Assistant Dean for
Graduate Studies
1801 North Broad Street
Philadelphia, PA 19122-6096
215-707-3252

Temple University Medical School has a proud tradition of training excellent clinicians. The curriculum at Temple is traditional, with the first two years of school devoted to the basic medical sciences with classes divided by discipline and the latter two years comprising clinical rotations. Temple's strong commitment to teaching is apparent in professors' and residents' dedication and enthusiasm for teaching students. Temple is located in North Philadelphia, a poverty-stricken area of the city, and has maintained a strong commitment to the underserved population in its neighborhood as well as strong academic and clinical programs. One of Temple's claims to fame is its heart transplant program, which has been the largest in the nation for several years, and, indeed, is part of the reason why Temple can afford to continue its commitment to the community without going into the red. In a city that has seen recent sea-changes in the medical system, Temple remains a strong and steady entity that is not losing sight of its commitment to education and to the community.

Temple offers an M.D.-Ph.D. program, and will be starting an M.D.-M.P.H. program in conjunction with the already existing M.P.H. program on Temple's main campus.

Admissions/Financial Aid

Temple is a state-associated university; as a result, Pennsylvania residents are given priority for admission. However, the remainder of the class is geographically diverse, with many out-of-state students, particularly from California, and even some international students. There is a diversity of ages, ranging from students entering directly after college to those in their mid-forties, with most students in their twenties. Last year, the entering class was composed of 18 percent members of minority groups and 38

percent women. Temple has a Recruitment, Admissions, and Retention Committee to recruit underrepresented students and to provide academic support to students experiencing difficulties. The School makes a strong effort to have all entering students graduate.

Unfortunately, Temple does not offer many individual scholarships. Seventy-seven percent of the student body receives financial aid, and this is mostly in the form of loans. Because Temple is state affiliated, the in-state tuition is less than that for non-Pennsylvania residents. Some School-sponsored scholarship money is occasionally distributed among the top ranks of the student body, cutting their tuition minimally. The average debt of students at graduation is $111,050.

Preclinical Years

Temple's curriculum is traditional in the sense that classes are separated according to discipline, such as biochemistry, anatomy, and physiology, and classes are largely lecture based. However, there is a trend toward increasing small-group, problem-based sessions and interactive computer-based learning in many courses in order to supplement the lectures. Anatomy, which is one of the most popular basic science courses, has no lectures but comprises lab work and interactive small-group sessions. The director of the gross anatomy and neuroanatomy courses is a legend at Temple for his uncanny ability to dissect out the smallest nerve in seconds and elucidate the anatomy. Moreover, his anatomy notes and dissection guide provide students with a thorough yet concise and understandable review of the material, which is indispensable.

The summer between the first and second years is a wonderful time to gain some experience in a field students may be considering or simply to widen their horizons in any manner that the structure of the first two years cannot provide. Many students participate in programs abroad, learn Spanish, or work in public heath, in the ER at Temple, or in basic or clinical research at Temple and elsewhere. One program that is especially popular is Bridging the Gaps, a citywide program in which medical students work with other allied health students in creating and managing primary-care and public health programs for underserved communities.

The second year is much more clinically oriented, with courses like pathology, microbiology, pharmacology, and pathophysiology. Throughout the basic science courses professors make links to clinical medicine, but this is most apparent in the spring pathophysiology course, which is taught by the best of Temple's clinical teachers, who lecture on their specialty. This is the course that most prepares students for the following clinical years.

Clinical skills are introduced gradually to students by way of a course titles Fundamentals of Clinical Care. In the first year, history taking is refined, and students have the opportunity to interview a standardized patient. In the second year, students learn physical diagnosis in small groups in the hospital and then perform a few complete history and physical exams, which are reviewed in detail with the preceptor.

Clinical Years

The most exciting part of medical school begins with the third year, when, despite two hard years of preparation, no one is ever totally ready for the clinical work of medicine. This is where it all comes together, where students put into practice what they have learned, and more often, relearned, in the context of actual patients. Temple University Hospital is an amazing place to learn medicine. Many of the patients at Temple present already in advanced stages of disease, and they are very generous in letting students be part of their care. Temple is buzzing with activity, but attendings and residents alike are generally very concerned about the education of medical students and take out a lot of time to teach students. Despite the initial discomfort at being barraged by questions, they soon learn that students do not forget the material that this method of learning forces them to glean. This is essentially the Socratic method of

teaching with an edge, and students quickly learn to appreciate its benefits or risk becoming very irritable and likely to miss out on what is definitely the best part of their medical education. Students are also kept very busy doing their part to keep the work moving, which entails a lot of scut work. The degree of scut work varies among sites and rotations, but this too is another part of education, where students learn what they can from each task, such as reading chest X rays and obtaining the results. Students are encouraged to hone clinical skills such as blood-drawing and other procedures; there is a lot of hands-on experience.

The degree of teaching, hands-on experience, and scut work varies from site to site and even from team to team, and different students have different wishes of their rotations. The various sites where Temple students rotate are slightly different in this regard and also in terms of their patient population, so most students find their niche. The sites range from Temple University Hospital, which is a tertiary care hospital and a Level 1 trauma center, to community hospitals in Philadelphia, such as Graduate Hospital in Center City and suburban Abington Hospital to hospitals in Reading, Bethlehem, Scranton, Johnstown, and Pittsburgh. Family practice sites range even further to as far as Erie and sites in New Jersey and Maryland. Temple recently opened its own Children's Hospital, which is connected to the main hospital. The attendings on the floors are pediatric hospitalists, generalists who work largely in the hospital setting. Temple Children's does not yet have a residency program, so the attendings are the students' primary teachers.

The third year curriculum is composed of required clerkships in medicine, pediatrics, surgery, ob/gyn, psychiatry, and family practice. The required courses in the fourth year are emergency medicine, neuroscience, and a subinternship in medicine, pediatrics, or surgery, and the remaining seven to nine blocks are electives, two of which may be away from the Temple system, domestic or abroad.

Temple students are well prepared for both primary-care specialties and specialized fields of medicine. Approximately half of the class enters primary-care fields. The Primary Care Institute oversees the medical student primary-care interest groups, facilitating their activities, such as pairing students with primary-care preceptors in the first two years of school. The relatively new Department of

Family and Community Medicine is also very active in expanding educational opportunities in primary care. Temple students normally score above the national average on the boards, and the School's reputation for clinical excellence prepares students well for their future ambitions.

Social Life

The medical school classes, about 180 students each, may not be as cohesive as at some other schools due to the fact that almost all students commute from various areas of the city, but it is a friendly atmosphere. Students do have a driven nature typical of most medical students, but rather than being competitive, they tend to work in groups and help one another with classwork and clinical work. The grading system is honors/high pass/pass/fail for all four years. Many students are involved in the multitude of student-run groups, from specialty interest groups to community service programs, which are especially popular.

Most students live in either Center City Philadelphia or nearby East Falls and Roxborough, a residential section of the city about 10 minutes away. Many students rent houses and apartments together. Housing is reasonably priced in Philadelphia, compared to nearby New York and Washington, D.C.—a one-bedroom apartment can be found for about $400 to $600, and group houses and shared apartments can cut down even further on rent. Parking is available on the streets surrounding Temple, but many students prefer to park in the lots run by the School. These run approximately $50 per month for the regular lot or $100 per month for the 24-hour garage (only available to students during surgery or ob/gyn rotations). So far there are no student discounts on parking, which is a constant source of frustration for students. Many students carpool to cut

expenses. There are also subway stops a few blocks away from either end of campus.

The security department at Temple is excellent. Temple security officers patrol the entire neighborhood, including the subway stops. The few blocks that Temple's health sciences campus occupies are brightly lit and well patrolled; however, the surrounding blocks are not as well lit or as safe, but security officers are available to escort students at any time of night. Security also provides classes on self-defense. The officers even invite students to train with them for the annual 10-mile Broad Street Run, one of Philadelphia's largest races, which passes right by Temple's campus.

Philadelphia has many different neighborhoods that should satisfy most tastes. There are places like Old City, South Street, and Manayunk for nightlife and numerous parks and museums for daytime distractions. Philadelphia is said to be undergoing a restaurant renaissance, with many new restaurants and cafés opening in the past few years. The cultural life of the city is vibrant, with a world-renowned orchestra and art museum, as well as an opera and ballet, a lively jazz scene, art galleries, theaters, and clubs. It is a historic city, with areas like Chestnut Hill that are lined with cobblestone streets and old houses, as well as the historic attractions of Independence Mall and Old City. The College of Physicians in Center City is the home of the Mutter Museum, where students can entertain visitors with exhibits of strange and grotesque medical curiosities. New York and Washington, D.C., are 2 to 3 hours away by car if students need a weekend getaway.

The Bottom Line

If students are interested in obtaining an excellent clinical education, Temple is a superb place to be.

TEXAS A&M UNIVERSITY HEALTH SCIENCE CENTER COLLEGE OF MEDICINE

College Station, Texas

Applications: 251
Size of Entering Class: 64
Total Number of Women Students: 87 (38%)
Total Number of Men Students: 144 (62%)
World Wide Web: hsc.tamu.edu/

Contact: Filomeno Maldanado, Assistant Dean for Student Affairs and Admissions
College Station, TX 77843-1244
409-845-7743

Founded in 1973, Texas A&M University System Health Science Center College of Medicine is largely unknown. While the College of Medicine may suffer from a publicity problem, it still offers a high-quality education. With an incoming class size of sixty-four, professors who know each student by name, and hands-on clinical experience with minimal scut work, Texas A&M's medical school is the state's best-kept secret.

Texas A&M ranks as one of the few medical schools that offers a tremendous amount of one-on-one faculty/student interaction. A&M received 1,420 applications for sixty-four places in the 1998 entering class. Acceptances are tendered on a monthly basis beginning in August and continue until the class is filled. The 1998 entering class consists of 97 percent Texas residents, 58 percent of whom are women and 6 percent of whom are underrepresented minorities. The mean college GPA is 3.70, and the average MCAT score is 9.7 for each subset.

A new Medical Science Scholars Program was recently initiated, in which high school students can be admitted to medical school and may complete both undergraduate and medical degrees in as little as six years. To apply, students must be Texas residents who are either National Merit, National Achievement, or National Hispanic Recognition Scholars.

Preclinical Years

A&M currently runs a conventional didactic format with laboratories. Problem-based learning (PBL) is incorporated in the second-year curriculum, with an introductory internal medicine course being completely PBL. Graded on a traditional A/B/C/F scale, the first two years can be stressful. Fortunately,

courses are not graded on a curve, so classmates are more than willing to help each other. Plans are being developed to phase in a new preclinical curriculum to encompass a systems-based approach. Scheduled to begin in August 2, the new curriculum is slated to be roughly half PBL and half traditional didactics and laboratories.

Particular strengths during the preclinical years are gross anatomy, neuroscience, and microbiology. Professors are so committed to teaching that they often hold extra small-group tutorial sessions. Genetics is the least favorite first-year class, and pathology is the most grueling experience during the first two years.

Students are exposed to patients early on. In the first semester of first year, a pass/fail Introduction to Patients course begins in which students learn to take complete histories from each other and then from volunteer patients with real illnesses. During second semester, a pass/fail Physical Diagnosis course guides students through their first examinations of patients. Students spend a half day once a week in clinics with local physicians during second year. Summer preceptorships in family medicine, internal medicine, and pediatrics are also available.

Humanities in Medicine and Leadership in Medicine courses are required during the first two years. These courses are well received but not taken as seriously because of their pass/fail grading status.

Clinical Years

The strength of the Texas A&M medical school is in the clinical clerkship experience. Students work at Scott and White Hospital (S&W) and the Olin E. Teague Veterans' Center (VA) for the most part, but there are also weeks spent at nearby Darnall U.S. Army Hospital, the Waco VA Hospital, and Driscoll Children's Hospital in Corpus Christi. Grading in each third-year core clerkship is A/B/C/F and is based on faculty/resident evaluations of the student, standardized national board exams and Objective Structured Clinical Examination (OSCE) or oral examinations. In the fourth year, students have the freedom to choose their electives, and the grading is pass/fail.

Before advancing to third year, students must pass USMLE Step I and be certified in Basic Life Support and Advanced Cardiac Life Support through courses provided by the school.

Internal medicine, a twelve-week rotation, is one of the more intense of the core clerkships. Six weeks are spent inpatient at either S&W or the Temple VA. As such, experiences and patient population/case mix vary considerably. S&W is a physician-run managed-care hospital and serves as the foremost tertiary-care center for the central Texas region. With the completion of a new addition to the hospital in 1998, the VA is aesthetically impressive, but services still run at a snail's pace compared to S&W. The remaining six weeks are spent outpatient at the Temple VA or S&W community internal medicine clinic.

Surgery is consistently ranked as one of the best clerkship experiences, and with good reason. While there are a few temperamental residents, surprisingly, there is not one malignant general surgical faculty member. Despite long hours, students generally feel appreciated as integral members of the team. The experience here is very hands on. Four weeks are spent at S&W, four weeks at Temple VA, and then four weeks of surgical electives. In the S&W experience, students may help close skin incisions. At the VA, it is not uncommon to hear about motivated and capable students participating significantly in procedures. During the four-week elective time, students can choose from all of the surgical subspecialties in two-week blocks. Plastic surgery at the VA. Students who endure the professor's parental rantings and perfect the square knot are rewarded with opportunities for minor procedures (under his guidance). The oral examination at the end of the surgery rotation is a huge pimp session, but students survive intact.

The obstetrics/gynecology clerkship is a six-week rotation. The obstetrics component has recently been shifted to 8-hour shifts at S&W, with students staggered throughout the day to maximize delivery opportunities. On average, each student helps deliver at least ten babies and participates in numerous cesarean sections. There are days built in at Darnall Army Hospital, where students also help deliver babies alongside midwives.

Pediatrics, family medicine, and psychiatry are all strong six-week rotations. An option to spend three weeks at Driscoll Children's Hospital in Corpus Christi is a new option in pediatrics this year. In the family medicine rotation, students often complain about the travel requirement; commutes to S&W community clinics can be as long as 50 minutes from the clinics. Psychiatry also requires some commuting to both the Darnall and the Waco VA. Additional clinical experience can be had at the student-run Martha's Clinic for indigent patients.

Like the preclinical curriculum, plans are being drawn up to modify the clinical experience. Internal medicine and surgery are to be combined into a twenty-four-week block called Medical and Surgical Basis of Patient Care, ob/gyn and pediatrics into a twelve-week block called Women's and Children's Health, and family medicine and psychiatry into a twelve-week block called Family and Mental Health.

Even with structural changes forthcoming, the clinical experience remains strong here. With minimum scut work, maximal hands-on training, daily didactic sessions, and a good blend of managed care and government hospital and clinic exposure, students can't ask for a better clinical experience.

Social Life

Texas A&M has a split campus—the first two years are spent in College Station, Texas, and the last two years are spent in Temple, Texas, 70 miles away. Both are safe cities with minimal crime, plenty of parking, and no traffic headaches.

College Station, as its name suggests, is a college town and home to the more than 50,000 A&M undergraduates and graduate students. It's a Southern kind of city in which pick-up trucks often outnumber cars at any given intersection and down-home friendliness oozes everywhere. The cost of living is a bargain, with nice two-bedroom apartments as low as $475 a month. There are ample restaurants. Entertainment is typical for a college town: numerous local bars and a Barnes & Nobles nearby. For students who prefer the outdoors, there are parks, golf courses, and the nearby Bryan and Somerville Lakes. The University draws cultural performances at its Rudder Auditorium, from international ballet companies to popular college music performers (e.g., REM). The George Bush Presidential Library is on A&M's campus. The student athletic center is amazing, equipped with a rock-climbing wall, an indoor track, several indoor and outdoor pools, beach volleyball, and so forth. Intramural sports are big among the medical students, and students consistently field competitive softball, soccer, and basketball teams. The students are generally pretty social, holding annual Cadaver Balls, Chili Cook-Offs, informal parties, and get-togethers.

Temple makes College Station seem like a burgeoning metropolis. A quiet, damp city (students can buy beer at the grocery store but they can't buy wine, and they need a Unicard to purchase alcoholic beverages in the local restaurants), this is the perfect place to raise a family. However, singles may find the lack of stimulation to be depressing. The restaurant selection is extremely limited. The upside to all of this is that students hardly notice the dearth of activities when they are busy with third-year clerkships. Also, housing is dirt cheap. Texas A&M offers apartments on the VA campus (less than 100 yards from the VA hospital) to all of its students, with spacious efficiencies starting as low as $150 per month and two-bedroom apartments renting for $240 per month. As far as social life, parties and baby showers are the norm, and community softball exists. Lake Belton is nearby for water sports. Morgans Point is just outside of Temple and is where people go to stock up on beverages. Singles quickly learn that Austin is just an hour's drive away.

The Bottom Line

With a small class size, Texas A&M offers affordable, top-notch, individualized teaching and extraordinary hands-on clinical training in a variety of clinical settings.

TEXAS TECH UNIVERSITY HEALTH SCIENCES CENTER SCHOOL OF MEDICINE

Lubbock, Texas

Size of Entering Class: 122
World Wide Web: www.ttuhsc.edu
Contact: Barbara Ewalt, Director of Admissions

3601 4th Street
Lubbock, TX 79430-2
806-743-2297

Deep in the heart of west Texas, sitting atop a caprock, lies Lubbock, home of Texas Tech School of Medicine and Buddy Holly. This town breathes red and black, with die-hard loyalty from the citizens of Lubbock to all Tech students. The medical school has seen many positive changes in the last couple of years under the guidance of Dr. David R. Smith, previously the Commissioner of Public Health for Texas. Although Texas Tech is considered a young medical school (25 years old), it has marched forward quickly in both research and clinical medicine, serving 40 of percent Texas. Texas Tech also offers M.D.-Ph.D. and M.D.-M.B.A. programs.

Although the population is approximately 200,000, Lubbock feels like an overgrown small town, with small-town advantages and disadvantages in regard to medical education. Some folks say that the friendliest people in the world live in west Texas. The attitudes of the patients students meet and the faculty and staff certainly support that. Patients often treat medical students as if they've had their M.D. for the last fifteen years. Most professors give out their home phone numbers along with the course syllabus. This makes for a very nonthreatening and noncompetitive environment in which to learn. For example, Dr. Bernell Dalley, Dean of Admissions and Professor of Anatomy, is famous for his three knocks on the podium during the anatomy reviews to emphasize "This item will be on the test."

Preclinical Years

The basic sciences are still taught in the traditional didactic manner for the first two years, but clinical preceptorships and suture clinics have been added to the first-year curriculum. In the preceptorships, students spend one afternoon per week shadowing a primary-care physician.

A three-month summer break follows the first year, and several optional activities are available.

Students may participate in a six-week-long primary-care preceptorship, for which they are reimbursed $500. Tutoring gross anatomy for the physical therapy students in the summer session allows students to earn $30 per hour in the following fall tutoring the medical students. (This is such a great way to make income that one fourth-year student actually took his wife to Rome for ten days on his tutorial earnings alone.)

In the second year, students learn history-taking and physical examination skills; they put this knowledge to use in the second semester with six hospitalized patients. Students appreciate the team-teaching course structure of Pathology II and Introduction to Clinical Medicine. Electives are offered in Spanish, ophthalmology, and anesthesiology—just to name a few—for interested students during the spring semester.

Standardized exams produced by the National Board of Medical Examiners, the same agency that administers the USMLE exams, are used for final exams. Students are ranked for the first time at the end of the two basic science years in quartiles. The top twenty-five students are given their exact rank. Texas Tech students have a 96 percent pass rate when they take the USLME Step I exam for the first time.

Clinical Years

Texas Tech School of Medicine divides students among three geographically distinct clinical campuses for the last two years: El Paso/Juarez (population 1,000,000), Amarillo (population 200,000), and Lubbock. After being accepted by the School, students state their first, second, and third preference for clinical location. They are then assigned a destination prior to the first year. Breaking the students into smaller groups allows for a great deal of hands-on clinical experience since students are not competing with peers to perform procedures. Third year is very structured, but the fourth year allows students three months of time in which to do what they choose—interview for residency spots, do additional rotations around the globe, or take a much-needed vacation. The remainder of fourth year comprises a subinternship in internal medicine, surgery, or pediatrics; two clerkships in family practice, obstetrics/gynecology, psychiatry, or pediatrics; one clerkship in neurology; and four electives.

On the Lubbock campus, clinical experiences are performed at University Medical Center (365 beds). Although all of the rotations are hospital based, ambulatory experiences are strongly emphasized and probably account for 40 percent of the total experience. The family practice rotation is a favorite among students and may be the reason that approximately 25 percent of graduates for the last four years have chosen to pursue family practice residencies. On the downside, neurology has been rated as relatively weak by most of the fourth-year students due to the limited amount of knowledge they feel is gained during that clinical experience.

The El Paso campus is noted for its strong Hispanic influence (many of the medical students become bilingual) and extensive clinical obstetrics experience (students participate in twenty to thirty deliveries during that rotation). Pediatrics is another favorite rotation on this campus, as these particular patients touch students' hearts and minds. Clinical experiences in El Paso occur at Thomason Hospital and William Beaumont Army Hospital (335 beds and 240 beds, respectively). For a rural/border health experience, this is definitely the place to go.

The smallest number of students choose Amarillo. Consequently, students at this campus receive a great deal of individualized attention from attending physicians and residents. Access to many rural physician practices provides a way to gain vast clinical exposure. Three hospitals provide clinical experiences in Amarillo: Baptist/St. Anthony Hospital (379 beds), Northwest Hospital (358 beds), and the VA Hospital (seventy-eight acute beds and 120 nursing home beds).

Eighty-one percent of the 1998 graduating class received their first-, second-, or third-choice residency match.

Social Life

The only downside to Lubbock is the social scene. However, fun can be found. The undergraduate campus has an unbelievable multimillion-dollar recreation center, where students can work out on treadmills or stair machines, in the indoor Olympic-size pool, or in one of the seven or eight aerobics classes offered each day. Intramural sports are very popular with the medical students and enable them to team up with classmates against the law students in the ever-popular Malpractice Bowl. Three wineries are located on the edge of town and are a great place for a first date. Within a 4-hour drive are the ski slopes of New Mexico, and within a 55-minute plane ride is shopping in Dallas.

For married students, especially those with children, Lubbock is a wonderful place to raise a family. All of the restaurants cater to families, and there are several large churches with active social calendars. The cost of living is low, and housing is very affordable, with a three-bedroom, two-bath, two-car-garage home ranging from $65,000 (previously owned) to $135,000 (new). The crime rate is extremely low, and students feel very safe here.

In the spring, the School hosts a Spring Training weekend for students that is filled with golfing, mud football, a real Texas barbecue/picnic, and a live country band. In April, the Texas Tech chapter of the Texas Medical Association hosts the City Lights Charity Ball, a black-tie event. It is an elegant evening of dining and dancing with local physicians and prominent political figures in order to raise several thousand dollars for local children's charities. Finally, at the end of the year, the physiology department hosts a crawfish boil and keg party for the first- and second-year students. The more flamboyant faculty members may even show up at this event.

Summers in western Texas are hot, but the dry climate makes it tolerable. Winters are not harsh, but Lubbock does receive occasional snow. In any case, the unbelievable sunsets definitely make up for the appearance of this flat western setting, which comes complete with tumbleweeds.

The Bottom Line

Texas Tech offers a super medical education with few distractions. The cost of living is low, the climate is good, and the people are friendly.

THOMAS JEFFERSON UNIVERSITY, JEFFERSON MEDICAL COLLEGE

Philadelphia, Pennsylvania

Tuition 1996–97: $26,770 per year
Applications: 9,979
Size of Entering Class: 223
Total Number of Women Students: 331 (37%)
Total Number of Men Students: 570 (63%)
World Wide Web: www.tju.edu

Contact: Dr. Benjamin Bacharach, Associate Dean for Admissions
Eleventh and Walnut Streets
Philadelphia, PA 19107
215-955-6983

Thomas Jefferson Medical College (JMC) was established in 1824 and founded on the unusual philosophy that medical students should be participants, under proper supervision, in the diagnosis and care of patients. JMC (known affectionately as Jeff) continues to foster this philosophy and allows students to have maximum amounts of responsibility during their clinical years. Since its establishment, Thomas Jefferson Medical College has grown to be the largest private medical institution in the country. Thomas Jefferson Medical College is part of Thomas Jefferson University, which runs programs in other allied health fields such as nursing and physical and occupational therapy. This allows for a multidisciplinary teaching experience for on-campus activities and clinical rotations.

Admissions/Financial Aid

Of the several thousand applicants, 1,000 are interviewed, and slightly more than 200 students matriculate each year. The 1998 entering class originated from ninety-six different colleges and universities and from twenty-nine states and Puerto Rico. Twenty-nine percent of the first-year class members are age 25 and above. Fifty percent of the students are women and 6 percent are underrepresented minorities. Last year, more than 17 percent of the freshman class had advanced degrees.

Thomas Jefferson Medical College is a private institution with a total yearly cost of about $40,000, including tuition, books, and living expenses. There have been small increases in tuition each year, which supposedly parallel inflation. There are few scholarships offered by Jefferson itself. Most students finance their education through student and government loans. This past year, students were more satisfied with their financial packages than in previous years. However, overall, financial aid is not Jefferson's strong point.

Preclinical Years

The first two years at Jefferson are dedicated to the teaching and memorization of the basic sciences. The basic core classes during the first and second year are not pass/fail but rather are letter graded. Many people have the notion that this fosters a competitive atmosphere; however, no matter which medical school students attend, there is always a group of competitive medical students. During the first year, the schedules include anatomy and biochemistry for the first semester, followed by histology and physiology during the second. All throughout the first year, students also take Doctors in Health and Illness, which is a course that focuses on the softer side of medicine. This course, with small group meetings, is an occasionally insightful class that allows for a chance to discuss medical, legal, moral, scientific, and social issues faced by physicians.

The first few weeks at Jefferson are scheduled to be light, with gross anatomy lab not beginning until the third or fourth week. This allows for free afternoons and evenings—to explore Philadelphia, to adjust to the shock of being in medical school, to build friendships, or to settle down. By the second semester, students usually have adjusted and fallen into a routine, which essentially continues into the second semester, with histology and physiology. While class time occupies much of the day, there is definitely time to participate in extracurricular activities. At the end of the first year, before the two-month summer vacation, there is a one-month intensive class in neuroscience. During this one month, students are truly entertained and taught by an enthusiastic and exceptional neuroscience faculty led by Dr. Brainard.

The second year at Jefferson starts with microbiology and pharmacology. The two courses are currently not well integrated; however, this is improving. Both courses require significant amounts of memorization. During the first semester, pathology is also scattered throughout. The pathology course presently is only a fairly taught class; however, it has potential. Most students have found that most of pathology is auto-tutorial. The second half of the year is highlighted by Introduction to Clinical Medicine (ICM). This is a course taught exclusively by clinical physicians that brings the first year and a half of medical school into a clinical perspective. It is not only an excellent preparation course for third-year clerkships, but it is also an excellent course for preparation for the boards.

During the second year, students also are required to take a sophomore seminar. These sophomore seminars are held once a week and are an opportunity to explore any aspect of medicine. Seminars cover topics that range from medical Spanish to alternative medicine to literature. Also during second year, there is a physical diagnosis class, in which the students meet with a clinician and learn and execute the various parts of the physical exam. Finally, students' December/January Plans need to be mentioned. This is the three-week period between first and second semester during both the first and second year, when classes such as medical ethics, biostatistics, nutrition, health and public policy, and genetics are taken. All of these courses are pass/fail. This is an extended vacation time for students, with few hours of class time and a zero to minimal workload. It is both an educational and a fun part of the JMC medical education experience.

Clinical Years

Jefferson Medical College is known for the clinical experience that it provides for its students during the third and fourth years. Jefferson has multiple affiliates in varied locations, which allows students to have rural, urban, and community office experiences. The clinical curriculum starts in July, approximately three weeks after the United States Medical Licensing Examination Step I.

During the third year, all students must complete six weeks of family medicine, six weeks of general surgery, twelve weeks of internal medicine, six weeks of pediatrics, six weeks of psychiatry and human behavior, and six weeks of obstetrics/gynecology. During the fourth year, students must complete a six-week combination of anesthesiology, orthopedic surgery, and urology; a six-week combination of neurology/neurosurgery, ophthalmology, and otolaryngology; four weeks of oncology and rehabilitation medicine; four weeks of advanced basic science; four weeks of inpatient subinternship in either internal medicine, general surgery, or pediatrics; six weeks of an outpatient subinternship in either family medicine, internal medicine, pediatrics, or psychiatry and human behavior; and twelve weeks of electives.

Students are exposed to a variety of populations and a variety of physicians, which exposes them to variations in disease as well as medical practice. Jefferson students are given as much responsibility as they feel comfortable undertaking. The teaching residents and attending physicians are, for the most part, excellent. Students who graduate from Jefferson feel competent and confident in beginning their intern year. Last year, more than 50 percent matched with their first choice of hospitals for internship or residency, and 73 percent obtained one of their first three choices.

Social Life

Thomas Jefferson Medical College has a variety of student-run extracurricular activities. The atmosphere at Jefferson is no more competitive than at your average medical school. In fact, with the large student body, there is a niche for everyone, with very successful and friendly group studying. There is a medical specialty society club for every discipline imaginable, along with other community service organizations and cultural organizations. For example, Jeff HOPE is a shelter clinic and health-care project created, managed, and run by students to provide accessible, high-quality, and dignified care to the homeless and medically underserved individuals. More than 90 percent of the student body participates in this amazing organization throughout their four years. Another student-run organization is Jeff MOMS, which pairs students with mothers-to-be to follow during the prenatal, labor, and postnatal experience, which provides the future mother with a support system and at the same time provides the student with a fulfilling and educational experience. Some other clubs include the International Medicine Society, Jeff Amigos, Jeff STATS, Married Students and Significant Others Association, and American Medical Women's Association.

Thomas Jefferson University is located in Center City Philadelphia. There is a lot to do within the cobblestone streets and corners of quaint, historic Philly. Recreational sites include the distal and proximal Irish, the Walnut Street and Forrest theaters, clubs on Delaware Avenue, the Philadelphia Art Museum, the Academy of Music, jazz clubs, and the trails in Fairmount Park for students who enjoy hiking and biking. Philadelphia also has multiple universities

and medical schools that provide an incredible number of resources and activities.

The Bottom Line

Thomas Jefferson Medical College is a prestigious institution that provides a strong and comprehensive medical education. While the basic science curriculum has its glitches, it does provide a good foundation for third and fourth years. The clinical years are strong and speak for themselves. The extracurricular activities are numerous, and JCM is actively involved in the surrounding Philadelphia community. At Jefferson, students are expected to work hard and study for countless hours, however, they are rewarded in the end with an excellent education and foundation for future ambitions.

TOURO UNIVERSITY COLLEGE OF OSTEOPATHIC MEDICINE

San Francisco, California

Size of Entering Class: 76
World Wide Web: www.SFCOM.edu
Contact: Office of Admissions

1210 Scott Street
San Francisco, CA 94115
415-292-0584

Because it is one of the newest osteopathic medical schools in the nation, Touro College of Osteopathic Medicine (TUCOM) is still developing as an institution. One of its greatest strengths is its location. The San Francisco Bay Area is a diverse and growing region that offers the diversity of more than 6 million people, major universities, and, perhaps most important, a tradition of openness to new ideas. It is a fantastic place for a new school.

In summer 1999, the school will move to its permanent campus on Mare Island, a retired naval base in the East Bay. This new campus has housing, a student union, a golf course, a pool, and all the trappings of a traditional college campus. This pioneering spirit is matched by the growing research programs and an innovative osteopathic medical curriculum.

Admissions/Financial Aid

For the 1998–99 school year, there were 2,000 applicants for a class of only seventy-six. The interviews take place in groups of three or four students, which has drawn both positive and negative comments. In general, the interviews are nonthreatening, and there is a great deal of student interaction, which the applicants reportedly enjoy. On the down side, it is more difficult for the faculty members to get to know each student who is applying. The average GPA was 3.4, and the average MCAT score was 27. Having people-oriented extracurricular activities is a big plus on the application. Research experience is also highly recommended.

Because TUCOM is a private school, no preference is shown for in-state applicants. The student body is relatively young and averages about 25 years of age, but a good number of students are older than 30, married, or entering medicine as a second career.

Most students are Californians but more than a quarter of the student body comes from elsewhere.

TUCOM's tuition averages about $24,000 a year. The cost of living is pretty high, especially if students choose to stay in San Francisco (rated the most expensive city in the country) and commute to the new campus. On-campus housing at Mare Island or in nearby Vallejo is much cheaper but prices for most other areas remain high.

Preclinical Years

TUCOM is only a few blocks from the University of California, San Francisco (UCSF), which allows for TUCOM and UCSF to share some of the top professors in the nation. With two years under its belt, TUCOM is making its move to Mare Island/Vallejo, and bringing in faculty members from all of the UC schools. This makes the basic science curriculum quite strong.

The courses are structured as individual subjects. First year includes yearlong classes in biochemistry, anatomy, and physiology. In addition, there is a semester-long course in histology and neuroanatomy in the fall and spring. Clinical correlates are brought in to each of the classes, with varying degrees of success.

Touro University was founded by a Jewish organization; as a result, classes are not held on Jewish holidays and school lets out on Fridays at 4, but this does not preclude the school from keeping students busy every other moment of the year. The school offers maximum lecture time: first-year students can expect to have classes at least 8 hours a day. Attendance, while officially required, is not enforced, and it is left up to the student's discretion which classes to attend. That is, of course, as long as students keep a good grade point average. The school is on the letter grade system (A–F), which the students hate and the faculty members plan to keep. Exams are varied, but expect one every Monday from 8 until 10 a.m. for the first year. First semester is not too bad, especially if students take a number of biology classes as an undergraduate. Second semester is considerably harder as class workload increases and more difficult courses, such as neuroanatomy, are added. The clinical courses in the first year are hit and miss. Physical diagnosis and clinical medicine courses are on track, but the OMM and community health courses have been under review. The biggest complaint: these two move too slowly and do not teach as much as the students want to learn. The problem is being worked on.

Second year is a combination organ system and basic science approach. The curriculum continues with strong and well-taught pharmacology, pathology, and microbiology/immunology courses for half the day, while the other half is clinical systems. This portion of the curriculum is not just a new approach for the school, it is a new approach to medical teaching. Students are introduced to clinical problems, with an emphasis on reviewing basic science information. It results in repetition of major medical concepts from the first year, which makes board review much easier, but there are a number of problems with the system. The most pressing problem is the quality of instruction; the variability between clinicians and lack of continuity between individual sessions make it difficult for students to learn all topics equally well.

Clinical Years

Currently, there are no third- or fourth-year students at TUCOM. The school has scheduled core hospital rotations in San Francisco, the greater Bay Area, Las Vegas, and the New York area. Students who come to TUCOM need to know that the clinical curriculum is still a work in progress.

Social Life

The biggest draw for applicants is the school's location. A 30-minute drive or ferry ride from Mare Island/Vallejo, San Francisco, suits anybody's taste, whether they are looking for a quiet night out or a taste of the lively club scene. There is an amazing variety of restaurants, from dirt cheap to outrageously expensive, from Vietnamese to Basque and everything in between. Dance clubs, Irish pubs, and live music of every kind are available seven nights a week. The museums are world class, the views are incredible, the parks are beautiful, and the beach is a stone's throw away. The winters are never really harsh, so students can plan on enjoying the outdoors twelve months of the year.

If students prefer to stay closer to campus in Vallejo, there is an eighteen-hole golf course located just behind the student lounge, allowing students to play a few holes after classes or a full eighteen on a Saturday morning. Just 10 minutes north of Vallejo is California's famous Wine Country.

Student events include a one-week orientation, Friday basketball throughout the year, and Monday bar nights after weekly exams. Outdoor activities include surfing, touch football, and ultimate Frisbee. The student government and clubs are highly active and are helping to shape the direction of the school.

The Bottom Line

TUCOM is a small, new school with a big ambition to promote osteopathic medicine in California. Students are ambitious and fun loving, and faculty members are focused on building a strong institution. Because the school is only two years old, the clinical curriculum is still being developed.

TUFTS UNIVERSITY SCHOOL OF MEDICINE

Medford, Massachusetts

Size of Entering Class: 168
World Wide Web: www.tufts.edu/med/
Contact: Thomas Slavin, Director of Admissions

Medford, MA 02155
617-636-6571

One of the key benefits of attending Tufts University School of Medicine is its location—Boston, a city rich in medical tradition. The medical School is located in downtown Boston, a short distance from the undergraduate campus in Medford. The School attracts a wide range of students from a variety of geographical and educational backgrounds. Roughly one half of the students are from California, with the rest of the students coming from all states across the country.

Admissions/Financial Aid

The most recent numbers on applicants, interviews, and admissions can be found in the application packet. The interview process is fairly informal, and most people have two interviews, which tend to follow the typical format—tell me more about yourself, your interests, your activities. A few interviewers attempt some tougher questions, but, overall, it is a low-stress experience.

Tufts has the distinction of being one of the more expensive medical schools; students who are on full financial aid graduate with approximately $160,000 of debt. The specifics about financial aid can be found in the application or by calling the financial aid office.

Preclinical Years

The curriculum at Tufts has deviated somewhat from the traditional. There is a good balance between the hard science courses and other medical school classes. There is also an opportunity to enroll in combined M.D./M.P.H., M.D./M.B.A., or M.D./Ph.D. degrees. The School of Nutrition is quite well known, and a nutrition course is offered during the second year.

Most notably, anatomy is not taken until the second semester, which is met with some mixed reviews. Some people like to ease into the other course

work first and tackle anatomy during the second semester, while others expect it to be a rite of passage for starting medical school.

The first two years consist of lectures in the morning and discussion groups and labs in the afternoons. Particular courses of note include pharmacology, anatomy, and epidemiology. Tufts offers a fairly extensive course in hematology during the second year, which students feel is a little excessive. Problem-based learning is utilized during both the first and second years as a way to incorporate more clinically relevant learning with the rest of the curriculum.

One afternoon a week is free. This time is spent in selectives. Selectives are clinical experiences that are arranged so students can see the relevance of their course work before their third and fourth years. Selectives range from shadowing a primary-care physician to gaining exposure to surgery in the operating room. There is a wide range of experiences from which to choose, including some interesting discussion-based sessions. Faculty members also accommodate individual interests and allow people to arrange their own experiences.

The exam structure has changed at Tufts, and exams are now taken in block form, with several tests from different classes taken on the same day, following a systems approach to learning. The grading system for the first two years is pass/fail/honors, which makes for a noncompetitive learning environment.

Clinical Years

One of the main strengths of Tufts is the range and breadth of the clinical years. Approximately ten hospitals are used for the clinical rotations, with the home base at the New England Medical Center, located in downtown Boston. Baystate Medical Center, located in Springfield, is another tertiary-care center through which the students rotate. In addition, students choose to spend their entire third year at Baystate, which allows them to avoid the hassles of choosing rotations through a complicated computer-based ranking system that confuses everyone.

The range of responsibilities depends on the particular rotation and hospital. Certain rotations are more rigorous, and students interested in a particular field may choose these experiences over others. Usually, third-year students are expected to take call, often in house, occasionally until 10 or 11 p.m. Required third-year rotations include surgery, internal medicine, pediatrics, ob/gyn, psychiatry, and a block of elective or vacation time. Fourth year is spent focusing on students' future field of interest, with students participating in subinternships, taking time to do visiting electives at other medical centers, and interviewing for residency. The bulk of this year is spent in electives and completing rotations of particular interest. There are only a few required rotations for fourth year. Fourth year is also an excellent time to travel and become involved in international electives. The schedule is flexible for interviews, and counseling is available through the dean of students or through your advisers. Students do well in the match, with roughly 80–90 percent matching in their top four choices.

Social Life

There actually is time to spend outside the classroom and labs. There are numerous clubs and organizations on campus, and the School is open to new sugges-tions. In addition, there are numerous opportunities for enjoying life in Boston. The medical school is located in the heart of the theater district, and students often receive discount tickets to shows. There are several museums, sporting teams, and outdoor activities to explore. Surprisingly, there is actually time to get to know the city quite well.

Housing prices are expensive, but cheaper neighborhoods can be found. Most areas are accessible by the T (the subway system), and monthly passes can be purchased at Tufts. Students don't need a car until their third year, although some people manage to avoid it entirely. Having a car certainly makes traveling to the outlying community hospitals easy. The dorm, Posner, is located just down the street from the campus, and the housing prices there are somewhat cheaper than elsewhere in Boston. Living in the dorm makes life easy, although some people feel that it is too close to school. Dental and vet students live here as well.

The Bottom Line

Tufts offers a well-rounded education and is particularly appealing to students who want to attend medical school in a large metropolis. Students do well in the match and feel well prepared for their residency training. Boston is a city that is filled with young adults, given the number of colleges and graduate schools in the area, and there are ample activities that benefit a wide range of individual interests.

TULANE UNIVERSITY SCHOOL OF MEDICINE

New Orleans, Louisiana

Size of Entering Class: 150
World Wide Web: www.mcl.tulane.edu/
Contact: Gayle A. Sayas, Administrative Assistant

6823 St Charles Avenue
New Orleans, LA 70118-5669
504-588-5187

Tulane Medical School, located in New Orleans, is a school with a rich history and many traditions. The School is located across the street from Tulane Hospital and Charity Hospital. Charity Hospital is shared with the Louisiana State University Medical School, which is just a few blocks down the street. Students find attendings, residents, and students from both schools at the hospital, and patients are assigned to be "L" or "T," depending on the day they wander into the system. It's a weird system, but it works. Like many things in the Crescent City, some of the quirkiest things are what give it the most charm.

Preclinical Years

Tulane was run in a traditional manner for a long time. There have been two major changes in the last ten years that have attempted to upset this tradition. First, there has been an effort to integrate as much clinical experience into the first two years as possible. Students are now assigned to an attending from the beginning of first year and are taught to do histories and physicals, first on standardized patients and then on real patients. This is integrated into a Foundations of Medicine class that spans the first two years and includes such things as ethics, statistics, ambulance ride-alongs, and volunteer work in community clinics. Overall, the response to this has been generally positive, especially to the activities that students get out of the library. A number of students also hang out in the emergency room to learn basic skills such as suturing and starting IVs. The response to the standardized patient program, however, is varied. Some feel it is too time consuming and are uncomfortable being videotaped, particularly in an artificial doctor-patient setting. Other students enjoy practicing on a fake patient before working on the real thing. Regardless of student opinion, faculty members are so sold on this program that they probably won't be changing much in the future.

The second major break from tradition involves classroom instruction. In the last three years, the preclinical curriculum has changed from discipline-based to organ-systems–based instruction and from weekly exams to daylong exams held once a month. The changes were implemented to keep the curriculum up to date with recent changes in medical education and also to prepare students better for the national boards. Tulane has not been historically above average in passing rates for USMLE Step I, but it is unclear if this system improves scores. Some people like the increased time between tests, but others prefer having more tests that cover less material at one time. It is likely that the new system will continue to be refined over the next few years.

The first two years are mainly for learning a lot of facts and taking a lot of tests. The first year is dominated by anatomy. The personalities of the lab instructors are distinct, and students often form an attachment to one particular person and follow them around from lab to lab. The lab practicals (a fancy word for more tests) inspire cram sessions that fulfill all expectations of what medical school can be. Students are never able to get that smell out of their clothes and hair, so they shouldn't wear anything they can't burn and shouldn't plan any big dates for a few months. Students are required to buy a microscope, but there are lots of good used ones that third years are trying to sell for $1,000 less than a new one.

The second year is more enjoyable for most students, as they have learned the ropes and are quite ready to tackle pathology, pharmacology, and neurosciences. Neurosciences is the only class in which attendance is required, due to the punitive use of surprise quizzes. It is a scary class because it is the only subject that is not taught as a makeup course during the summer and so requires that anyone failing it must actually repeat the whole year. Students will understand this fear when they are asked to examine a slide of a brain that looks like a blizzard on a broken TV set and then are asked to distinguish fourteen different tracts and name the level of the cut.

Nearly every student subscribes to the note service, which pays classmates to tape classes. Old tests have traditionally been available for most classes through the Owl Club—students understand what this is once they have been there, since this was the tried and true (and legal) way of preparing for tests in the old system. It remains to be seen if this system is useful in the new integrated testing format. Students who do poorly on a test receive a note in their mailboxes offering free tutoring and help in that specific subject.

Clinical Years

Third-year students are encouraged to take an increasing amount of responsibility for their patients as the year progresses. At times, this breeds a lot of internal conflict, as students get anxious about exams and want to leave the wards to study. Most residents and attendings are sympathetic and try to balance students' responsibilities with their exam schedule.

The third year is divided in half. The big blocks consist of three months each of internal medicine and surgery, and the little blocks consist of two months each of pediatrics, ob/gyn, and neurology/psychiatry. Students can take big or little blocks first and can choose the order of each discipline within the blocks. Certain rotations may be done at different hospitals, which allows students to tailor their third year to their preferences. For example, general surgery may be done at Charity (for loads of trauma and good letters of recommendation for residency), Alton Oschner Hospital (for a call-free month with lots of teaching), Pineville Hospital (rural but a lot of suturing experience), or Touro (a private hospital where students don't have to steal scrubs).

Fourth year is flexible and allows for interviewing and away rotations. Many students take advantage of the combined M.D. and public health program that costs nothing extra if students complete it during the four years they are in medical school. This is

particularly useful if students are interested in tropical medicine, one of the School's strongest departments. A number of students travel abroad, either as part of standing exchange programs or through their own planning.

Match day is the climax of medical school, and graduation is more of an epilogue. Envelopes are handed out in alphabetical order, the results are read, and, afterward, everyone eats cake and drinks punch or champagne. Tulane students do extremely well in the match, with up to 90 percent getting one of their top three choices. This is due to a reputation for clinical competence and realistic counseling by the deans. Tulane has traditionally been a surgery powerhouse, with a significant number of students entering both general surgery and the subspecialities. In recent years, there has been a shift toward primary care. For last year's match list, visit the School Web site.

Social Life

Tulane's student body is always interesting, with a fair number of students who come from nontraditional backgrounds. The deans are quite student friendly and are always on the lookout for that person whose life experiences may have prepared them for medicine in ways that college life alone could not have.

Life in New Orleans is a unique experience. The city has an endless supply of bars to explore, fine food to sample, and historical sites to visit. Students also find themselves near the top of their friends' to-visit list. Regardless of their classroom experience, students leave with memories of late nights in the Quarter, evading armed robbers on Tchopitoulas Street, and sailing on Lake Ponchartraine.

The Bottom Line

Tulane is a school that is strong in the clinical aspect of medicine and has a lot of resources available to those interested in tropical medicine, research, surgery, or emergency medicine. Students work hard, but the faculty and administration genuinely care about them.

UNIFORMED SERVICES UNIVERSITY OF THE HEALTH SCIENCES F. EDWARD HÉRBERT SCHOOL OF MEDICINE

Bethesda, Maryland

Applications: 3,422
Size of Entering Class: 165
Total Number of Women Students: 227 (29%)
Total Number of Men Students: 563 (71%)
World Wide Web: www.usuhs.mil/

Contact: Janet M. Anastasi, Graduate Program
Coordinator
4301 Jones Bridge Road
Bethesda, MD 20814-4799
301-295-9474

The F. Edward Hérbert School of Medicine at the Uniformed Services University of the Health Sciences is a school with a ridiculously long name and even worse acronym (USUHS). In order to make its name shorter, the School now refers to itself as the Uniformed Services University, or USU for short. USU is the nation's federal health sciences university.

Admissions/Financial Aid

All students at USU are commissioned officers in one of the three branches of the Armed Forces (Army, Navy, or Air Force) or the U.S. Public Health Service and receive a salary. Unfortunately, the Public Health Service has not funded student slots at USU for several years, but that will hopefully change in the near future.

USU is a tuition-free institution.

Matriculating students at USU tend to be older than other medical students across the country. The average age at matriculation is around 26. More than 35 percent of students are married. Women comprise approximately 30 percent of each class. In general, students are happy (a salary tends to do that) and fitness oriented. All students are required to meet the physical fitness and weight standards of their respective service. Despite a traditional letter-grade system, competition among students is scarce. Students at USU understand that they will be working closely with their classmates for many years after medical school.

Preclinical Years

The academic schedule during the first two years is surprisingly lenient. Because of the military's emphasis on family time and the high proportion of married

students within each class, classes are generally finished by 11:30 a.m. on Monday, Wednesday, and Friday. On Tuesday and Thursday, classes usually run until 4 p.m. In typical military fashion, classes start early (7:30 a.m.) every day. The drawback to this lenient schedule is an extended school year. While students' friends at other medical schools are at the beach by mid-May during the first academic year, for USU students, class is extended through the end of June.

The first academic year is dominated by gross anatomy, neuroanatomy, histology, biochemistry, and physiology. Dr. Rosemary Bourke's neuroanatomy class is a particularly well-taught course, and generations of military physicians can only recall a single neuroanatomical structure—the "bing bongs." In addition to the standard first-year courses, several military-specific classes are added to the schedule. Military studies serve as an introduction to military medicine, teaching students the organization and methods of health-care delivery for each. In addition, students learn basic combat medical skills and military applied physiology in preparation for a one-week field training exercise at the conclusion of the first year.

The summer between first and second years is a busy one. In addition to attending the weeklong field training exercise, students must complete a four-week-long summer experience at a destination of choice. This experience is designed to give students an opportunity to get a taste of the real military. Popular destinations include Army Airborne training, tours on Navy ships, and the Air Force's Top Knife program, in which students spend lots of time wearing flight suits and hanging out around jets. Some students choose less adventurous experiences, including research around the USU campus.

As with other medical schools, the second year at USU is far more challenging academically. Before the tan has faded from summer, pathology, microbiology, and, later, pharmacology make students yearn for the sun.

Clinical Years

Clinical exposure is limited in the first two years. Introduction to Clinical Medicine begins in the spring of the first year, and students are taught the fine art of interviewing patients, both real and fake. In the second year, students graduate to physical exams in the fall and full-scale history and physicals in the spring.

The clinical years of medical school are spent at major military medical centers across the country. Third and fourth years are divided into eight 6-week rotations and ten 4-week rotations, respectively. Third-year rotations include internal medicine, ambulatory internal medicine, surgery, surgical subspecialties, pediatrics, psychiatry, family medicine, and obstetrics/gynecology. In the third year, students go out of town for several rotations. Popular out-of-town locations include Tripler Army Medical Center in Honolulu, San Diego Naval Hospital, David Grant Air Force Medical Center near San Francisco, Madigan Army Medical Center near Seattle, and Wilford Hall Air Force Medical Center in San Antonio. Students are reimbursed for expenses such as lodging and travel that are incurred during these rotations. The fourth year offers more flexibility, although there are several mandatory rotations, including emergency medicine, military contingency medicine, and neurology.

Social Life

Located in upscale Bethesda, Maryland, USU is inside the famed beltway surrounding Washington, D.C. The School is on the campus of the National Naval Medical Center. The National Institutes of Health and the National Library of Medicine, a popular hangout for first-year students three days before the due date of the medical history paper, are just across the street from the Naval Hospital.

USU's location inside the beltway has tremendous advantages. It's only a few minutes from two of the largest military medical centers in the world, the National Naval Medical Center and Walter Reed Army Medical Center. The School commonly receives guest lecturers from the National Institutes of Health, the Armed Forces Institute of Pathology, and other world-renowned institutions. Yet the School is only minutes from great restaurants, clubs, museums, and political spectacles. However, all is rosy in Bethesda. The traffic around D.C. has recently been recognized as the second worst in the nation, behind only Los Angeles. There is no student housing, and rent in D.C. is far from affordable, even with a salary. The weather around the nation's capital is sweltering in the summer and cool in the winter, which is much too varied for students from California.

Despite these few drawbacks, life at USU is amazingly good. Students' images of crawling under barbed wire through the mud while studying pathology are quickly shattered as they enter the student lounge area, complete with a pool table, Foosball tables, and stately wooden lockers. In addition to the salary and zero tuition, students are issued just about every book they ever need in medical school. All courses also provide students with detailed lecture notes, which largely supplant the need to read textbooks. Many students claim that the majority of their free books remain in shrink-wrap throughout medical school. Students are also issued their own personal medical equipment, including a stethoscope, otoscope, and sphygmomanometer.

Graduates of USU are obligated to serve on active duty in the military or Public Health Service for seven years. Time spent in postgraduate training (i.e., internship, residency, or fellowship training) does not count toward fulfilling this seven-year obligation. The majority of USU graduates decide to make the military a career. After twenty years of service, military members are eligible for retirement with generous compensation.

The Bottom Line

In summary, the opportunity to attend medical school tuition free while being paid a salary is tremendously appealing. However, students choose to attend USU because of their commitment to serve the nation. Uniformed service members deserve the finest health care available, in any environment and at any time, and it is a tremendous privilege and honor to be their physicians.

UNIVERSITY OF ALABAMA AT BIRMINGHAM SCHOOL OF MEDICINE

Birmingham, Alabama

Tuition 1996–97: $22,722 per year
Applications: 1,984
Size of Entering Class: 165
Total Number of Women Students: 221 (37%)
Total Number of Men Students: 384 (63%)

World Wide Web: www.uab.edu/uasom/
Contact: Dr. William B. Deal, Jr., Interim Dean
UAB Station
Birmingham, AL 35294

In recent years, the University of Alabama School of Medicine (UASOM) has built a reputation for innovative medical training in a superb research environment. The School has consistently been ranked among the leading twenty-five research-oriented medical schools by *U.S. News & World Report*. The kidney transplant program is ranked number one in the world, and the UASOM Department of Medicine is ranked third in total direct dollars of support from the National Institutes of Health (surpassed only by Johns Hopkins and the University of California at San Francisco). An added incentive to attend UASOM is the city of Birmingham, which offers inexpensive living, safety, and an international community in a climate that is hard to surpass.

Preclinical Years

The UASOM preclinical curriculum follows a traditional two-year format. The first two years are primarily spent in basic science courses, with a mixture of lecture and small-group and computer-based learning. Letter grades (A, B, C, and F) are awarded for each course, and all tests are closed book.

The cornerstone of the first year is gross anatomy, which employs case-based teaching in conjunction with weekly lectures and is routinely voted as the best course by the students. Since the switch to the case-based format in 1996, students have scored well above the national average on the anatomy portion of the Step I boards. Other highlights of the first year include a clinical nutrition course (one of few such courses in the nation) and a three-month neuroscience course, both of which are considered very strong by the students.

The second year includes courses in pharmacology, general pathology, microbiology, immunology, and virology and is concluded by a five-month-long course in correlative pathology. The correlative pathology course is engineered to synthesize the material of the first two years and provides a useful review for the Step I boards. The relatively new Introduction to Clinical Medicine course, which continues throughout the first and second years, attempts, somewhat awkwardly, to provide a foundation for physical diagnosis and bedside skills. This course is currently under new management, and students are more positive about its content this year than in previous years.

There is a three-month hiatus between the first and second years. Many students take advantage of this time to pursue research opportunities within the medical center or to study abroad. A favorite with students is the UASOM-sponsored trip to Gambia that occurs yearly during this time.

Clinical Years

Formal clinical training begins in July of the third year, shortly after completion of the Step I boards. Approximately forty students switch permanently to the two branch campuses in Huntsville and Tuscaloosa, while the remainder of the students are based permanently in Birmingham. All students are required to complete rotations in the traditional areas of internal medicine, obstetrics/gynecology, pediatrics, psychiatry/neurology, and surgery and a month each of family medicine and rural medicine.

At the Birmingham campus, students rotate through the University Hospital as well as the Veteran's Hospital, Cooper Green (a county hospital), and the Children's Hospital, all located within walking distance of each other. Opportunities for electives are also available at several community-based hospitals in the Birmingham area. Many of the Birmingham-based students opt to fulfill one or two of the required third-year rotations at a branch campus. Surgery and obstetrics/gynecology are favorites to complete at a branch campus because of increased hands-on exposure and less rigorous schedules.

To complete the rural medicine elective, students have the opportunity to choose from a wide variety of locations throughout the state. For obvious reasons, rural medicine spots on the Gulf Coast of Alabama tend to be favorites with students who elect to complete this rotation during the summer months.

The fourth year is used primarily for elective opportunities, with only four months reserved for required rotations. Many students take the opportunity to study abroad; UASOM has links to elective programs in Switzerland and Germany, and students are encouraged to pursue other international opportunities. Traditionally, UASOM students do extremely well in the residency match process, and in 1999, 65 percent of UASOM students (compared with 50 percent nationally) matched at their first-choice residency program.

The major weakness of UASOM is Volker Hall, the building that houses most of the lecture rooms, student services, and student lounge, which is renowned for its lack of natural light, limited study space, and poor acoustics. However, a $40-million renovation of Volker Hall is scheduled for completion in 2002. Included in the new project are significantly improved student facilities and study space. In addition, the architects in charge of the project have assured the students that the remodeled building will have at least one window.

Like most state schools, the bulk of the UASOM student body is composed of Alabama residents. However, there is more diversity among the students than might be expected. UASOM has shown a strong interest in older students and students who have pursued other careers prior to their interest in medical school. Current students include a former symphony violinist, a former Hollywood screenwriter, former pharmacists, former dentists, and former engineers.

Social Life

Unfortunately for Birmingham, the first image that usually comes to people's minds at mention of the city are the race riots of the 1960s. Birmingham has worked hard to overcome this image, and with the recent opening of the Civil Rights Museum and the leadership of an African-American mayor, many believe that the city has moved beyond its tragic heritage.

Birmingham is an extremely livable city for students. Housing is affordable, traffic (with minor exceptions) is almost unheard of, and the weather invites outdoor activities most of the year. Favorite student hangouts include a coffee shop that is open only when the owner feels like it (which luckily is most days) and a collection of bars, dance clubs, and restaurants within easy walking distance of the medical school. Other student favorites include canoeing at nearby Oak Mountain State Park and weekend runs to the Alabama beaches, which are approximately 5 hours away.

The Bottom Line

The University of Alabama School of Medicine offers a strong academic and research environment in a city that is pleasant and affordable. With the completion of the newly refurbished Volker Hall in the next few years, the University of Alabama School of Medicine promises to continue to build its reputation as a first-rate institution.

UNIVERSITY OF ARIZONA COLLEGE OF MEDICINE

Tucson, Arizona

Tuition 1996–97: $8,434 per year
Applications: 1,097
Size of Entering Class: 100
World Wide Web: www.ahsc.arizona.edu/com. shtlm/

Contact: Dr. Shirley Nickols Fahey, Associate Dean for Admissions
Tucson, AZ 85721
520-626-6214

You can tell the medical school in Arizona is different the very first day of orientation. After a half day at the Arizona Health Sciences Center (AHSC), the whole group of new first years travels an hour away to a retreat site in the desert. Here students spend the next couple of days getting to know new classmates, all about beginning medical school, and what to wear to gross anatomy (a T-shirt you are not too fond of and scrub pants). Also introduced in the first days of medical school is Arizona's dedication to training primary-care physicians, community service, and maintaining a diverse student body.

Admissions/Financial Aid

Unfortunately for those people who don't have residency in Arizona or aren't from a Montana or Wyoming program, there is no need to even send an application to this school. This is strictly a state school and applicants from other states are not even considered. However, if students are from Arizona, they would be missing a great opportunity by not applying.

When students mail their application materials, they can rest assured that the Admissions Committee is not going to look solely at their grade in organic chemistry and their MCAT scores. The committee is interested also in volunteer work, what extracurricular activities students have been involved with, and students' lives before applying to medical school. The age of incoming students ranges from 21 to 51; many have pursued other careers and have other graduate degrees. Minority students make up a growing part of each incoming class as the school continues to strive to represent the population of Arizona.

If applicants choose to interview at the University of Arizona, they have an information session about the school at the beginning and then

receive a list of the interviews they will be having that day. Applicants not only have three interviews with different physicians in the hospital (usually at opposite ends of the hospital), but they also are scheduled to see a physician in the community. Speaking to so many people allows applicants to learn as much as they can about the program and also lets the school take a good look at them from some different angles.

Tuition is not as much as a private school but is still a hardship to most people. The financial aid office is dedicated to getting enough money for everyone. There are many state and medical school scholarships and loans available to supplement government funding. The staff is always accessible and very helpful, especially with shortages in the middle of the semester.

Preclinical Years

The first two years at Arizona are in a lecture format, with small-group supplementation. There is a midterm/final system, with a big block of exams about every ten weeks. The grading system is pass/fail/ honors, with any score above 90 percent earning honors. There is usually no grade curve, which tends to foster a sense of cooperation among classmates to try to get everybody into the honors range. One of the downfalls of the organization of the first two years is the small amount of time off students receive. First years start in July and generally only receive five to six weeks off between the two years. They then get another four to five weeks off to study for boards, but after boards students jump directly into third-year rotations with only three days off.

First-year courses include the usual anatomy, biochemistry, physiology, neuroscience, histology, and genetics. Almost all of these first-year courses are well taught, with anatomy being the standout and physiology and genetics often being weak. Norm, one of the anatomy instructors, is so dedicated to teaching anatomy that he has turned his body into a living cadaver. He is able to isolate and flex any muscle on his body. He also holds review sessions every week in lab to go over new material. Neuroscience is another good one. Not only did Dr. Nolte write the book that you use for the course, but he also has designed an interactive computer program (Hunting the Wild Asparagyrus) to teach neuroanatomy structure and function.

The second year includes pathology, microbiology, and pharmacology. All of these courses are good, especially pathology, a yearlong course. The entire department is dedicated to having students excel on the pathology section of the USMLE. There are not only the usual lecture, lab, and slides but also regular reviews during the course and before boards and the threat of an oral exam at the end of each ten-week unit. During this exam, students are given three specimens and must answer questions posed by the professor.

Throughout the entire two years, students take Social and Behavioral Sciences (SBS) and Preparation for Clinical Medicine (PCM). SBS introduces you to all the touchy-feely aspects of being a doctor with a combination of lectures, small groups, and visits to different sites. It is team taught by the Department of Psychiatry and of Family and Community Medicine.

PCM allows students to start learning clinical medicine as soon as they start medical school. They begin first semester learning history taking in a small-group setting, which is taught by attending physicians, and physical exam in groups of four, which is taught by fourth-year medical students in the PCM Clinic, a group of fully equipped exam rooms in the medical school that are designed for teaching. Also in the first year, students begin learning directed exams with the Patient-Instructors (PI), laypeople trained to be patients. Each PI has medical problem that is presented to students in the way a patient might present in the clinic. Students are then evaluated on their examination and diagnosis skills. Clinical training continues in the second year with physician precep-tors. Students typically spend an afternoon a week with their preceptor seeing patients.

Clinical Years

The clinical years at Arizona are split into the required rotations of the third year and the electives of the

fourth year. Because the University of Arizona is the only medical school in the state, students are able to rotate through almost any of the big hospitals in Tucson or Phoenix. About one third of students choose to do their entire third and fourth year in Phoenix, keeping in touch at the Phoenix satellite campus.

Medical students are given a large amount of responsibility on their rotations and are often expected to function as interns. With this responsibility comes the chance to get a lot of clinical experience and not as much scut work as students might expect. In Tucson, the main hospitals are the University Medical Center (UMC), the VA, and the Tucson Medical Center (TMC), a private hospital. These are all busy hospitals but students tend to get to do more at the VA and have to go through a few more layers at the other two. Because students rotate through so many hospitals, they are sure to see a wide variety of patients with many different problems.

Arizona places a high priority on primary care, and this is apparent in the required rotations. There is a required family practice rotation as well as a month of clinics incorporated into the medicine rotation. There is also a required rural rotation, to be done in either the third or the fourth year. In the fourth year, there are currently no requirements except to complete at least eighteen weeks of clinical rotations and eighteen weeks of rotations that are directly supervised by Arizona faculty members, a total of thirty-six weeks overall. The rest of the time is free for interviews, travel, vacation, or anything else students want to do before the grind of internship.

Although there is no scheduled counseling for interviews and the match, each student meets with the Dean of Students before the application season. About half of Arizona graduates choose to stay in the state, and the other half scatters around the country, with the majority staying in the West. About 80 percent get one of their top three choices.

Social Life

Tucson is a medium-size town with a lot of old West history. What most people love about the city is all there is to do outdoors and the temperate climate.

Students can mountain bike, hike, rock climb, and play outside pretty much year-round. Tuscon is also a college town, so there are enough nighttime places to appeal to everyone, especially downtown and on Fourth Avenue. There is also more culture than one would expect because of the influence of those affiliated with the University. It is easy and not too expensive to find a place to live in Tucson, either in the cheaper places close to the campus or further away for those with families.

The Bottom Line

If applicants are Arizona residents and are looking for a solid medical school that does not cost and arm and a leg, this is the place for them. Faculty members are caring, and the education is exceptional. Students who graduate from Arizona often remember the school for the surprisingly nurturing atmosphere they found and the high-quality medical education they received throughout their four years.

UNIVERSITY OF ARKANSAS FOR MEDICAL SCIENCES COLLEGE OF MEDICINE

Little Rock, Arizona

Tuition 1996–97: $17,006 per year
Size of Entering Class: 150
Total Number of Women Students: 246 (35%)
Total Number of Men Students: 448 (65%)
World Wide Web: www.uams.edu

Contact: Tom South, Director of Student
Admissions
4301 West Markham
Little Rock, AR 72205-7199
501-686-5354

The University of Arkansas for Medical Medical Sciences (UAMS) is Arkansas's only institution dedicated solely to graduate medical education. As such, it is instrumental in the education and training of many of the state's physicians and other health-care professionals. More than 50 percent of the College of Medicine's graduates eventually practice in the state after finishing their postgraduate training.

From the moment they take the Medical Student Oath and the Dean places their first white coat around their shoulders during the White Coat Ceremony at the end of Freshman Orientation, students of the UAMS College of Medicine are considered members of the medical profession. During the next four years, these students share experiences unique to medical training. They develop a sense of community and commitment to each other and form friendships that carry them through their professional careers.

Admissions/Financial Aid

Getting into UAMS varies in difficulty yearly. The College of Medicine is required to have a class of 150 each fall at registration; therefore, competitiveness varies depending on the pool of applicants. By state law, UAMS must limit the number of students with out-of-state residency status it accepts into each class. Of the 150 students admitted each year, usually about 140 are Arkansas residents, and most of the others also claim strong ties to the state.

All Arkansas residents who apply to UAMS are invited to visit the campus on one of several Saturdays designated as interview days. Nonresidents may or may not receive this invitation. Aside from being interviewed by two faculty members (usually one

preclinical and one clinical), applicants get the opportunity to ask current medical students questions during student-guided tours and receive some helpful information about school policies and financial aid.

Relative to medical institutions nationwide, UAMS offers one of the lower costs for attendance. Financial aid is a must for most students and is relatively easy to obtain. Aside from loans, the school offers a number of partial scholarships and has a strong community match program. In this program, an individual agrees to practice in a certain community in exchange for the community financing his or her medical education.

Preclinical Years

UAMS continues to have a fairly traditional curriculum, with the majority of the first two years devoted to the basic sciences. Lectures (but not labs) are rarely mandatory, and some students find that they learn better on their own. For one course a term, classes can, and usually do, pay someone to take notes, which other members of the class can buy. Grades during these years are determined using a traditional letter-grade scale. While there are gunners (students who will do anything to get an A) in each class, most students learn the 'I used to be a straight A student' attitude and the benefits of group studying very quickly.

Freshman year is dedicated to the normal structure and function of the human body—anatomy, physiology, genetics, and biochemistry. Gross anatomy is consistently a favorite of students, especially since the opening in 1996 of a new state-of-the-art laboratory with computers for every other bench, or every eight students. There is a three-month vacation between the first and second years, during which many students participate in a rural preceptorship program that allows them to work with primary-care physicians around the state and gain some hands-on experience. Other students spend the time doing research, working and saving a little money, or just enjoying their time away from the books. During second year, the curriculum turns to the study of the nature and function of disease states—pathology, microbiology, behavioral science, and pharmacology. There is much less lab time during this year, and students find they spend a lot more time in the library and in study groups.

To provide some patient interaction during the first two years, in 1997 the administration started an Introduction to Clinical Medicine course, which runs throughout the freshman and sophomore years. This course gives students the opportunity to practice interviewing skills and physical examinations on both standardized (actors trained to play patients with specific illnesses) and actual patients. There is about an eight-week break between the second and third years, but it is not necessarily vacation time. All students are required to take Step 1 of the USMLE before they start their junior year, and this is traditionally when they take it.

Clinical Years

Third year begins in early July, marking the close of seemingly endless days of classes and labs, weekly tests, and late-night studying. During their third year, all students rotate through required clerkships (family practice, geriatrics, internal medicine, neurology, obstetrics/gynecology, pediatrics, psychiatry, surgery, and surgical subspecialties) on a lottery basis. Most of these rotations occur at the University Hospital of Arkansas, the Veterans Administration Hospitals in Little Rock and North Little Rock, Arkansas Children's Hospital, and the Area Health Education Centers (AHECs) around the state. Grades are still given on the standard letter scale, but they have a large subjective component.

Surgery and obstetrics/gynecology are well-known for their long and early hours and generally have a reputation of having less understanding and more demanding supervisors. However, most students enjoy learning and practicing suturing and delivering babies. Students also enjoy their month of family medicine. Many do this rotation at an AHEC outside

of Little Rock, which gives them a break from the university setting and the opportunity to experience a more community-based practice. In 1998, UAMS established a required geriatrics rotation. Because this rotation was disliked by many members of the first class to complete it, faculty members are working actively to improve the clerkship. It does, however, provide students with exposure to palliative care, nursing home visits, and the transitional care unit setting, which have not been a part of the traditional medical school curriculum.

Senior year marks the end of required clerkships. Students are also allowed to choose selectives to fulfill the requirements of spending four weeks in primary care and four weeks as an acting intern. The rest of the year is open for students to schedule electives of their choice—some students even spend some time in Africa or Australia. The best part is that all clerkships are now pass/fail. There are also four extra weeks built into the year, which some students take as vacation to interview for residencies and others use to study for Step II of the USMLE. The school has a required senior course the month before graduation, which deals with business and ethical issues. It also allows members of the senior class to obtain ACLS certification and to spend some time back together as a group.

Dean Richard Wheeler and his staff are a great help with the logistics of applying for residency and are always willing to discuss career choices with students. The number of graduates choosing residencies in primary care has continually risen in recent years, but many still choose specialty fields.

Social Life

Medical school certainly demands a lot of time and energy, but students still find time to take a break from the books and wards. Little Rock is the capital and largest city in Arkansas, which makes it the ideal site for much of the entertainment and culture in the state. Symphony orchestra concerts, Arkansas Travelers baseball games, touring Broadway productions, Razorback football (at a student discount price), and national concert tours are only a few of the possibilities. There are also a number of school-sponsored activities, from dances such as Cadaver Ball and Skit Dance to intramural football and class picnics to nights at the comedy club and movies. The annual Volunteer Fair sponsored by the College of Medicine offers a different type of study distraction, and many students take advantage of this opportunity to get involved in the community. While housing is available for both single and married students in the dorm on campus at very inexpensive prices, most students prefer to spend a little more and rent an apartment or house nearby. Rates are fairly reasonable, and a variety of housing is available.

Little Rock has a reputation of being a violent city when compared per capita to other cities in the nation. None of the hospitals where students receive the majority of their training is located in a very safe neighborhood. However, the security staff is good (except, of course, when they are writing parking tickets in the middle of the day), and students rarely feel uncomfortable on campus.

The Bottom Line

UAMS offers a wonderful medical education for residents of the state of Arkansas, but admission for out-of-state residents is extremely difficult. The curriculum remains fairly traditional, but it does offer some patient contact during all four years and is integrating much more computer-based education into the first two. The students whose names appear on Senior Wall testify to the wonderful education they received at UAMS and to the many opportunities they have had since then.

UNIVERSITY OF CALIFORNIA, DAVIS, SCHOOL OF MEDICINE

Davis, California

Tuition 1996–97: $9,384 per year
Students Receiving Financial Aid: 80%
Applications: 5,401
Size of Entering Class: 93
Total Number of Women Students: 176 (42%)
Total Number of Men Students: 239 (58%)

World Wide Web: www-med.ucdavis.edu/
Contact: Edward D. Dagang, Director of
Admissions
Davis, CA 95616
530-752-2717

Founded in 1968, University of California, Davis (UCD) School of Medicine has been overshadowed by its older sisters, particularly University of California, San Francisco, and University of California, Los Angeles. But it offers affordable education that has been ranked as high as second in *U.S. News & World Report*'s comprehensive category. Davis, where the main undergraduate campus and most medical school teaching and research facilities are located, offers escape from the congestion and cost of living in the Bay Area and southern California.

UCD matriculates 93 medical students per year. In 1998, 49 percent of these students were women. The initial pool of more than 4,000 applicants is reduced to approximately 700 to be interviewed by a formula combining GPA and MCAT scores. The average age of entering students is approximately 25, with some older than 35. Interviews consist of one faculty and one student interview, and both carry equal weight with the admissions committee. UCD has a tradition of actively recruiting minority students, and this philosophy will likely continue despite policy changes from the UC administration. Minority applicants are generally interviewed by minority students.

First-year students volunteer their couches for applicants visiting Davis to interview. Staying with them saves money and provides an excellent chance to get the inside scoop on the School.

The majority of students come from the University of California (UC) undergraduate system, particularly Los Angeles, Davis, Berkeley, and San Diego. Many applicants have participated in unique experiences such as Peace Corps service, work experi-

ence in another profession, or obtaining advanced degrees (such as the M.P.H. and Ph.D.). Although all matriculating students call themselves California residents, a small but significant number are not; rather, they moved to California (or at least got a California P.O. Box) a year or so before applying.

California resident tuition at UCD is approximately $9,900 per year (nonresident tuition is more than $19,000). Combined with the area's reasonable (by California standards) cost of living, UCD School of Medicine is certainly the least expensive California medical school to attend and probably one of the ten cheapest schools to attend in the country. Approximately 85 percent of students receive financial aid, and the average indebtedness of 1998 graduates was $58,000. A long list of scholarships and grants is distributed by the financial aid office, although most have specific requirements regarding career plans, ethnicity, gender, religion, parental occupation, and level of destitution. All students with financial need are able to get adequate aid through grants and deferrable loans (e.g., Perkins), and many take out nondeferrable loans such as HEAL.

Preclinical Years

The curriculum at UCD is fairly typical in overall structure: two years of basic science followed by two years of clinical rotations. The curriculum may be spread in various ways over five years in order to accommodate research or personal needs (such as pregnancy); this option is growing in popularity (15–25 percent of students participate).

During the first two years, courses are quite structured, with a tremendous amount of in-class time. Most courses, especially during the second year, mix didactic and problem- and case-based teaching approaches. Computers are integrated into the several courses with case simulations and photo files. Half-day-per-week clinical experiences (preceptorships) begin in the first quarter and continue through second year. Student-run "free" clinics offer additional clinical opportunities.

Pathology is generally regarded as the most controversial and grueling basic science course. It trains students on the level of pathology residents. Some students love it and some hate it. Other courses vary in quality, from exceptional to adequate. Fortunately, students are elected to the curriculum committee, and their input is taken seriously.

USMLE Step I exam scores have always been very good, with several students scoring above the 90th percentile. The average score is 220, and the pass rate has been 100 percent for the last three years.

Combined degree programs are available. The M.D./Ph.D. program currently offers two competitive fellowships per year but may be expanded. Still under development is an M.D./M.H.A. dual-degree program. Coordination with other advanced degrees is possible with M.S., M.A., M.B.A., and M.P.H. (with UC Berkeley School of Public Health) programs.

Clinical Years

The medical school location, adjacent to one of the nation's best veterinary medical schools and teaching hospitals, enhances research and teaching. The main teaching hospital, the 485-bed UCD Medical Center, is located 15–20 minutes east of Davis in the rapidly growing state capital, Sacramento. It was ranked among the nation's top hospitals in seven specialties by *U.S. News & World Report*'s 1998 "America's Best Hospitals" and houses a high-volume trauma center. Other teaching institutions include Kaiser Hospitals, Sutter Hospitals, Highland Hospital (Oakland), David Grant Medical Center (Travis Air Force Base), and a multitude of private practice clinics across northern California. All of the institutions in the Sacramento area are part of an intensely competitive, highly evolved managed health-care marketplace.

The morale of the house staff (resident physicians) at the School's teaching hospitals is high, and this translates into excellent resident-student interaction (i.e., teaching). Most applicants do not appreciate the significance of this until their third-year clerkships.

Students do some (but not excessive) scut work and have opportunities for meaningful patient involvement. However, the level of that involvement depends largely on the student's team. Opportunities for procedures, such as placing IVs and suturing lacerations, during clinical rotations can be spotty and poor at times. But a required fourth-year emergency department rotation partially rectifies this.

The third year consists of eight weeks each of medicine, surgery, pediatrics, psychiatry, and obstetrics/gynecology. In addition, an eight-week clerkship called Primary Care Plus consists of four weeks of family medicine and two weeks each of urology and orthopedics. Students can elect to defer either psychiatry or obstetrics/gynecology to the fourth year, enabling them to take eight weeks of electives during the third year.

Medicine and surgery are felt to be the best clinical rotations, and obstetrics/gynecology and Primary Care Plus (PCP) the worst. Obstetrics/gynecology receives its low marks due to the low obstetrics volume and unhappy residents; PCP is disliked by students due to a painful weekly conference and a commonly held feeling that family practice is being forced upon students. Nevertheless, the Family Practice Department is strong at UCD.

Fourth-year requirements include emergency medicine (four weeks), neurology or neurosurgery (two weeks), physical medicine and rehabilitation (two weeks), otolaryngology (two weeks), ophthalmology (two weeks), and bioethics (two weeks). Eighteen additional weeks of "selectives" are required, leaving fourteen weeks of vacation/elective time. The fourth year is flexible and offers ample opportunity to customize the curriculum, to take a vacation, and to do rotations at other schools. This is vital for checking out other institutions and making residency contacts. One of the best required fourth-year clerkships is emergency medicine, and many students enter that field.

Some students complain about the lack of a formal mentor system. Professors are usually willing to offer mentoring support to students, but these relationships must be sought independently. Nationally recognized clinical academicians are available for advice, research opportunities, and, importantly, getting residency-ensuring letters of recommendation. More than half of UCD graduates pursue primary-care careers. But every year specialty-minded students successfully match in competitive fields like orthopedic surgery, radiology, and otolaryngology.

Social Life

Most students live in Davis for the first two years, but a few commute from as far away as the Bay Area. Davis is 90 minutes east of San Francisco and 15 minutes west of Sacramento. Although its population has grown to approximately 55,000, Davis still clings to its rural small-town feel, with an authentic twice-weekly farmers' market and a functioning downtown shopping area. Davis hosts the usual college town assortment of bookstores, cafés, and pizza restaurants but conspicuously lacks a full-size shopping mall. Parks and pools are plentiful, and many programs for children are available from the city's Parks and Recreation Department.

Night life in Davis is timid, with only a few clubs. Most action occurs at undergraduate fraternities. Many medical students find time during the first two years to play on intramural sports teams. Davis's good weather and flat geography have made it the bicycle commuter's paradise. In fact, class breaks on the main campus emerge as two-wheeled rush hours. Bike paths and friendly road surfaces are abundant, and several intersections feature bicycle-specific traffic lights and turn lanes. Students should beware of bike cops who can and do issue bicycle speeding tickets.

Approximately half the students move to Sacramento, the California state capital, for the third and fourth years. Rent there is generally cheaper than Davis. Safe and dangerous areas neighbor the medical center and are within blocks of each other. The Sacramento area is steeped in gold mining and trains, and related historical sites are abundant. The California State Expo is held annually in Sacramento, and the River City has a reputation as an overgrown cow town. Professional sports teams include the Sacramento Kings NBA team, the Knights indoor soccer team, and occasional visits by the San Jose Sharks NHL team. "Generic" is the term students use to describe night life in Sacramento. Many bars and clubs can be found, but most feel the scene lacks the character of San Francisco or Los Angeles. Gambling and great skiing are 2 hours away at Lake Tahoe. The many rivers in the area offer excellent rafting and kayaking.

The weather is conducive to most outdoor activities almost year-round. In the Sacramento Valley, summers are hot and dry, with average July highs of 95 degrees. Cool evening breezes from the bay can dampen the summer heat. Spring and fall climates are perfect. The abundant grasses and farming in the valley wreak havoc on seasonal allergy sufferers. Winters are short and mild, with average January highs in the mid-50s and an average rainfall of 16 to 24 inches. But snow and skiing is abundant in the nearby Sierra Nevada about 1½ to 2 hours away.

The Bottom Line

UCD School of Medicine is a perfect school for thrifty Frisbee-throwing, bicycle-riding sun lovers who want comprehensive training at a well-respected medical school. But those who crave nightlife and urban expanses may find themselves lonely.

UNIVERSITY OF CALIFORNIA, IRVINE, COLLEGE OF MEDICINE

Irvine, California

Tuition 1996–97: $9,384 per year
Applications: 4,700
Size of Entering Class: 92
Total Number of Women Students: 212 (42%)

Total Number of Men Students: 287 (58%)
World Wide Web: meded.com.uci.edu/
Contact: Dr. Thomas Cesario, Dean
Irvine, CA 92697

Originally founded more than 100 years ago as an osteopathic medical college in Los Angeles, the California College of Medicine was purchased by the regents of the University of California in the 1960s. Since that time University of California, Irvine (UCI) has dropped the osteopathic roots of the program and is one of the five allopathic medical schools in the University of California system. Few people outside of California have heard of UCI, and it is the least well-known of the UC medical schools. For this reason, it is consistently outside the top twenty-five in the *U.S. News & World Report* rankings. Nevertheless, at the end of four years, students feel they received a good education and find great comfort that their loan payments are less than half of what their friends have to pay for attending school in the chilly northeast. As a result, entrance is competitive, with average MCAT scores in the 10s.

Preclinical Years

Like most medical schools, the first two years consist of the dry basic sciences. The first-year curriculum consists of anatomy, biochemistry, physiology, microbiology, histology, and neuroscience. Attendance at each course is variable and depends on the quality of the lecturer. By the end of the year, there are only about twenty students in the microbiology lectures, as many students find it more efficient to read the texts (or go to the beach) during the day rather than sleep in the lecture hall. By comparison, physiology and neuroscience are usually well attended. The second-year curriculum consists of pharmacology, pathology, and mechanisms of disease. These courses are well received by the students and well taught by faculty members.

Students learn mostly from study groups and teamwork on projects. In general, students tend to work well together. Part of this stems from the honors/pass/fail grading system. This markedly reduces the stress associated with letter grades and also to reduces competition between students.

Clinical Years

The third-year curriculum is fixed: ten weeks each of medicine and surgery, nine weeks of obstetrics/gynecology, and eight weeks each of pediatrics and psychiatry. Most of the rotations are divided between UCI Medical Center, which is essentially a county hospital, and the Long Beach VA Medical Center. Some students do their pediatrics or obstetrics at the Long Beach Memorial Hospital, a private hospital that serves a mixed community. A diverse mix of patients can be seen at UCI, while at the VA, students learn the effects of age, alcohol, and tobacco on the human body.

The most exciting rotation is surgery, especially for students who request rotating through the trauma service. The hours are long, but the teaching by senior residents is great, and opportunities to learn procedures abound. The surgeons at UCI are compulsive. They expect students to know clinical medicine, but they teach a great deal as well.

The medicine and pediatrics rotations are relaxed, and the services are slow enough that students have time to read about patients. The downside to this is that students do not have enough of a patient volume to see more than one or two presentations of any disease. On the obstetrics/gynecology rotation, students have the opportunity to learn from some of the most prominent physicians in the field. Despite the UCI fertility scandal several years ago, when allegations of mishandling human embryos led to the collapse of an excellent reproductive endocrinology division, the remaining divisions still have some of the best physicians in the field. The gynecology/oncology division is prominent; thus, students spend three weeks on this service. The labor and delivery service is light, and students generally deliver fewer than five births. It is on this rotation that students develop endurance for staying up all night and being criticized the next day. Psychiatry rounds out the third year, with eight weeks of time split between the VA and UCI. The experience varies depending on whether students are assigned to consults or inpatient wards. Generally the experience is good, with weekends off so students have time to read their DSM-IV.

The fourth year has many requirements: neurology; radiology; physical medicine and rehabilitation; a subinternship in medicine, surgery, or pediatrics; an ICU month; and more surgical electives. Despite this, students still have more than ten weeks off for vacation. Most of this time is consumed by residency applications and interviews. UCI students perform fairly well in the residency matching program, typically getting one of their top choices. Most choose to stay within California. A few go off each year to prestigious academic institutions, but most stay at local programs that offer more in the way of lifestyle rather than intense residency experiences.

Social Life

UCI is located in conservative Orange County, California, approximately 10 minutes from the beach. The area is a haven for surfers, soccer moms, mountain bikers, and sunbathers. A 1-hour drive takes students to Los Angeles, the mountains, or San Diego. The area has great restaurants, safe streets, and shopping malls. The School does offer subsidized graduate student housing for those who do not wish to pay the pricey rents in Irvine. The more adventurous may choose to share a small house in nearby Newport Beach.

The admissions office is accepting of nontraditional students, and most classes have a few students whose ages range from 30 to 40. Historically, the student population is diverse. Unfortunately, recent changes in affirmative action policies in California have led to a significant drop in minority enrollment throughout the UC system. Recent years have seen the demise of several good outreach programs.

The Bottom Line

UCI is a place for California residents who wish to stay in California. Students choose UCI because the education is good, the beaches are great, and the price is right.

UNIVERSITY OF CALIFORNIA, LOS ANGELES, UCLA SCHOOL OF MEDICINE

Los Angeles, California

Applications: 6,195
Size of Entering Class: 121
World Wide Web: www.medsch.ucla.edu/

Contact: Admissions Office
405 Hilgard Avenue
Los Angeles, CA 90095
310-825-6081

University of California, Los Angeles (UCLA), is a high-profile university in one of the most high-profile cities in the world. It attracts top-notch clinicians and researchers to its many hospitals. As a result, being a UCLA medical student can be quite awe inspiring, but it can also be difficult to get some personal attention. The ideal student for UCLA is an independent learner, one who is willing to take advantage of the many opportunities available. The School's other strength is its location. It sits between the beaches and mountains and offers glitz and glamour. It also sits within a diverse patchwork of ethnically diverse communities, which provides a wide range of clinical experiences.

Admissions/Financial Aid

It is difficult to gain acceptance to UCLA. There are 121 students in each class, selected from 5,244 applicants. The majority are from California, but there are nearly twenty-two out-of-state students. Twenty percent of the class is composed of underrepresented minorities, and 46 percent of the class are women. UCLA students are joined by students from Drew Medical School for the first two years and by University of California, Riverside, students in the final two years. This effectively increases the class size to 143 students at any given time. Because UC, Riverside, students join for the last two years, they are poorly integrated into the class.

Ninety percent of the students receive some form of financial aid, with an average indebtedness of $56,000. The financial office determines need using parental income, even for students who are independent. This leaves some members of the class in much more debt than others ($125,000 versus $25,000).

Preclinical Years

During the first two years at UCLA, students filter through voluminous lecture handouts from the basic science courses. The quality of these courses runs the gamut, and many students are forced to use their own discretion when it comes to class attendance. The house is always full for pharmacology, taught by recent Nobel Prize winner Dr. Louis J. Ignarro. He has received ten Golden Apple awards, granted by the students for outstanding teaching. Anatomy and neurology are also generally well received by the students. Unfortunately, the doctoring course, which ranks lowest in student popularity, has mandatory attendance. Doctoring meets twice a month to cover material outside of the basic sciences, such as medical ethics or medical legal issues. Although the mission of the class is appreciated, the course itself tends to evoke fury and frustration. UCLA integrates problem-based learning into the curriculum with the Clinical Approach to Basic Science (CABS) course. Students also enjoy early clinical exposure during their first two years, with a special emphasis on primary care.

UCLA's pass/no pass grading system fosters a cooperative learning environment, though it usually takes an entire semester for students to shed the competitive nature they acquired as undergraduates. The merits of this system continue to be debated by the medical education committee, and there is the danger that it could be changed at any time.

Between the first and second year, there is ample opportunity for research and international medicine. Many students choose to go abroad for medicine/language programs. There are excellent local outreach programs as well.

Clinical Years

Medical students tend to be treated quite well on the wards. In fact, some say that they are coddled. Call schedules tend to be light, students are often excused from the wards for didactics, and scut work is considered unacceptable. Most students take great comfort in their school's concern for their personal well-being. A student who enjoys the concept of old-school hierarchy and discipline may not feel that UCLA is the place for them.

Students rotate through several affiliated hospitals, which offers a wide range of clinical experience. At UCLA Medical Center, students see very rare diseases but get little hands-on training. Meanwhile, at the West Los Angeles VA or at UCLA–Harbor Hospital, students are given more autonomy, more procedures, and more exposure to "bread and butter" medicine. The patient population ranges from the homeless and poor to the rich and famous. Spanish skills come in handy, particularly at Olive View Hospital. Because students can choose where to do each rotation and because the hospital system is so diverse, students are able to tailor their education to their interests. One unfortunate consequence of this is that students may go many months before seeing classmates. All of the clerkships tend to be well received, though the obstetrics/gynecology rotation is the most grueling in terms of hours and workload. Many also complain that they do not get enough deliveries while on the rotation.

During the third and fourth year, students are generously allotted sixteen weeks of vacation. These weeks can be scattered throughout the two years or hoarded until the very end for a long vacation. There are also several interesting electives that serve as "little vacations" from the rigors of medicine. Some of these include medicine and the media, literature and medicine, East-West medicine, and the Spanish elective.

Social Life

The School is located in Westwood, 10 minutes from beautiful stretches of beach. On weekends, students can hike the Santa Monica Mountains, visit Palm Springs, tour Vegas, or ski Mammoth. Surfing and in-line skating are popular year-round outdoor activities. Interesting restaurants and world-famous museums are abundant in the city. Students often organize group field trips to the Getty Museum or to see the L.A. Philharmonic. Some enjoy Hollywood, while others prefer the local feel of the beach towns. Sports fans can get season tickets to UCLA football and basketball games. Despite these attractions, some students cannot put up with the city's "plastic" feel, its congested freeways, and the influence of Hollywood.

The class tends to be young and quite social. Classmates enjoy playing intramural sports, forming bands for the talent show, and planning ski trips together. Students make the most of what little free time they have.

Students choose to live all over the metropolitan area. Initially, most students live near campus in Westwood Village or Brentwood, where the cost of living is relatively high. Once the clinical years begin, many people scatter to the coastal towns. Hollywood, Palms, and the Valley seem to be other popular options. UCLA does offer graduate student housing for those interested.

The Bottom Line

UCLA is a highly respected medical institution with some expert teachers and diverse clinical opportunities. It is located in a superb environment and is comparatively cheap. It offers all of the perks of a university in a big city, while providing year-round sun. It is better for independent learners, who can find their way around the huge medical center.

UNIVERSITY OF CALIFORNIA, SAN DIEGO, SCHOOL OF MEDICINE

La Jolla, California

Size of Entering Class: 122
Total Number of Women Students: 200 (41%)
Total Number of Men Students: 288 (59%)
World Wide Web: medicine.ucsd.edu/

Contact: Office of Admissions
9500 Gilman Drive
La Jolla, CA 92093-5003
619-534-3880

University of California, San Diego (UCSD) is a difficult school to get into and an even more difficult place to leave. Students become accustomed to the warm climate, sun, beaches, deserts, and mountains.

Admissions/Financial Aid

Given the large number of premedical students in the state, MCAT scores and GPAs tend to be the primary selection factors in financial aid. In recent years, as the state has mandated a larger output of primary-care physicians, students expressing an interest in generalist careers have probably had the upper hand, though lab-based research is still the lifeblood of the medical school.

The student body is primarily composed of native Californians and recent transplants, most of whom came to the University for the location. Though academic interests tend to be limited to the sciences, students invariably have a broad number of athletic interests. A good handful of classmates, for example, will walk into class having surfed that morning. Students tend to be young, with an average age between 22 and 25. Only a small number of students are older than 30.

Of note, the UC system recently passed a ban on all affirmative action policies. The School is attempting alternative methods of recruitment and has been reasonably successful at rebuilding the mostly Hispanic minority population.

The application process is standard and includes the AMCAS, secondary application, and interview. The interview day is fairly loose, and interviewers usually stress outreach and information rather than resume dissection. Tuition, as with all the UC branches, is reasonable, and financial aid tends to be quite plentiful.

Preclinical Years

In 1968, the School's founders, mostly Harvard and Yale Medical School expatriates, designed a curriculum based on the principle that students need a unified approach to medicine, solidly grounded in the basic sciences. As such, the first quarter begins with cell biology and biochemistry (CBB), an amalgam of six graduate school–oriented classes. Physiology is taught alongside pharmacology. Anatomy is reserved for second year. Pathology and microbiology are taught in unified four-month blocks at the end of the second year.

CBB often leaves students bewildered and frustrated. The teaching is consistently average, and the material dry. Most classes are lecture based, though organ physiology and pharmacology incorporates case-based approaches in piecemeal fashion. Class times, moreover, tend to be long (at least 4 hours per day), and exams even longer and usually highly detailed multiple choice. Students are introduced to clinical medicine early on (the first week) on Saturday mornings, where they interview patients.

The highlight of the year is the third trimester's basic medical neurology. The consistency and quality of the teaching improve considerably in the second year, with anatomy and microbiology being the high points. Relying on the note taker is essential, given that lecture time seems to expand to the fill to the day. Despite the long hours in class, students are rewarded with ample vacation time between trimesters and a number of research and clinical opportunities between first and second year. Even more important has been the development of three free clinics by UCSD students in the past two years. These clinics are staffed entirely by medical students and give first- and second-year students the opportunity to do histories and physicals well before the School has scheduled them into the curriculum.

Anatomy in the second year helps consolidate the principles of physiology taught in the first year and helps set the stage for organ systems–based pathology in the next semesters. Since pathology and microbiology finish only three weeks before the boards, UCSD students tend to do extremely well in these subjects, which comprise the bulk of the exam.

Clinical Years

The bad rap on UCSD over the years has been its clinical training. Part of this reputation is myth. Because so few UCSD graduates leave the West Coast for residency training, many academic institutions are unfamiliar with the Schools' graduates. When looking at *U.S. News & World Report*'s list, students can note the difference in rank between scientific reputation (near the top in NIH funding and research output) and residency director evaluation (somewhere in the middle). Were more graduates to look elsewhere for their training, this discrepancy would likely disappear.

The criticism about clinical training is also based partly on fact. San Diego has the highest HMO penetration in the nation, and students tend to see only a limited number of patients because there are only so many hospital beds in town. UCSD has been quite proactive in this regard and, in the past several years, has greatly expanded the number of opportunities at non-University sites. In fact, students probably get as much exposure to the "real world" of medicine as any other medical school. One third of the internal medicine rotation and one half of the pediatrics rotation are devoted to outpatient care. Throughout third year, students participate in a primary-care rotation; for one afternoon each week, they see their own patients in a private family or internal medicine clinic. It is a unique opportunity that few schools offer.

Patient exposure is reasonably broad, though each hospital has its unique character. UCSD Medical Center in Hillcrest has ample county medicine catastrophes (such as HIV, injection drug use, alcoholism); the VA hospital has hypertension, diabetes, and vascular disease, and the Balboa Navy Medical Center has more middle-class problems. Teaching tends to be best at the VA and Navy, while scut work dominates at Hillcrest.

All third-year clerkships must be done in San Diego. During the fourth year, however, students have no specific required clerkships. They must do three rotations at UCSD (an inpatient month, an outpatient month, and a primary-care month), but the rest of the time can be spent at other hospitals or working on the Independent Study Project (ISP). The ISP, a requirement to graduate, is a minithesis that can be done on any topic related to medicine. Grading tends to be lax, and topics are reasonably flexible. Students generally spend anywhere from one to two months to one to two years working on it, depending on their level of motivation.

Social Life

Though not a perfect school, UCSD is at least in a perfect place for medical school. San Diego offers every type of outdoor and indoor entertainment. A further bonus is Baja, California, with its long white sands, cheap beer, and fish tacos less than 30 minutes away.

Each class has its own committee designed to organize social events, of which there are several. The first-year orientation is a weeklong party put on by the second-year students, and other events include a Halloween Party, Dance on San Diego Bay, and the Spring Talent Show, a time for raucous first-year students to lampoon faculty and classmates.

Students tend to live on or close to campus for at least the first two years. La Jolla, unfortunately, is not a student town, and most tend to congregate in the series of overpriced, semiluxury apartments that circle the campus. Others live in campus housing, which, though a bit difficult to secure as a first-year student, is of good quality, quite accessible, and inexpensive. After the first two years, students tend to disperse a bit more, with some choosing the beach and enduring the long commute and others forsaking the water for the convenience of downtown San Diego (near the main hospitals).

The Bottom Line

UCSD, with its location and inexpensive tuition, makes it an irresistible location for school. Though traditionally geared toward the sciences, the School has recently emphasized real-world medicine, making it a great choice for budding generalists.

UNIVERSITY OF CALIFORNIA, SAN FRANCISCO, SCHOOL OF MEDICINE

San Francisco, California

Tuition 1996–97: $9,384 per year
Students Receiving Financial Aid: 87%
Applications: 5,508
Size of Entering Class: 153
Total Number of Women Students: 340 (56%)
Total Number of Men Students: 272 (44%)

World Wide Web: www.som.ucsf.edu./
Contact: Kathleen Ryan, Admissions Officer
Parnassus Avenue
San Francisco, CA 94143
415-476-4044

Located in one of the country's most progressive and culturally vibrant cities, the University of California, San Francisco (UCSF), School of Medicine offers top-notch medical training at an affordable price. Whether students are interested in primary care, super-specialized tertiary care or research, or just want to enjoy some breathtaking views while studying in the library or dissecting a cadaver, UCSF offers something to satisfy professional interests and goals.

Preclinical Years

The first two years of medical school at UCSF are designed to provide the scientific foundation for the practice of clinical medicine. Classes are arranged in a traditional quarter system, with an eight-week vacation slotted between the first and second years. First-year courses include anatomy, cell and tissue biology, biochemistry, physiology, epidemiology, genetics, behavioral science, and neuroscience. The second year consists of pathology, pharmacology, immunology, microbiology, growth and development, and psychiatry. Most courses are given in a combined lecture, case seminar, and laboratory format, and exams are typically administered two or three times per quarter.

Students receive moderate exposure to clinical medicine during the preclinical years, mostly through an integrated two-year course entitled Foundations of Patient Care. During the first year, students acquire basic skills in patient communication and practice by taking histories from real patients, while the second year introduces clinical disease mechanisms, physical exam skills, and medical diagnosis. A yearlong clinical preceptorship during the second year helps students bridge the gap in their skills from the classroom to the bedside, as significant time is devoted to examining real patients and shadowing practicing physicians.

In the midst of an ever-changing health-care marketplace, a first-year course also introduces economic, governmental, ethical, and legal issues in medicine. A separate three-year curriculum is offered to a small number of students through the University of California at Berkeley–UCSF Joint Medical Program, which requires a separate application.

UCSF students are typically very happy during the preclinical years because the teaching is fantastic, the classes are all pass/fail, which maintains student cohesiveness and morale), and every Wednesday is a day off. Classes are only held four days per week, which gives students an extra day to explore personal interests, spend time with their significant others, or improve their golf games. Other nice touches include an entire cadre of teachers who go above and beyond the call of duty to help students learn anatomy, pathology, or neurology into the wee hours of the morning before a midterm, a Medical Scholars Program in which second-year students help first-year students learn anatomy and physiology, a student-run Homeless Health Clinic, a variety of elective offerings (ranging from AIDS health policy to medical Spanish to emergency medicine), and an outstanding USMLE review series taught by a faculty "Dream Team" (several are authors of popular Boards Review texts) during the spring of second year.

The first two years culminate with the USMLE Step 1 exam, for which students are given a two- to three-week study period. UCSF students consistently score well above the national mean for the exam, with few or no failures.

Clinical Years

Overall, the clinical experience at UCSF is tremendous, with exposure to a wide variety of patients as well as an appropriate balance between hands-on learning and teaching. Beginning in the third year, required and elective clerkships are scheduled in two-week through eight-week blocks. Required rotations include medicine (eight weeks), surgery (eight weeks), pediatrics (six weeks), obstetrics and gynecology (six weeks), psychiatry (six weeks), family and community medicine (six weeks), surgical subspecialties (four weeks), neurology (four weeks), anesthesia (two weeks), medical ethics (two weeks), and an additional five months of elective rotations. In the last month of the fourth year, all students must also take a course in the mechanisms of disease and advanced cardiac life support. Unlike the first two years, the third and fourth years are graded as honors/pass/fail, based on clinical evaluations.

One complaint about the current curriculum is that the large number of required clerkships (fifty-six weeks) limits time for scheduling electives. In addition, the curriculum is currently under evaluation, and additional emphasis on ambulatory care may be added to reflect the practice of most graduates. Also noteworthy is that the recent merger between UCSF and Stanford Health Services appears unlikely to affect the UCSF and Stanford medical schools, which remain distinct entities.

As UCSF's flagship teaching hospital, Moffitt-Long Hospital provides exposure to a variety of challenging cases and medical "zebras." San Francisco General Hospital, a public hospital, and San Francisco Veterans Administration Hospital are popular with students seeking a more hands-on approach. Students rotating at these hospitals also see more "bread-and-butter" medicine. The clinical experience is rounded out by UCSF–Mt. Zion Hospital, a community/university hospital, as well as a group of affiliated hospitals, including Kaiser San Francisco (an HMO setting), California Pacific Medical Center (a private setting), and Children's Hospital of Oakland, which help ensure that students see diverse patient populations.

The School places a strong emphasis upon education, which means that clerkship directors see to it that students receive organized didactic instruction and do not spend excessive time performing scut work or taking call. During third year, inpatient call averages every fourth night and ends at 10 or 11 p.m., although students frequently volunteer to take overnight call.

Social Life

Nestled in the heart of San Francisco and the Bay Area, UCSF offers a dazzling array of cultural, social, and recreational activities. Weekends and Wednesdays off during the first two years provide ample opportunity for students to ski and gamble in Lake Tahoe, taste wines in Napa Valley, roam the Monterey coastline, or explore San Francisco's numerous restaurants, nightclubs, museums, and cafés. Another popular destination is Golden Gate Park, which is located adjacent to the medical center and includes several museums, and miles of running/biking/skating trails.

Housing and parking in San Francisco can be expensive, particularly in the current tight real estate market. UCSF is situated in the Inner Sunset district, one of the cheaper parts of town (one-bedroom apartments rent for approximately $800 per month) that is still safe. The majority of students live in duplex apartments located within walking distance of the school. Furnished campus housing, located a 5- to 10-minute shuttle ride away, is available at reasonable rents for both single and married students. Single students, however, find this option less than ideal because it often requires shared bedrooms.

The Bottom Line

UCSF offers students a great education, a great city, and a great price.

UNIVERSITY OF CHICAGO PRITZKER SCHOOL OF MEDICINE

Chicago, Illinois

Applications: 8,220
Size of Entering Class: 104
Total Number of Women Students: 201 (48%)
Total Number of Men Students: 222 (52%)
World Wide Web: www.uchicago.edu/u.acadunits/
BSD.html#pritz

Contact: Dr. Norma Wagoner, Dean of Students
5801 Ellis Avenue
Chicago, IL 60637-1513
773-702-1939

Located on a Gothic campus along Chicago's historic Midway Plaisance in the lakefront neighborhood of Hyde Park, the University of Chicago (U of C) has received international attention as a top research institution. This intellectual university has had the first sustained nuclear reaction and more Nobel laureates than any other American institution, with eleven in physiology and medicine alone. The academic atmosphere is intense and cerebral but completely unpretentious. The dress is casual to urban-hip, and there are no grades or class rank at the University's Pritzker School of Medicine.

Preclinical Years

The School's approach is academic and interdisciplinary. The dichotomy of the preclinical years at Pritzker is this: the experience is intense but pass/fail. The committee on education has in the past few years proven so responsive to student recommendations that the curriculum proceeds with few or no complaints. The course work is dominated by an in-depth and comprehensive consideration of health and disease. Anatomy is taught as human morphology, which fuses the relevant portions of embryology and tissue histology with classical anatomic study. So intellectual is the approach of this course that a renowned paleontologist teaches head and neck anatomy with an evolutionary perspective. The School's Dean, who holds a Ph.D. in anatomy, walks the lab illustrating the most confounding chambers of the body with smooth alacrity.

Another unique and highly rated course is medical ethics, taught by faculty members from the nationally renowned MacLean Center for Medical Eth-

ics. Clinical exposure is not neglected, as students are assigned a physician, a resident, and a senior student preceptor group in the first year for history taking on the medical and psychiatric wards. No barriers exist between students and professors, and the year is highlighted by the best of the teaching faculty of the Biological Sciences Division.

Students work hard, but the drive is internal and the stress is minimal. In the sixteen-week summer following first year, students pursue intramural research on the school dole or off-campus study on prestigious national fellowships or abroad. Others work in the surrounding community.

The second year focuses on disease with clinical pathophysiology (CPP), microbiology, and pharmacology. Grades are pass/fail. The grading system allows for tight collaboration and friendships within lab groups, and studying is significantly more productive. The taste of patient care through physical diagnosis is a perfect primer for the third year.

Clinical Years

In the third year, students undergo twelve intense months of hands-on patient care. Responding to health-care trends and student requests, there is an increasing presence of outpatient-weeks medicine, obstetrics and gynecology, pediatrics, family practice, psychiatry, and surgery. A new affiliation with nearby suburban MacNeal Hospital, as well as a network of group practices extending deep into rural Indiana, gives interested students a chance to broaden their primary-care experience. The majority of time is spent at the University of Chicago Hospitals and the state-of-the-art Duchossois Center for Advanced Medicine (DCAM).

At the U of C hospitals, students wear long white attending coats. Though not immediately grasped by students, the decision to enshroud even the most junior members of inpatient teams in this symbol of aged clinical wisdom reflects the absolute regard in which senior faculty members hold students, as well as the expectations on student knowledge and performance. Students at Pritzker are given the first contact with emergency room patients, new outpatients, and a primary responsibility in the care of their inpatients on most ward services. The responsibility is awesome, and the education is unparalleled. Among students and residents, the camaraderie is high, and only rarely are students relegated to menial tasks.

The third year is the only year where performance is graded as honors/high pass/pass/or fail. Though the transcript still shows only pass/fail, the Dean's letter sent to residency programs offers more detailed grades as well as excerpts from evaluations from attendings. Grading is fair as a consequence of the small teams on which students play an integral role.

The fourth year is largely elective, with time set aside for subinternships in each of the specialty services and a small basic science requirement. Though the fourth year is spent largely on interesting electives, research, and match-related activities, students take advantage of programs in international medicine, with trips to Kenya and Central America, as well as to European medical centers. Eighty-five to 95 percent of Pritzker graduates match at one of their top four choices.

Social Life

Chicago is a youthful town, to the point where a student's budget offers access to virtually the whole city. Most students spend their first year living on campus in historic, lakefront Hyde Park. Spacious on-campus apartments range from $350 to $700 per month. Hyde Park's fully functional nightlife ranges from theater to cinemas to great ethnic restaurants to the best blues and jazz clubs in the city. Many students then migrate north to explore living in other Chicago neighborhoods. Lincoln Park is a large young-postgraduate lakefront village with all-night lounges, pubs, and clubs. Bucktown and Wicker Park are two adjacent neighborhoods on the West Side, which is the home of the visual arts and independent rock. Most akin to the East Village in New York, Bucktown differs in one key regard: a renovated 2,500-square-foot apartment costs $1,600 per month.

The Bottom Line

Students at Pritzker, a world-class medical school without grade pressure, can enjoy themselves,

UNIVERSITY OF CINCINNATI COLLEGE OF MEDICINE

Cincinnati, Ohio

Applications: 996
Size of Entering Class: 156
Total Number of Women Students: 204 (53%)
Total Number of Men Students: 179 (47%)
World Wide Web: www.med.uc.edu/htdocs/
  medicine/uccom.htm

Contact: Linda Moeller, Director, Graduate Affairs
PO Box 210091
Cincinnati, OH 45221-0091
513-558-7343

Medical students attending the University of Cincinnati College of Medicine (UCCM) will be adding their names to a roster of one of the oldest academic health centers around. Begun in 1819, it is the tenth-oldest in the nation and the oldest west of the Allegheny Mountains. It was established by Dr. Daniel Drake over a drug store in Cincinnati.

It is not just the historical aspect that makes this medical college unique. Its graduates and faculty members include some very impressive names, such as Leon Goldman, M.D., who graduated in 1929 and is considered the father of Laser Medicine, and Albert Sabin, M.D., the well-known developer of the first oral polio vaccine.

The College of Medicine started the ball rolling, and other institutions joined to make this one of the leading academic health centers in the nation. These include the Colleges of Nursing and Health, Pharmacy, and Allied Health Science and the Hoxworth Blood Center. Each offers medical and health-care students outstanding opportunities to explore different experiences in patient contact, research, and unusual options of training in primary care.

If research is where students want to be, the University of Cincinnati's medical college should be their choice—it is preeminent. It is connected with some illustrious institutions in medical research, such as the Children's Hospital Medical Center, which is the affiliate for pediatric training and research and the largest children's hospital in the United States. Medical students conduct research projects that can be benchmarked against the other 125 colleges of medicine in the country. They've been conducting research there for sixty-five years. Among fields presently underway are basic research emphasizing developmental biology and the transcriptional regulation of gene function, clinical research, clinical effectiveness and health services research, development of new prevention, and health promotion approaches.

The UCCM has scored major achievements in securing research funds. Of Ohio institutions, the College of Medicine and Children's Hospital Medical Center get top billing in the National Institutes of Health research funding and are among the top third in outside research funding in the nation. The Children's Hospital Research Foundation, whose members are also College of Medicine faculty members, in 1997, received more than $26 million in grants, which allowed College of Medicine students to take advantage of the Children's Hospital's volume of patients who offer experience in both rare and common conditions.

The College of Medicine, which received $60 million in grants in 1997, was the recipient of an $8-million award to develop a cardiovascular research center as well as a $7.5-million grant from Procter & Gamble for a pulmonary research division.

With such support, students interested in research have a number of facilities with different specialties in which to pursue their interests with the College of Medicine faculty members' active encouragement. Immediately following their first year, students have several options to explore their research interests. Between years one and two, they can participate in a summer research program, while yearlong research experiences can be taken between years two and three. Seniors can opt for research as an elective.

Admissions/Financial Aid

The College of Medicine offers a Medical Student Research Fellowship Program in which students who have completed their first (and occasionally their second year) of medical school conduct research and analyze data for ten weeks. They not only get to work alongside distinguished faculty members involved in projects that interest students, but they also receive a $2,500 stipend.

Students interested in short-term projects can conduct research during the summer. The College offers another summer program that links first-year students with physicians practicing family medicine.

For applicants interested in attending the University of Cincinnati College of Medicine, a strong early decision program might induce them to think seriously about it. Students who know without a doubt that they want to attend can take the MCAT in April or submit scores from previous administrations of the test to apply for early decision. By October 1, students have a final decision that either offers them acceptance or defers their application for further consideration. These early decision students get a head start with an early transition to medical school and special privileges, such as being able to look for housing ahead of everyone else and having easy access to the Director of Medical Student Financial Aid.

More than 80 percent of enrolled students receive some form of financial assistance. Since the College of Medicine has been around so long, it has substantial scholarship and student loan endowments for students who can show real financial need. About 80 percent of students come from Ohio, and Ohio residents are given preference. In 1997, 4,280 applications were received, of which 156 students were admitted. Of those, 42 percent were women and 15 percent were underrepresented minorities.

Preclinical Years

Not content to rest on past accomplishments in medical education, the College of Medicine has seriously revamped its curriculum for years one and two. It is basic science information in an integrated systems-based program, which focuses on the relationship between structure and function and promotes student activity as opposed to sitting in a classroom taking lecture notes. While this does not mean that students are not frantically scribbling while a professor is talking, the new emphasis is on basic science information that is applied to clinical situations. For instance, students participate in case-based learning and small-group conferences.

First-year students hardly get a chance to fill their first notebook with lecture notes before they are immediately thrust into hands-on training with patients in an Introduction to Clinical Practice that begins in their first weeks. The College asked students what they think of this program, and students responded that it is clearly a winner. In addition to learning about the normal structure, function, and development of the body, students are exposed to basic interviewing skills, history taking, and physical examinations. In the second year, they focus on the basics and mechanisms of human disease and spend a half day per week with patients.

Clinical Years

Year three brings even more clinical experiences, and the greater Cincinnati area offers a variety of places for students to work with its diverse population. Third-year students take a strong core of clinical material, as well as core and selective clerkships, which combine clinical service work with classroom work. One interesting required class is Efficient and Cost-Effective Clinical Decision Making. This is an interdisciplinary course that draws upon many faculty and staff members from a variety of departments and hospital services.

Most students do their clinical training at the University Hospital, Veterans Administration Medical Center, Children's Hospital Medical Center, Christ Hospital, and Jewish Hospital.

By year four, students are active members of a health-care team and work with physicians in the Acting Internship in Internal Medicine. Looking back at this class, graduates say it was a superior help in their transition into residency. It is easy to see why: students are given primary-care patient responsibility for outpatients, under the watchful eyes of first-year residents, senior residents, and an attending physician. In 1998, 24 percent of the students took programs in Cincinnati.

The College of Medicine offers a Physician Scientist Training Program that leads to a combined M.D./Ph.D. degree. Students in this track get full financial support, including a stipend of $15,500 plus tuition and health insurance.

Social Life

Cincinnati is a strange town. Where else would you find a Flying Pig Marathon? *WKRP in Cincinnati* once called it home. There's good reason why Cincinnati was dubbed the Queen City and was voted a most livable city in the U.S.—probably because of the river, the rolling hills, and historic architecture. For those not into old gracious houses, there's a big Oktoberfest and the Cincinnati Bengals and the Reds. To really impress someone, take them to dinner at the Omni Netherland Plaza, Cincinnati's premier hotel, which is listed on the National Register of Historical Places. As far as native cuisine, you can find Celtic to Sri Lankan restaurants.

The University-owned apartments are limited and most medical students rent. For two nights in spring, books are tossed aside as students dig deep into their reserves of creative energy and come up with skits, slideshows, and elaborate numbers that range from the hilarious to the ridiculous.

Off times are not all for fun and games. The medical school encourages outreach opportunities with a Blood Drive, a Health Care for the Homeless Mobile Health Van, and a Preventative Medicine at Homeless Clinics.

The Bottom Line

Students at the University of Cincinnati College of Medicine are in the thick of an institution that rests on the past wisdom of an illustrious history in medicine. However, it also has a reputation of looking forward into the future with groundbreaking medical research in the heady environment of the nation's elite medical facilities.

UNIVERSITY OF COLORADO HEALTH SCIENCES CENTER SCHOOL OF MEDICINE

Denver, Colorado

Applications: 2,454
Size of Entering Class: 132
Total Number of Women Students: 246 (46%)
Total Number of Men Students: 293 (54%)

World Wide Web: www.uchsc.edu/sm/sm/
Contact: Dr. Richard Krugman, Dean
4200 East Ninth Avenue
Denver, CO 80262

Located in beautiful Denver, moments from the Rocky Mountains, the University of Colorado Health Sciences Center (UCHSC) has been training physicians and providing health care since 1883. The School also houses a diverse range of research, from basic to clinical, and offers an excellent M.D./Ph.D. program. The primary focus is on providing strong clinical training and a broad experience to prepare physicians for work in the real world. In 1998, *U.S. News & World Report* ranked UCHSC fourth in the nation for primary-care training.

Admissions/Financial Aid

The majority of students are Colorado residents, although approximately 15 percent of the 130 places are available to applicants from out of state. The class is, on average, about 50 percent women and 8 percent members of minority groups. The typical student has been out of college for a few years; their average age is 26–27, and they often enter medicine after pursuing a different career. A few are married. Most are outdoor oriented, with interests in mountain biking, rock climbing, or running marathons. This creates a more relaxed student body and brings many different perspectives to group discussions. Bonding with fellow students begins at orientation and continues with parties, group hikes, bike rides, and ski trips.

Preclinical Years

The first two years follow the standard didactic format, with long days and many lectures. Grades are honors/pass/fail, with about 10 to 15 percent of students getting honors. One nice feature of the first two years is that student representatives for each course are responsible for gathering student input and helping to generate constructive changes for the

courses. The faculty members really care about the quality of the teaching, and things do change in response to student concerns. The School has worked hard to integrate problem-based learning. This is achieved through researchers who discuss how their scientific work impacts specific patients, small groups that dissect real cases, and the primary-care curriculum.

The first trimester is taken up by anatomy. Fortunately, it is taught by an excellent and enthusiastic staff. This is followed by physiology and neurobiology, which are widely regarded as two of the more difficult classes. Other classes, however, tend to leave students frequenting the student-run note service, especially biochemistry, genetics, and embryology. Students are placed in the office of a community doctor for half of a day per week. Most students tend to enjoy the experience early on, though their interest wanes with time. One particular concern has been that the preceptors do not seem to teach enough about physical examination skills.

In the second year, the material is more focused toward clinical medicine, with even more use of problem-based learning and better integration of course material. Pathology is an important course and is well taught; the final is comprehensive and takes place right before Boards. Pharmacology is wide ranging and often obscure. The winter quarter is the most intense of the first two years, with courses in neurology and human behavior.

There are many opportunities outside of the basic sciences. There are interest clubs that range from informal after-hour meetings to lectures and hands-on training. Many students volunteer at Stout Street, a homeless clinic run by students, or with the Salvation Army. Both are supervised by enthusiastic attendings and offer plenty of hands-on experience. There are also elective courses on Medicine in Literature, Ethics, and Medical Spanish. During the summer between first and second years, many students obtain jobs in research or clinical settings. There are scholarships to support work with private doctors in small towns or with the Health Service Corps.

Clinical Years

One of the most distinctive things about Colorado is the AHEC program, which was established to expose students to what it is like to live and work in small towns and to foster interest in primary care. Sites in the required clerkships have been arranged all over the state. Students work one-on-one with an attending and depending on their abilities, are given more responsibility and independence than students at the traditional settings in Denver. The hours, especially for rotations such as surgery and obstetrics/gynecology, are much improved. Students may get to be first or second assistant in a surgery. Spots in this program are popular and are determined by lottery. The School reimburses food and lodging costs so that finances are not a burden.

This is not to say that the sites in Denver are not enjoyable. There are multiple hospitals with a diverse patient base (Spanish is helpful but not essential) that offer a variety of experiences: a county hospital (trauma, alcoholism/substance abuse, and infectious disease), a nationally renowned Veterans Hospital (COPD, cardiac disease, and diabetes), a tertiary-care university hospital (transplant, zebras, and some good primary care), a free-standing Children's Hospital, and two managed care hospitals (broad spectrum). Students are encouraged to take responsibility and be the doctor for their patient. Teaching is emphasized and tends to be quite good, though the experience is heavily dependent on the attending and residents, who can make experiences sublime or painful. Obstetrics/gynecology is typically the least popular experience because of the hours and the often-bitter residents and faculty members.

Attempts to change this rotation have begun, and recent reports are more favorable.

Hands-on experience is plentiful, particularly in the ER rotations. Students get good outpatient experience in pediatrics, medicine, surgical subspecialties, and family medicine. Generally, students complete all but one or two of their requirements in the third year, and the fourth year is open for electives. Students have twelve weeks of vacation over the third and fourth years that allow them to schedule interviews, travel, or take family time. There are also good resources and connections for setting up electives abroad or at other institutions.

Then comes the residency match. The School has a good reputation, and the faculty and residents are good sources for information about other programs in their fields. According to the dean's office, Colorado students do well, with most matching at one of their top three choices. Usually, approximately 40–50 percent choose primary-care residencies, and a fair number stay in Colorado to complete their training.

Social Life

While Denver does not offer the excitement and diversity of New York City or Los Angeles, there is a little of everything. Denver is one of the microbrewery capitals of the world, and there is an almost endless selection of beers to try. The downtown is undergoing a revival, with multiple sports stadiums, restaurants, and cultural attractions. Abundant trails for in-line skating, biking, and running and the mountains are about 40 minutes away.

There is no student housing, so students tend to live all around the area. The School is set in an older residential neighborhood, so there are affordable places within walking and biking distance. A few students choose to live as far away as Boulder.

The Bottom Line

Students who are relaxed outdoor enthusiasts and who want an excellent education, a relaxed atmosphere, and year-round sports activities enjoy UCHSC.

UNIVERSITY OF CONNECTICUT HEALTH CENTER SCHOOL OF MEDICINE

Farmington, Connecticut

Students Receiving Financial Aid: 82%
Total Number of Women Students: 168 (50%)
Total Number of Men Students: 169 (50%)
World Wide Web: www.uchc.edu/
Contact: Keat Sanford, Assistant Dean and Director

263 Farmington Avenue
Farmington, CT 06030
860-679-3874

The University of Connecticut (UConn) School of Medicine is relatively new among this nation's medical institutions. In 1961, the groundwork for the future home of the University of Connecticut Health Center was initiated in Farmington, Connecticut. This health center was built on a hill approximately 8 miles west of the state's capital, Hartford, and is the current home of the University of Connecticut School of Medicine, the School of Dental Medicine, and the University of Connecticut Health System.

The School of Medicine's mission is to provide outstanding health-care education in an environment of exemplary patient care, research, and public service. Although UConn graduated its first physicians in 1972, the School prides itself on being flexible and innovative in its methods of education. For example, UConn recently changed to a problem-based learning approach using the newly renovated Multi-Disciplinary Laboratories (MDLs). In addition, UConn places medical students into clinical settings in the community within the first weeks of the first year.

For the class of 2002, UConn received more than 2,200 applications, for an eventual class size of seventy-seven students, including two M.D./Ph.D. and three M.D./M.P.H. candidates. The composition of this most recent class is 86 percent residents of Connecticut, 45 percent women, and 18 percent members of underrepresented groups. Sixty-nine percent of the class came from undergraduate institutions that are classified as most or very selective, and 78 percent were science majors, with nine students also having advanced degrees or certifications. The average GPA of incoming students is 3.56, and the average MCAT score is 30.5.

The selection process for prospective students includes a day on campus, with two faculty interviews and a chance to meet with the admissions director. Interspersed through the day are lunch and a tour of the medical center with current students. Students can also sit in on one or two classes to observe what the new curriculum offers and witness how the faculty truly enjoys spending time with UConn's bright, inquisitive minds.

Preclinical Years

The class of 1999 was the first class to graduate with a new curriculum, and the results have been impressive. The performance on Step 1 of the United States Medical License Examination (USMLE) improved by 10 points (approximately one half standard deviation), and the failure rate dropped to 1 percent. The first two years of the medical school curriculum still offer the same basic medical science concepts in a new presentation. The emphasis is now on problem-based learning, integrated with ambulatory experiences and disease prevention.

The first year is based on the organ systems, while the second year stresses the mechanisms of disease. The lecture format still exists, but its predominance in the curriculum has been minimized. Smaller, more interactive groups are now the main forum. Groups of eight to fifteen students are paired with a faculty member, and everyone is expected to contribute to the discussion. UConn's medical and dental students participate in the same basic medical science curriculum over the first two years. This means that approximately 120 students (about 80 medical and 40 dental) are included in this lecture and group interaction.

Examinations are pass/fail and are graded on a curve. There is no further separation of the students among the pass group, and there is no minimum percentage of students who must fail. After the exams have been completed, students may be offered free tutoring from upper-level students if problem areas have been recognized. Likewise, if parts of the curriculum are deficient, the faculty members are responsible for making the appropriate changes.

The first year begins with biochemistry and molecular biology. Then, students begin examining the human body by looking at the organ systems individually. For example, as the basic physiology of the respiratory system is taught, students also go through the anatomical dissection of the respiratory system. This approach works well, especially with the new Multi-Disciplinary Labs. The anatomy labs are separate from other classrooms, are for students only, and have state-of-the-art ventilation systems. Thus, UConn enables students to actually see what they are learning about, rather than forcing them to remember what they saw earlier in the year.

The first year is followed by a two-month summer break. While there are plenty of opportunities for research within the health center, the only specific requirement is to be ready for the second year of medical school. As in the first year, lectures and small, interactive groups are utilized as the medium for the learning process. The mechanisms of disease are the focus of the nine months of second year. Again, the subjects are separated as uniformly as possible into an organ-systems approach, in which the relevant physiology and pathology are emphasized. This is good preparation for the boards. Also included in the second year is pharmacology.

Students get a few weeks off at the end of the second year to study prior to taking the USMLE Step I. UConn's new curriculum is preparing its students better for this test than in the past, enabling students to become more competitive for the residency slots they desire. After the test, there are also a few open weeks before students start the third year.

Clinical Years

The third-year curriculum has also been recently restructured. The year is separated into three 16-week blocks, with two weeks utilized for Multi-Ambulatory Experience Programs (MAX). Before the third year, the eighty or so medical students select their desired order of these blocks. Two of the three 16-week blocks are designated ambulatory, while the third is inpatient. The main inpatient hospitals are John Dempsey (UConn Health Center), Hartford Hospital, St. Francis Hospital (in Hartford), and New Britain General Hospital. The ambulatory experiences utilize the previously mentioned hospitals' clinics as well as the offices of practicing physicians in the surrounding community.

For the inpatient experiences, students rotate through surgery, internal medicine, psychiatry, obstetrics/gynecology, and pediatrics in various hospitals. The two ambulatory blocks take place in the outpatient clinics of internal medicine, family medicine, pediatrics, obstetrics/gynecology, surgery, and psychiatry. After each ambulatory block, faculty members and students discuss their experiences, and the students present interesting clinical scenarios to broaden their classmates' education. Unfortunately, there does appear to be a paucity of inpatient learning. Nonetheless, UConn's performance on the clinically oriented USMLE Step II improved with this new curriculum. UConn's class of 1998 was the first class to participate in this new clinical curriculum, and their performance improved by an average of 11 points when compared to the previous class.

The fourth year includes more electives and more freedom to pursue personal interests. Faculty members treat students more as peers. The only requirements are a month each in a subinternship, the emergency room, and one of the intensive care units. A whole month is set aside for residency interviews.

Beginning late in the third year, medical students start to receive information and counseling regarding the residency match process from many sources within the UConn School of Medicine. The dean and the faculty write numerous letters on the students' behalf and help students pursue specific avenues to achieve their goals. The class of 1998 had 64 percent and 19 percent match at their first and second choices, respectively.

Social Life

During the first two years, the atmosphere at UConn is similar to that in college, with various class theme parties funded by the medical school, such as the Halloween party and the holiday dance. There are also funded parties at various students' homes/apartments.

Students are also involved in helping each other through such venues as free tutoring provided by upper-level students and free counseling for drug and alcohol abuse. Student-assisted groups run programs for high school and college students who are interested in a career in medicine and are members of minority groups. There are numerous research opportunities. In the clinical years, some disciplines, such as pediatrics, medicine, and surgery, hold scholar groups, where students can meet with potential mentors and impress each other with presentations.

The bar scene in Hartford offers happy hours, pool and Foosball, and dancing (1970s music included). Boston and New York City are both within 2 hours by car, and two new casinos in Connecticut are an hour away. Hartford also has indoor and outdoor concert venues and theaters for Broadway productions, ballet, and other stage performances.

Sporting events center on UConn. Medical students can be included in the lottery for men's basketball tickets and view any other UConn sporting event at the student rate. Hartford also has minor-league hockey (the Rangers). The Hartford Civic

Center offers professional tennis events. On the outskirts of Hartford are a professional golf tournament and three double-A baseball franchises (the New Britain Rock Cats, Norwich Navigators, and New Haven Ravens).

About a mile from campus is a reservoir for mountain biking, exercising, or lying in the sun. Some students set aside time for touch football, basketball, Ultimate Frisbee, and soccer. Local gyms also offer discounted rates for students.

Students have easy access to the Connecticut and Rhode Island shoreline during the warmer months as well as high-quality ski slopes throughout New England during the winter. For those who enjoy the fall, a drive to pick apples in Connecticut is quite beautiful as the leaves change color during September and October.

The Bottom Line

The University of Connecticut School of Medicine offers a high-quality education within a new, exciting framework. The students are as eager to learn about medicine as they are to experience their New England surroundings.

UNIVERSITY OF FLORIDA COLLEGE OF MEDICINE

Gainesville, Florida

Tuition 1996–97: $28,098 per year
Applications: 3,245
Size of Entering Class: 116
Total Number of Women Students: 311 (46%)
Total Number of Men Students: 368 (54%)

World Wide Web: www.med.ufl.edu/
Contact: Dr. Mohan K. Raizada, Associate Dean
for Graduate Education
Gainesville, FL 32611
352-392-5461

The faculty and administration at the University of Florida (UF) are overwhelmingly concerned with the quality of education, and the curriculum is constantly evolving as a result of student feedback. The teaching, with a few exceptions, is excellent, and graduates are well received throughout Florida, which makes UF the ideal choice for anyone considering living in the area.

The Program in Medical Sciences (PIMS) is a one-year cooperative effort in medical education between the Florida State University (FSU) and the University of Florida College of Medicine and has its own admissions process. The goal of the program is to train primary-care physicians to work in rural and underserved communities. The students spend their first year on the FSU campus in Tallahassee and then move to Gainesville to join the UF medical students at the start of the second year. The PIMS year is twelve months long, in contrast to the nine-month first year in traditional medical schools. The program starts in June.

The didactic component of the PIMS year parallels that taught at the University of Florida but is spread over three extra months, allowing a much slower pace. Students feel that they have a chance to take their time and really learn anatomy well. Since there is no medical school in Tallahassee, the classes are often taught by Ph.D.'s instead of M.D.'s, which means that they can be a bit dry and lack clinical correlation. The small class size (30 students) makes faculty and staff members extremely accessible for questions and discussion. The program emphasizes clinical skills, and PIMS students get more clinical experience than they would at traditional schools by serving in local health clinics for migrant workers, working with primary-care physicians, and completing a semester-long preceptorship at the Family Practice

Residency Program at Tallahassee Memorial Regional Medical Center.

The biggest concern that most PIMS students have is the transition from the first to second year because they have to physically relocate from Tallahassee to Gainesville and join the UF class. Students worry about how they will fare academically and socially in the new setting. Some students reported feeling weaker in certain subjects, such as biochemistry and genetics, compared to their UF counterparts, and some felt socially isolated at first. Overall, the transition goes smoothly, and, by the spring semester, everyone has gotten used to each other and to the workload. Whatever disadvantages the PIMS students felt during the second year are more than counteracted in the third year, when they ease gracefully into patient care thanks to all of their clinical experience.

The PIMS program is unique, and it is not for everyone. The class is small. There are no upperclassmen from whom to ask advice, seek inspiration, or borrow texts. Not being in a major medical center means limited access to clinical research and a medical library. PIMS suits students who are interested in primary care in a rural or underserved community and want an intimate and slower-paced learning environment.

Admissions/Financial Aid

As with most medical schools, admission to UF is not easy. The school's quality and outstanding price make it the most selective medical school in Florida and, along with the warm location, make it the choice of many qualified applicants over the more prestigious private institutions of the northeast. In 1998, UF had more than 2,000 applicants for seventy-five available places (an additional twelve students matriculate through the University Junior Honors program). Of the eighty-seven matriculating students, 58 percent are women, and 7 percent are members of minority groups. The average age of the entering class is usually 23–24, ranging from as young as 20 (mainly Junior Honors students) to early 30s; a majority of students have led interesting past lives before entering medicine. Tuition is inexpensive ($10,000 per year), and the standard financial aid is supplemented with various scholarships and grants on an individual basis.

Preclinical Years

Of the many factors that make the preclinical education at UF unique, the first-year faculty members deserve the most credit. The first semester is taught in blocks, with anatomy, histology, radiology, and examination skills meticulously synchronized and taught by professors who have dedicated their lives to educating first-year medical students. (There is no embryology course. Some embryology is mixed in with anatomy.) Professors are constantly available in and out of class, including during the weekends, for extra help and review sessions. This makes learning these subjects feel more like a team sport, with much support, encouragement, and fun along the way.

The first semester is over by Thanksgiving. Students spend the remaining weeks before Christmas in a primary-care preceptorship shadowing a family practice physician or pediatrician in an underserved area of Florida. The early clinical exposure is beneficial.

January is spent in a monthlong intensive immersion into neuroscience, in which students can be found poring over brain slices, studying tracts and pathways, and naming lesions well into the night. Most students agree in retrospect that they learned a lot during this time and were well prepared for the wards. The high point of spring semester is physiology; the low points are biochemistry, genetics, human behavior, and Keeping Families Healthy. The decline in course quality is accompanied by a decline in intensity.

Second-year students should be prepared for 8 hours per day in lecture halls, 6-hour exams, and pathology. When pathology finally ends in February, it is quickly replaced by pharmacology, along with some other classes such as epidemiology and ethics.

When the year ends, students begin studying for the Boards. The pass rate for the Boards is 99 percent. Fortunately, all that time in pathology pays off, and studying is really reviewing. One criticism some students had is that they felt weak in pharmacology, for both the Boards and clinical clerkships.

Clinical Years

In general, the residents and faculty members in Gainesville love to teach and are good at it. Students primarily work at three hospitals, which allows for a variety of patient populations. Shands, the main teaching hospital, is primarily a tertiary-care center, which allows exposure to a variety of relatively rare disorders and subspecialists who are world renowned. Across the street at the VA hospital, students do a lot of work that the nurses don't want to do, but in exchange they get a lot more hands-on experience. Students also spend eight to twelve weeks of their third year at the University Medical Center in Jacksonville, which is a community-based hospital in the heart of the city. This is the only place to get true trauma exposure. While students are usually hesitant to give up their homes for several weeks of life in dorms, most report enjoying the Jacksonville experience. They do a lot of procedures, experience little of the hierarchical attitude usually present at medical institutions, and get free meals. On the downside, the quality of the residents and faculty at the hospital is generally considered inferior. The nice thing about this setup is that students get to experience working in an academic as well as a community-based hospital, and this experience is a help when it comes time to choose a residency program.

No single rotation or department is unanimously loved or hated by students, primarily because the quality of the experience depends mainly on the team a student works with. The rotation that students constantly complain about is Interdisciplinary General Medicine, a six-week rotation in which students are exposed to the gamut of subspecialty clinics. Students feel that the constant change of environment (generally a different clinic every day, and sometimes two in the same day) makes meaningful learning difficult. However, the clerkship directors have been extremely receptive to student complaints and suggestions and are currently reworking the system.

Social Life

UF students are a friendly and diverse bunch. The majority of students are noncompetitive. Most classes maintain a strong sense of unity, with classwide activities planned several times per semester. Postexam parties are common, but there are other social outlets as well. One popular activity is Latin dancing (a novelty for those not from the Miami area).

The warm weather allows a high level of physical activity, with a variety of intramural sports teams in each class. Medical students are also artists, musicians, journalists, politicians, and entrepreneurs.

UF is located in Gainesville. College football is popular. The town lacks a vibrant young professional community as is found in larger cities. It also seems to have few social and cultural outlets. The closest cities are Orlando, Tampa, Jacksonville, and St. Augustine, and flights out of the tiny local airport are limited and costly. On the other hand, Gainesville has virtually no crime, pollution, or traffic, and the cost of living is inexpensive. Students can affordably live within a 5-minute walk of the medical center. The weather is warm, and various natural springs, lakes, trails, and rivers are nearby.

The Bottom Line

For students interested in primary care, community service, and warm winters, UF provides a solid education at an inexpensive price.

UNIVERSITY OF HAWAII JOHN A. BURNS SCHOOL OF MEDICINE

Honolulu, Hawaii

Tuition 1996–97: $24,635 per year
Size of Entering Class: 58
Total Number of Women Students: 184 (52%)
Total Number of Men Students: 169 (48%)

World Wide Web: medworld.biomed.hawaii.edu
Contact: Sherrel L. Hammer, Interim Dean
2444 Dole Street
Honolulu, HI 96822

The founders and shapers of the University of Hawaii John A. Burns School of Medicine (JABSOM) in Honolulu think of the Hawaiian islands as a tightly knit community that they are called to serve. The medical school's mission is to train physicians to provide for the health-care needs of the people of the state of Hawaii and beyond, into the Pacific Rim.

JABSOM began in 1967 as part of the University of Hawaii's Pacific Biomedical Research Center, teaching basic science in a two-year program. Six years later, it had grown into a four-year school, and it graduated its first class of M.D.'s in 1975. Less than twenty-five years later, a Harvard University survey recognized the School as a leader in reforming and improving medical education.

Though it is part of the University of Hawaii at Manoa, which has 20,000 students, the medical school is relatively small; it admits fifty-eight students each year and possesses a single building on the Manoa campus. However, the School has successfully integrated itself into the Hawaiian islands community. The catalog calls the medical school a commuter campus, which in Hawaii takes on a whole different connotation.

To foster this sense of community, the School of Medicine joined with a program called Community Partnerships with Health Professions Education. The purpose of this group is to form connections with community health centers throughout the islands that create a synergy of medical care, education, and research. In the process, medical students become intimately familiar with the needs of the community.

Another example of JABSOM's awareness of the ties it has to the community is a new research initiative in conjunction with the University of Hawaii's Athletic Department that will focus on sports

medicine and rehabilitation. Hawaii is a popular destination for tourists, sports trainers, and athletes, and this new initiative will provide greater research, education, and preventive medicine that ultimately will benefit athletes and tourists as well as the general public.

Admissions/Financial Aid

Because of the medical school's connection to its surroundings, first preference to the fifty-eight seats in each beginning class is given to Hawaiian residents and to those likely to practice medicine in the state of Hawaii upon graduation. An exception is made for residents of Montana and Wyoming, as those states have no medical schools of their own and have an arrangement with the University of Hawaii. Another exception is a Visiting Seniors program, in which medical students in their last year of medical school at other universities can be considered for enrollment.

JABSOM prides itself on its racial and cultural mix, which represents the rich east-west amalgam of the Hawaiian islands' population. Students from disadvantaged backgrounds are actively recruited and supported through the Native Hawaiian Center of Excellence, which was begun in 1991 and is funded by a grant from the United States Department of Health and Human Services. The grant's purpose is to increase the number of native Hawaiian physicians.

One program, IMI HO'OLA (Those Who Seek to Heal), targets possible students who might not be completely ready to face the competitive nature of medical school, particularly in the areas of language, math, and science. Twenty students are chosen for this program annually from Guam, Micronesia, the Republic of Belau, the Republic of the Marshall

Islands, the Commonwealth of the Northern Marianas, American Samoa, and other American Pacific islands.

Similarly, KULIA (Strive to Reach the Summit), opens eight positions in each freshman class to Hawaiians, Filipinos, and Pacific Islanders who are from socioeconomically disadvantaged backgrounds or who are members of groups that are underrepresented in medical school.

The financial aid office works by the same principles in giving need-based and federal loans.

Preclinical Years

As would be expected with such a strong commitment to serving the greater community, JABSOM's curriculum emphasis is on primary-care medicine and cross-cultural psychiatry. Biomedical research is equally important.

Problem-based learning took root at JABSOM in 1989 and has flourished since then. The more formal way of teaching medicine was replaced by small tutorial groups of students who deliberate about health-care issues. The School believes strongly that this method of teaching encourages overall learning and retention. Students are expected to be self-motivated, critical thinkers who are able to evaluate new data and use what they have learned in the real world. JABSOM calls this program the M.D. Training Program.

Problem-based learning takes place in small tutorial groups and outside of the classroom in the community. Twice a week, a faculty member meets with five to six students for about 3 hours. Aside from laboratory exercises, demonstrations, and library research, students learn basic science by solving clinical problems.

This emphasis on problem solving means that students start developing clinical skills right away. During the first two years, students have a Clinical Skills class, which brings them into contact with patients, and an interdisciplinary class called Community Medicine. Their classroom learning is spread out into affiliated community hospitals and clinics, especially in the second of their first two years.

Clinical Years

Though JABSOM doesn't operate its own teaching hospital, it understands the benefits of taking students into surrounding hospitals and health centers. The medical school is able to invest its resources in com-

munity medicine, research, and cutting-edge equipment and facilities, as well as human resources. Students are plugged into real-life learning situations, develop relationships with community physicians and other health professionals, and become part of the everyday environment of a working clinic. Interdisciplinary training comes through working together with other students in public health, nursing, and social work.

Third-year students take seven-week clerkships in each of the following: family practice, surgery, obstetrics/gynecology, pediatrics, and psychiatry. A special program for six to twelve students—the Longitudinal Clerkship—gives students experience with their own patients, who run the gamut of health from well to acutely ill. For the six months of the Longitudinal Clerkship, students follow their patients' progress. Clerkships areas include obstetrics/gynecology, pediatrics, psychiatry, and surgery.

By year four, students must have thirty-five weeks of required course work, which include emergency medicine, senior seminars, and twenty-eight weeks of electives.

JABSOM has received international recognition for research in human fertility, human heredity, comparative genetics, evolution theory, infectious disease, pharmacology, and cross-cultural psychiatry. Pathology and etiology of disease are ongoing areas of research excellence. Hansen's disease is also a component of this research, as are AIDS and Kawasaki Disease.

The School of Medicine is also involved in research of tropical medicine, communicable diseases, and cross-cultural psychiatric issues. JABSOM's research excels in the area of infectious diseases, particularly in the search for a malaria vaccine. Among all U.S. medical schools, JABSOM students gain experience with the broadest range of infectious diseases.

Social Life

There are probably few U.S. universities at which students can rent a surfboard and fins, a car rack, and a large cooler at the student center. Students can sign up for dance classes in Afro-Caribbean jazz, beginning hula, or introduction to Tahitian dancing. There is also a new windsurfing class.

The hotels and trans-Pacific companies bring tourists and businesspeople to Hawaii from around the world. As a result, Honolulu offers a full range of entertainment, nightlife, and great food. Most JABSOM students live off campus and join the rest of the University of Hawaii's student body for on-campus activities. As the major higher educational institution of the Hawaiian islands, the University of Hawaii is a cultural and sports center for the islands.

The Bottom Line

The University of Hawaii's John A. Burns School of Medicine's location has a lot to do with its strength in

research and education. Its commitment to meeting the health-care needs of the state of Hawaii's multicultural population makes it a unique center of training for physicians, biomedical scientists, and allied health workers who are prepared to fan out to the far regions of the Pacific.

UNIVERSITY OF ILLINOIS AT CHICAGO COLLEGE OF MEDICINE

Chicago, Illinois

Tuition 1996–97: $37,758 per year
Applications: 6,895
Size of Entering Class: 300
Total Number of Women Students: 538 (36%)
Total Number of Men Students: 946 (64%)

World Wide Web: www.uic.edu/depts/mcam/
Contact: Gerald S. Moss, Dean
601 South Morgan Street
Chicago, IL 60607-7128

The University of Illinois at Chicago College of Medicine is the largest medical school in the country, matriculating approximately 300 students every year. Half of these students attend the campus in Chicago, and the other half are divided among Urbana, Peoria, and Rockford. Each campus offers a different focus and has its unique strengths and weaknesses. The campuses are unified by a common application.

The Chicago campus is located in the medical district adjacent to the University of Illinois Hospital, Rush-Presbyterian–St.Luke's Medical Center, and the legendary Cook County Hospital. The school is easily accessible by public transportation and is 5 minutes west of downtown Chicago. The University of Illinois at Chicago (UIC) also offers the Urban Health Program, which actively recruits and ensures retention of students who are members of minority groups.

The Urbana campus is located about 3 hours south of Chicago. Urbana, with its twin city Champaign, is home to the primary University of Illinois undergraduate and graduate campus. Urbana-Champaign is primarily a college town, making research this campus's strength. It is home to most of the University's Medical Scholars Program (MSP) participants, who pursue a Ph.D. in any major offered on the campus or an M.B.A. or J.D. along with their M.D.

Peoria is a smaller city in central Illinois. Students assigned to this campus complete their first year at Urbana and then come to Peoria for the next three years. Peoria (with Chicago) also offers the Urban Health Program.

Rockford is a small city located a little over an hour outside of the Chicago area. Rockford offers the Rural Medical Education Program (RMED), which is intended to encourage students coming from rural areas to return to rural practice in primary-care fields.

There are no financial incentives built into the RMED program (other financial aid is available), so there is no written agreement to practice in a rural setting.

After being accepted to the University of Illinois College of Medicine, students submit a campus preference. The assignments come in the mail a few weeks later (determined on a first come, first served basis). Students assigned to the Chicago campus complete all four years in Chicago. The remainder complete their first year at Urbana and then part ways for the next three years. Of graduating seniors, 61 percent enter training programs in primary-care fields, and 52 percent remain in Illinois for residency. Results of the match are consistent with the national average, with the vast majority of students matching at one of their top three choices.

Preclinical Years

The first two years at the Chicago campus comprise a traditional basic science curriculum, with most lectures taught by Ph.D.'s. Only about half of the class actually attends all of the lectures; a well-established note-taking system (co-ops) offers a description of the lecture topic and transcribes what was said in class. All classes are pass/fail, and the top 10 percent of every class get honors. Since there are no grades, the faculty makes sure that the tests are challenging, and the number of students who fail tests is greater than expected. However, there is ample opportunity to make up these tests, and less than 10 percent of the class repeat the year (although this number is higher than at most other schools).

Although a good number of students never make it to lecture, the first year at the Urbana campus is quite strong. Nationally renowned researchers present the required curriculum while educating students on cutting-edge research. Recently, in response to student complaints, the curriculum was modified to make it more clinical, especially in immunology, microbiology, and neuroscience. The second semester of the second year is devoted to Introduction to Clinical Medicine. This course includes training on history and physicals, clinical problem solving and work-ups of hospitalized patients. This semester also affords students adequate time to study for USMLE Step I.

The first-year curricula at the Urbana and Peoria campuses are the same. An advantage of coming to Peoria for the second year is that the vast majority of classes are taught by clinical faculty members; however, a number of these faculty members teach and test at a clinical level that is too advanced for second-year students. The second year in Peoria is demanding, with challenging, clinically oriented tests every month. On the other hand, during the second year there are three 1-week blocks during which students are assigned to a primary-care clinic in or around Peoria. These weeks serve as a much-needed break from the classroom rigors of second year.

The first-year curriculum at the Rockford campus matches those of the Urbana and Peoria campuses. The second year at Rockford is taught almost exclusively by clinical faculty members. This results in practical lectures, especially given the clinical direction in which the USMLE Step I is heading. A unique feature of the second year curriculum at Rockford is the clinical exposure. Students are assigned to one of three University clinics in the Rockford area, which serve a largely indigent population. Students are required to work at these clinics once a week and develop their own patient pool. Students are largely responsible for their patients. For example, if a patient becomes pregnant, the student not only provides prenatal care but is also paged when the patient goes into labor and delivers the baby with attending supervision. These experiences make the second year in Rockford refreshing.

Over the past four years, the school has made a significant attempt to make the basic science years more clinical, but this has been only marginally successful. Clinical pathophysiology, taught the second year, is one of the best classes and is taught almost entirely by clinical faculty members. With lectures, small groups, and labs, this class succeeds in making basic science information clinically relevant. Also, the Longitudinal Primary Care Program, in which all incoming students are matched with a primary-care

physician in the Chicago area whom they follow for at least the first two years of school, was started recently. For various reasons, approximately 5–10 percent of the class fails the USMLE Step I, but most of them pass it the second time they take it in October.

Clinical Years

UIC probably has more affiliated hospitals than any other medical school in the country. In addition to the University Hospital (430 beds), students rotate at Cook County (848 beds), Christ (792 beds), Lutheran General (608 beds), Mercy (522 beds), Michael Reese (523 beds), Ravenswood (462 beds), St. Francis (250 beds), West Side VA (217 beds), and a number of other smaller sites, including Great Lakes Naval Base (for psychiatry). Most rotations are available at all of these sites, and students can easily graduate having spent minimal time at the University Hospital. The clinical experience is the one of the strengths of the Chicago campus. Students take the USMLE-produced standardized subject exams at the end of each rotation and are well prepared for the USMLE Step II. Students also take clinical tests (with mock patients) at the end of some of the rotations.

Rotations for students at the Urbana campus are spread between two community hospitals, the VA hospital in Danville, and various outpatient clinics. The only residency programs available are in internal medicine, family medicine, and colorectal surgery. This means that students do not have to deal with residents but work directly with attendings. On some rotations, the student is directly responsible for the inpatient service. A highlight is the surgery rotation, which is well above average as a learning and hands-on experience. The MSP program is not well integrated; most students complete each degree separately, often working on their other degree between the second and third years of medical school. As a small community, Urbana does not offer the breadth of clinical experience seen at most tertiary-care centers. Overall, the clinical training is sound for medical students.

Students at the Peoria campus rotate primarily at St. Francis Hospital, with a few rotations at Methodist Hospital (336 beds). St. Francis is a large city hospital with residents in most specialties. A strength is the internal medicine rotation, which offers some excellent pathology. More importantly, though, the internal medicine residents and faculty members are very excited to teach and make an obvious effort to make each student's time there an incredible learning experience. By contrast, the rotation in surgery can be malignant, and the teaching is below average. The fourth year in Peoria offers adequate elective time, with a few requirements in radiology, neurology, medicine, and surgical specialties. Most graduates from Peoria go into a primary-care field, and students do quite well in the match.

Students at the Rockford campus rotate at Rockford Memorial (490 beds), St. Anthony (254 beds), and Swedish American hospitals. During the third and fourth years, students continue to work at the clinic that was assigned during the second year; this takes priority over any other responsibilities. The clinical experience in Rockford is unique in that there are few residents at these hospitals, allowing students to function as interns on most rotations and work directly with the attendings. When there is an admission, the student takes responsibility for the patient and then calls the attending. Even on the surgery rotation, students are assigned to a surgeon and follow her or him around. This results in more reasonable hours and more hands-on learning; students first assist on most surgeries. The fourth year allows two months of discretionary time. Besides the usual handful of requirements, RMED students are required to spend four months on a family medicine rotation at a rural site. Even though an RMED student is allowed to pursue a career in another specialty, RMED should probably be avoided unless the student is sure that he or she will pursue family medicine.

A recently instituted change in the fourth-year curriculum has made a number of specialties mandatory, such as radiology, dermatology, orthopedics, anesthesiology, otolaryngology, ophthalmology, urology, and neurology. The goal is to ensure that all graduating students have a basic understanding of the breadth of medicine. A negative aspect of these requirements is that there is less time for electives.

Social Life

Chicago includes a vast diversity of cultures. Winter is cold, with temperatures hovering around and below freezing, although since 1993, winters have been relatively mild. Housing in Chicago has been getting more expensive but is reasonable compared to other similar cities, such as New York, Boston, and San Francisco. Chicago offers infinite possibilities in nightlife (neighborhood bars, dance clubs, and jazz

and blues), dining (from Italian to Malaysian), and culture (the Art Institute and other museums).

Urbana and its twin city Champaign house a large student body of undergraduates. The community is diverse, and housing and food are inexpensive. The cities have a number of small bars and coffeehouses. Both St. Louis and Chicago are within 2 hours and fill any gaps in social or cultural life. Big Ten sports are popular.

Peoria is a lot larger than most people think. There are a couple of bars frequented by medical students. This city is close to Chicago, Springfield, and St. Louis. Housing and food are inexpensive, and for those with children, there are good schools and parks.

Rockford is a good alternative for those wanting to live in a smaller city in proximity to a large city. Rockford is a fairly multicultural city, with a variety of restaurants and bars. While there are a few neighborhoods that to tend get unsafe due to gang activities, this is a good city to live in, for the most part. Housing is inexpensive. Outdoor activities such as fishing and mountain biking are easily accessible from Rockford.

The Bottom Line

Students have complaints but gain excellent clinical experience. Graduates from this campus are well liked in residencies, since they are well trained and work hard.

Urbana is an academic haven that offers a good clinical education. This is a good option for students who want to do more than just clinical medicine as part of their career.

The second year in Peoria can be trying, as the clinical faculty struggles to teach at the level of second-year students. On the other hand, this same faculty is an asset when it comes to the clinical third and fourth years. Peoria has a good mix of urban and rural exposure.

Rockford is the most student-friendly site, with a unique opportunity to train in a highly clinical environment. Most students from Rockford match in primary-care fields, but a small number each year match at competitive residencies in other specialties.

The University of Illinois is a state school and hence mired in red tape. Each campus has a unique focus, but the application process is collective. Students save money and graduate as good clinicians.

UNIVERSITY OF IOWA COLLEGE OF MEDICINE

Iowa City, Iowa

Applications: 3,600
Size of Entering Class: 175
World Wide Web: www.medicine.uiowa.edu

Contact: Tom Taylor, Director of Admissions
Iowa City, IA 52242
319-335-8305

The University of Iowa is a large university located in Iowa City, approximately 250 miles west of Chicago, the nearest big city. This area of the country is not well known by everyone, but those who spend any time there will agree that Iowa City has much to offer. The small-town atmosphere, combined with thousands of students and one of the largest teaching hospitals in the United States, provides a unique setting for those in the medical field to develop their skills.

Admissions/Financial Aid

Each year, approximately 170 students enter their first year of medical school at the University of Iowa. Eighty percent of the students are residents of Iowa, and 30 percent of the graduates continue their careers within the same state. Although the demographics seem to favor the Midwest, diversity is a strong emphasis in the recruitment of students, and with such a large class size, there are people interested in nearly everything. Forty percent of the students are women, and only half of the students have undergraduate degrees in biology. Students' peers may be writers, runners, musicians, or football players.

In-state tuition is about $9,000, while out-of-state tuition is about $24,000. Meeting the financial burden of medical school can be difficult, and students continue to praise the Financial Aid Office for its help.

Preclinical Years

The first two years of study are focused on the basic sciences—biochemistry, anatomy, histology, physiology, pathology, and pharmacology. However, a recent reorganization of the entire curriculum has incorporated case-based learning. The clinical correlations allow students to gain a valuable perspective on the practice of medicine early in their careers. Another emphasis of the new curriculum is small group ses-

sions. There are still auditorium-based lectures, but classes frequently break up into small groups, which makes the University's 1:1 teacher-student ratio a reality and the class size much smaller.

All training occurs in or near the hospital so that staff members and other resources are close by. The library, which lies immediately between the University and Veteran's Administration (VA) hospitals on the west side of the Iowa River and divides the undergraduate campus from the health sciences campus, is also located nearby. In addition to four floors of books and journals, the library contains a large computer facility for the computer-based courses taught in the first two years. The computer facility is also for individual use and is utilized often in the first two years. Reviewing the current literature is a constant theme in the new curriculum, and although many students complain, they excel in their ability to refer to primary papers during the clinical years.

Clinical Years

The clinical experience at the University of Iowa is first rate. Iowa is well known for its top-ranking ophthalmology, orthopaedic, and otolaryngology departments, but medical students receive solid training in every rotation. The breadth of talent at the University of Iowa is the School's greatest attribute.

The University of Iowa Hospital and Clinics (UIHC) is without a doubt one of the nicest hospitals in the country. It has grown at an impressive rate, while older sections of the hospital are well maintained. The facilities and support staff are excellent. UIHC contains more than 800 beds and serves as the only tertiary care center for a large geographic area. The VA hospital is a monolithic structure typical of other VA hospitals—a functional brick building. Although not aesthetically impressive, it is maintained at high standards and, like the UIHC, has good facilities and a good support staff. The patient population is slightly different from the UIHC, which adds to the experience of medical students.

Iowa has a strong emphasis on primary care, and about 25 percent of the students eventually pursue careers in family medicine. UIHC is very much a tertiary care center, but the ambulatory medicine experience is enhanced by student rotations at a number of small community clinics throughout the state. More than half of the students match with their first choice and more than 80 percent go to one of their top three choices.

Social Life

The University and VA hospital are right across the street from one another, and most of the basic science research occurs in or near the hospital. The business center of Iowa City is east of the river and has several good coffee shops, restaurants, and boutiques. There is a free bus system that takes students across the river to the center of Iowa City in less than 10 minutes, but riding a bike is by far the fastest way to get around campus.

Driving is harder than you would expect. You cannot drive to class or the business center of Iowa City and expect to park right in front of your destination. There is not enough parking. Students either live in the vicinity of the hospital or commute by bus. There are medical fraternities within walking distance of the hospital. The fraternities are an inexpensive place to live with a meal plan and are a good option if you are not particular about what you eat and you want to meet other people.

Sports fans can enjoy Big 10 football and basketball, along with the thousands of fans that flood the area during home games. If you enjoy the outdoors, there are two lakes north of Iowa City, a recreational reservoir and smaller lake for sailing and fishing. Iowa City is a great place to run or bike, and those who do will quickly learn that Iowa is not as flat as some people say. Everything from aerobics to swimming can be enjoyed at the Fieldhouse, a sports and fitness facility right next to the hospital.

If you get bored of Iowa City, Chicago is only a 4-hour drive away. Of course, you can go anywhere from the airport in Cedar Rapids, which is 30 minutes north of the campus. It has only one terminal but at least four different airlines operate flights to Denver, Minneapolis, Saint Louis, and Chicago before connecting to other destinations.

Iowa City offers almost every kind of weather. Rain washes the snow away in spring, and when the sun comes out, everyone seems to be outside. The summer is quite warm and humid, while the fall brings cooler temperatures and the changing of the leaves' colors. The winter is bitter cold at times with subzero temperatures but snowfall is usually reasonable.

The Bottom Line

The University of Iowa College of Medicine offers students a solid training in basic sciences and clinical medicine. Iowa City is an easy place to live, especially for those who love the outdoors.

UNIVERSITY OF KANSAS SCHOOL OF MEDICINE

Lawrence, Kansas

Students Receiving Financial Aid: 92%
Applications: 1,570
Size of Entering Class: 175
Total Number of Women Students: 280 (40%)
Total Number of Men Students: 423 (60%)

World Wide Web: www.kumc.edu/som/som.html
Contact: Peggy Heinen, Admissions Coordinator
Lawrence, KS 66045
913-588-5283

Change is good. Students who believe in this mantra may find that the University of Kansas School of Medicine is right for them. Two years ago, the School installed a new Dean and restructured the entire curriculum. The changes in the curriculum have provoked a bitter debate among students and faculty about the "right" way to teach and learn.

Admissions/Financial Aid

Students who have an interest in University of Kansas are usually prototypical type-A premed students who need to size up the competition of Kansas residents. Although these options are not mutually exclusive, it is the individual who possesses one third of these qualities whom the admissions committee seeks. Although more nonresidents actually apply (approximately 66 percent of total applicants), only 8 to 12 percent are granted an interview. Stated another way, even though Kansas residents and those with Kansas ties comprise only 33 percent (approximately) of the total applicant pool, roughly 90 percent of these candidates are interviewed. The entering class directly reflects this interviewing selectivity, with close to 90 percent of 175 calling themselves Kansas residents.

The student body is highly diverse, with a blend of ethnicities (15 percent are members of minority groups), ages (ranging from recent college graduates to those who have already paid off their college loans from the earnings of their previous careers), and experiences. The ratio of women to men is approximately 2:3.

Preclinical Years

The current curriculum was installed in fall 1997. It primarily affects the first year of medical school, but there were also many changes to the following years'

programs. The first year is traditionally reported as the most difficult and, not surprisingly, the least enjoyable of the four years at the School of Medicine. Unfortunately, the change in the curriculum has not done much to dispel this reputation.

The first year is broken into blocks, which are based on systems (cellular, cardiovascular, respiratory, gastrointestinal, endocrine, urinary, etc.). Each of the classes attempts to follow the designated block system and to integrate itself within each block; for example, the cardiovascular block includes classes on physiology (conduction curves, electrical potentials, etc.), cell and tissue biology (histology of the cardiac muscle and the vascular system), biochemistry (protein structure of hemoglobin and oxygen transport), and gross anatomy (the thorax and the dissection of the heart and related structures). This method of cross integration works well with some blocks and rather poorly with others. One of the biggest complaints students have is that certain blocks get too little overall time scheduled. The result is that lecture hours are increased to cover all the subject matter before a prearranged deadline. Unfortunately, the end of each block also ends in a mad rush, with exams for all four classes crammed somewhat unnecessarily into only two days.

Introduction to Clinical Medicine (ICM) offers a respite from the harsh science curriculum and links students to a practicing physician during both the first and second years. This relationship helps make the didactic information more relevant and serves as a welcomed light at the end of the tunnel. Physical Diagnosis, a second-year class, serves as a nice link between the clinical skills learned in the first year and the differential diagnosis that is critical to the clinical years.

Overall, the rest of the classes in the second year are better taught and better integrated. Pathology is the gem of the second-year lectures. It is difficult but is the best organized and structured course of the preclinical years. This correlates to a high attendance in lecture as well as exceptional performance by the majority of students, in spite of the 94 percent cutoff for a "superior" (which is equivalent to an A).

Because of the many changes in the curriculum, the School has become quite fanatical about surveying student opinion. Whether this data is actually taken seriously, though, is somewhat up for debate. Most students become accustomed to not only the sheer quantity but also the nonpotency of the majority of these surveys. Many students have become apathetic and feel they just have to get through the basic science years. It does not help that whatever changes are made only effect the next year's class.

In addition to the surveys, certain departments hold sessions for students to meet directly with course directors. To these departments' credit, much of the constructive input is incorporated and implemented with some degree of immediacy. Students also have the opportunity to voice their concerns via e-mail. E-mail seems to be the best way to address major concerns, such as the number, length, and content of the small-group experiences, and also to address minor matters such as exam information.

Clinical Years

After the completion of USMLE Step I, the class is split into two camps until graduation. The majority of students remain in Kansas City to complete their clerkships and electives. Approximately 50 of the 175 students, however, relocate to Wichita. The decision to attend the sister campus in Wichita for the clinical years is made on a personal level; unfortunately, the student is inexplicably forced to make this decision in the spring of the first year. Some believe that Wichita offers a more intimate education because the overall number of students is smaller. Others move away because they have friends or family in the area. There is no significant difference in the quality of education or information presented between the Wichita and Kansas City campuses—the experience is dependent upon what the student puts into it.

The majority of students seem satisfied with their clerkships and feel that their patient exposure and clinical experience is broad enough. Students find the family practice rotation the most hands-on. This is most likely due to the strong slant toward primary care (especially family practice) presented from the first day of orientation. A majority of University of Kansas School of Medicine graduates go on to residencies in primary care.

Social Life

Hard numbers aside, classmates are relatively easygoing and enjoyable to be around in and out of the lecture hall. Most students defy the traditional cutthroat mentality that students may have become accustomed to during premed classes. Study groups form readily, and helpful review sessions break out relatively spontaneously among students prior to exams. However, as with any collection of individuals placed in a lecture hall, noticeable cliques inevitably form, as do the territories that these cliques carve out in the lecture hall seating. However, the general "us versus them" attitude that the students adopt regarding the professors and the administrators (especially in light of the new curriculum) has a way of bringing these cliques and the class together as a unit.

The Bottom Line

The University of Kansas School of Medicine has recognized the deficiencies in the traditional medical school curriculum and has committed itself to the noble goal of making the preclinical years more comprehensive and unified. Students who are interested in this grand plan should bring their voices, ambition, and patience and a red pen.

UNIVERSITY OF KENTUCKY COLLEGE OF MEDICINE

Lexington, Kentucky

Tuition 1996–97: $20,923 per year
Size of Entering Class: 97
Total Number of Women Students: 216 (38%)
Total Number of Men Students: 355 (62%)
World Wide Web: www.comed.uky.edu/medicine/
welcome.html

Contact: Dr. Carol Elam, Assistant Dean for
Admissions
Lexington, KY 40506-0032

For three of the past four years, the University of Kentucky (UK) College of Medicine has been ranked one of the top five primary-care medical schools in the country. After receiving a grant in 1992 from the Robert Wood Johnson Foundation, the school has implemented important changes to its curriculum, including a greater focus on small-group learning and early clinical exposure. Students are mostly pleased with the curriculum, and most of the faculty members heed student suggestions for changes. Students come from urban and rural areas, are mostly Kentucky residents, and include students from as far away as Belarus and New Zealand. More than half of UK's students are interested in primary care, and many are especially interested in rural practice. However, in a given year, UK graduates enter nearly every medical specialty.

Preclinical Years

One of the most common praises given to UK by preclinical students is that classes average only about 24 hours per week the first year and about 28 hours per week the second. Students with families appreciate just how active a parent and/or spouse they can be in the first year and, to some extent, the second.

The atmosphere is friendly and noncompetitive, but the letter-grading system in most classes, based strictly on percentage scores, tends to promote an over-awareness of grades. Gross anatomy and histology lead off the first year. The anatomy faculty is top notch and very helpful, but the written exams are convoluted. ("They could ask me how to get to my apartment and I'd get the answer wrong," one student quipped.) Biochemistry and neuroscience are the other

highlights of the year, the former for the wit and high expectations of the professor and the latter for elegant instruction.

Small-group classes in the first two years include Healthy Humans and Physicians, Patients, and Society. Students refer to these as alphabet classes, either because of their popular acronyms or because of their perceived lack of difficulty. Introduction to the Medical Profession provides students with the opportunity to learn history-taking and physical exam skills in the first two years and includes twelve write-ups in the second year.

A large array of electives is offered on a pass/fail basis, and research can be performed between the first two years, but most students choose to take a relaxing break. Two of the biggest gripes about the preclinical years are the lack of parking close to the school, for which there is no relief in sight, and the lack of study space. The study space problem has been ameliorated somewhat by a new $55-million library less than ½ mile from campus and will be improved further when the renovation of the medical center library is complete in a few years.

Clinical Years

Students do most of their training in the third and fourth years at UK Hospital (a 473-bed facility) and the adjacent Veterans Affairs Hospital. In addition to these sites, the medical school has relationships with hospitals and voluntary faculty members throughout the state, especially in the central and eastern regions. UK is especially proud of its Sanders-Brown Center for Aging and the Lucille P. Markey Cancer Center, both of which offer research and clinical opportunities for medical students.

The third year includes two months each of medicine and surgery along with one-month rotations in other disciplines, including one month of primary care and another of primary-care pediatrics. In addition, a one-month, off-site rotation in primary care in rural Kentucky is required. While on this rotation, students participate in grand rounds and problem-based learning sessions with their peers in Lexington, using videoconferencing.

The rural rotation is the favorite of most students because of light hours and a good atmosphere for learning offered by helpful voluntary faculty members. In contrast, the most exhausting third-year rotation is two weeks in gynecological oncology, which is constant work from 4 a.m. to 8 p.m. each day, not including reading time. Students have mixed but mostly positive views on other rotations. One common complaint is that the high number of scheduled student activities during the surgery rotation makes it difficult to participate in many procedures. For students especially interested in psychiatry, the rotation at Eastern State Hospital is enjoyable and in-depth.

The fourth year is more flexible, with room for three months of elective rotations. Most students find time for a vacation before graduation. Approximately 90 percent of the class of 1998 matched in one of their top choices.

Social Life

Lexington is often referred to as the world capital of horse racing and college basketball and features a surprisingly wide variety of restaurants and bookstores. The Appalachian Mountains lie just a few hours to the east, and Kentucky is dotted with numerous state parks and resort areas. While many students lament that they are too busy to have a life, nearly everyone acknowledges that Lexington is a good place to live.

Popular class leisure activities include group outings to local bars and restaurants, UK basketball and football games (with tickets purchased through the helpful student affairs office), and weekend skiing, hiking, and camping trips. Once a year, the first-year class sponsors a Lampoons Night, and all four classes gather for the Caduceus Ball.

Housing in Lexington is inexpensive, ranging from $350 to $450 for a one-bedroom apartment to $550 to $700 for a spacious two-bedroom duplex or house. Housing near campus costs about the same as in other parts of town. There are many places to live within a 10- to 15-minute walk of the medical center. Graduate housing is also available through UK, although few students choose that option.

The Lexington economy is vibrant, with unemployment under 2 percent. Crime is not much of an issue. For student couples and single parents, the state offers a child-care subsidy program that pays for most of day care or preschool.

The Bottom Line

For Kentucky residents leaning toward primary care, the choice of UK should be a no-brainer. But those considering specialization should also give it a very close look.

UNIVERSITY OF LOUISVILLE SCHOOL OF MEDICINE

Louisville, Kentucky

Tuition 1996–97: $23,150 per year
Size of Entering Class: 137
Total Number of Women Students: 365 (49%)
Total Number of Men Students: 375 (51%)

World Wide Web: www.louisville.edu.medschool
Contact: Dr. Donald R. Kmetz, Dean
2301 South Third Street
Louisville, KY 40292

The city of Louisville is home to the Kentucky Derby, the Falls of the Ohio, and one of the oldest medical schools in the country. Founded in 1837, the University of Louisville (U of L) School of Medicine joined the state university system in 1970 and has trained more than 40 percent of the state's physicians. Although both U of L and the University of Kentucky have the mission of training physicians to serve the commonwealth, the U of L tends to produce more specialists and to attract more students with an interest in surgery. Most students are from Kentucky. However, the student body remains surprisingly diverse and includes many students who are returning home from distant colleges and others who are from the Louisville area.

Preclinical Years

U of L was home to Abraham Flexner, author of the groundbreaking *Flexner Report*, which recommended two years of classroom education followed by two years of clinical training. The School has only recently changed from a very traditional curriculum to a more problem-based learning and primary-care emphasis. The changes have most keenly affected the preclinical years. One of these changes is the addition of the two-year-long course Introduction to Medical Practice, now in its third year. It has received mixed reviews thus far and is still being refined. There is also a new clinical neurosciences course that has taken the place of the old neuroanatomy and behavioral sciences courses.

Traditional courses, such as gross anatomy and immunology, are still around, as are traditions such as the student-run transcription service (scribes). U of L provides transcripts of lectures for a modest subscription fee, a money-making opportunity for students who transcribe these lectures, and a rich source of

revenue for the student government, which in turn throws outstanding parties.

Grading at U of L is pass/fail, although students are ranked. Many students find the combination stressful. Despite the School's rigorous and competitive reputation, many support systems exist. Free tutoring, arranged through the student affairs office, is usually excellent.

The Health Sciences Library houses many useful resources, including software and videotapes; however, this is at the expense of study space, especially at exam time. Lots of study space is available, however, in unit labs, the student lounge, and empty classrooms. A great place to study is at the law library on the main campus.

Special opportunities available during the summer between the first and second years include both clinical and basic science research on the medical campus and Medical Education and Community Orientation (MECO) rotations, which allow students to study and participate in the delivery of health care in underserved counties. A stipend is provided for housing, food, and transportation. Most students find their MECO experience to be one of the most rewarding in medical school and form close relationships with their mentors. Many students choose to use this last summer off for travel and rest.

Clinical Years

The clinical experience at U of L is one of the curriculum's greatest strengths. In addition to serving the needs of the Louisville area, affiliated hospitals serve patients for specialty care who were referred from Indiana, West Virginia, Illinois, and Tennessee. The Kleinert and Kutz Hand Care Center provides microvascular surgery and attracts patients from across the nation. Hospitals available for rotations include University Hospital, the Veterans Administration (VA)

Medical Center, Norton's Hospital, Jewish Hospital, and Kosair Children's Hospital. Patient populations served and amenities vary widely.

The clinical learning experience has a strong tradition of "see one, do one, teach one." Students are expected to become proficient in procedures before graduation, and some are even comfortable placing central lines. Students are given a lot of patient-care responsibility, often being the first to assess a patient, write a note, and make recommendations; their work is checked by the residents and attendings who write the orders. Students take call with their team (sometimes as often as 24 hours on, 12 hours off) on rotations such as trauma surgery. Individual rotations vary, but the tenor of most interactions among the hierarchical strata is quite formal, particularly in general surgery. Rotations in underserved counties, in contrast, are more informal.

There are plenty of electives to choose from. Two outstanding experiences are transplant surgery and emergency medicine. Louisville also offers many opportunities in specialty pediatrics, including cystic fibrosis clinics and autism spectrum research.

Social Life

Louisville provides a surprising amount of activities for its size. It is home to the Louisville Orchestra, the Louisville Ballet, the Actors Theater of Louisville, and the Kentucky Center for the Arts. Students often usher at these places so that they can see shows for free. Bardstown Road and Frankfort Avenue are home to a number of restaurants and shops.

The health sciences campus features a large-screen television and exercise equipment, and the main campus offers a full-amenities gym. Free personal counseling is available, and the Louisville Medical Student Auxiliary provides programs for spouses of students to meet and commiserate. Also, the Louisville medical community has a strong tradition of professional courtesy, so many local physicians do not charge students for their services.

Compared to the rest of Kentucky, Louisville's cost of living is expensive, but it's very reasonable compared to that of the rest of the nation. Room, board, and miscellaneous expenses are estimated by the financial aid office to be $13,302 per year. The University does own a small apartment complex near the campus, but most students find apartments or homes in nearby neighborhoods and drive to the campus.

The Bottom Line

U of L provides a strong medical education in both cutting-edge tertiary care and rural primary care.

UNIVERSITY OF MARYLAND SCHOOL OF MEDICINE

Baltimore, Maryland

Applications: 352
Size of Entering Class: 145
Total Number of Women Students: 43 (43%)
Total Number of Men Students: 58 (57%)
World Wide Web: www.som1.umaryland.edu/

Contact: John Mollish, Director, Graduate
Admissions and Records
520 West Lombard Street
Baltimore, MD 21201-1627
301-405-4198

The University of Maryland School of Medicine, now 192 years old, is the fifth-oldest medical school in the United States and the first to institute a residency training program. The School of Medicine is home to the oldest building in the Western Hemisphere in continuous use for medical education (Davidge Hall). The University of Maryland is also on the cutting edge of incorporating computers into medical teaching. Medical students have laptop computers and Internet access in the newly renovated multilabs and the recently completed Health Sciences Library, one of the largest medical libraries on the East Coast. Maryland is credited with having the first online mednote service, and students can download lecture slides and audio from the Medscope Web page. Maryland's block program allows students the opportunity to get involved in an endless list of community programs and intramural sports or to watch an Orioles game at Camden Yards.

Admissions/Financial Aid

Admission is competitive. The 1997–98 first-year class had a total of 4,121 applicants (3,088 out of state, 1,033 in state); of those, 511 were interviewed, and there were 144 new entrants (18 out of state). Students are encouraged to apply early. Accepted students had an average GPA of 3.62 and an MCAT average of 10; 47 percent of the students matriculating were women, and 15 percent were members of minority groups. Two second-year medical students serve on the admission committee, and a student and a faculty member or two faculty members usually interview prospective students. Compared to most state schools, Maryland is expensive, with tuition and fees at $12,890 in state and $24,378 out of state. Students are provided with scholarships and grants that average

$5,884 per year, and the majority of the remaining costs are filled by loans or help from family members.

Preclinical Years

While medical school can be intimidating at first, at the University of Maryland, fears quickly turn into a desire to learn with a new laptop and a course in medical informatics, which gives students information on accessing medical data through today's technology. Maryland encourages a problem-based approach to medicine and offers early clinical exposure through patient interviews.

With a block curriculum in place, the anatomy department is a student's first link to medical education. The staff is eager to teach and sets the tone for the open relationship between faculty members and students that characterizes learning at Maryland.

After anatomy, blocks of biochemistry, behavioral science, neuroscience, and physiology begin. Biochemistry is one of the harder courses, but open-book exams alleviate some of the difficulty. Neuroscience is generally easier, while physiology is more difficult.

Within each block, students attend lectures (2 hours a day), small groups, and problem-based learning (PBL) sessions. Small groups may consist of specialized teaching sections, problem-solving workshops, or clinical case discussions. In PBL, cases are presented, and unanswered questions become research topics, which students present at the next meeting. The small groups are low-key and informative. All learning is supplemented through computer integration and online services.

The first year is highlighted by a longitudinal course in Introduction to Clinical Practice. This course is effective in giving students early exposure to patient care and history taking.

During the second year, MSII's become buried in blocks of microbiology and pathophysiology and therapeutics. The workload increases, but the subject matter becomes more clinically relevant. The second year is a bit slow, but Maryland students form a cohesive class with a common goal of passing the boards and beginning work in the hospital.

Clinical training in physical diagnosis also takes place throughout the second year. Pairs of students meet with preceptors who give them hands-on training in history taking and physical exams.

Clinical Years

In general, the third-year clerkships are outstanding. Students are considered integral members of the team and are responsible for patient care. Attendings and residents are eager to teach and are reprimanded for "scutting" students.

Most clerkships are offered at University Hospital, the Baltimore VA, and Mercy Medical Center. In addition, obstetrics/gynecology and pediatrics can be done at two other hospitals in the area. This provides for a diverse patient population ranging from the underserved to the affluent.

While on service, evaluations are less dependent on the student's preexisting knowledge than on the desire to learn, work hard, and be a team player. Each clerkship contains an exam as part of the grade.

The strongest clerkships are medicine and surgery. While on surgery, students may really get involved or may have to resist the temptation to help. Call-on surgery is every fourth night, and students usually get some sleep. The exception is shock trauma, in which students play an active role in managing acute traumas. A separate four-week course in subspecialty surgery (such as plastics, ENT, etc.) is also required and can be taken in one of the elective blocks.

The medicine clerkship consists of two inpatient montsh and one outpatient month. There is no overnight call but students take new admissions and do formal presentations. A lecture series is complemented by weekly teachings. In the spirit of primary care, students also attend a biweekly primary-care clinic and are lectured in preventative medicine throughout the third year.

The fourth year consists of two subinternships, which prepare students to enter their internships with confidence. Fourth-year students must also complete three more electives and spend two months doing rural medicine. Most students do their rural medicine in Maryland, while some prefer to travel to locations as diverse as Indian reservations and as far away as Alaska.

Finding a job is one of the most important tasks of the fourth year, and the dean's office at Maryland is always helpful. The deans are superb in career counseling and are serious about getting students into the programs of their choice. Residency directors hold Maryland graduates in high regard.

Social Life

An orientation program called Human Dimensions in Medical Education (HDME) fosters the transition to medical school. Students spend a week in western Maryland, where they have an opportunity to interact with fellow classmates, upperclass students, and faculty members in a very informal atmosphere. On the first day of school, the Medical Alumni Association welcomes students with a continental breakfast and an evening gourmet pizza party. Later in the year, students take part in a white-coat ceremony, where they are adorned with their short whites and parents get a firsthand tour of the School. Maryland can be competitive before exams, but students always find ways to relax with intramural sports, weight lifting, or aerobics at the gym, which is one block from school. Students can participate in Sympathetic Tone (an a cappella singing group), submit poetry or art to the *Equilibrium* student magazine, or create skits at the annual Follies. Baltimore offers many restaurants, including Thai, Afghanistan, and Italian. The Inner Harbor, a 5-minute walk from campus, offers the Hard Rock Café, Barnes & Noble, and Pier Six Music Pavilion. Housing prices range from $300 per month in nearby Ridgley's Delight to $10,000 per month for one-bedroom luxury lofts. Housing is plentiful in the suburbs. Campus police officers are abundant, and there is a free van service for students.

The Bottom Line

The University of Maryland is an outstanding medical school. Students learn while having fun. Student input counts at Maryland, and the School is responsive to problems (students meet with the dean on a monthly basis). By doing well, students can ensure positions in the most competitive and prestigious residency programs.

UNIVERSITY OF MASSACHUSETTS MEDICAL SCHOOL

Worcester, Massachusetts

Applications: 958
Size of Entering Class: 100
Total Number of Women Students: 218 (52%)
Total Number of Men Students: 204 (48%)
World Wide Web: www.umassmed.edu

Contact: Dr. Jane Cronin, Director of Admissions
55 Lake Avenue North
Worcester, MA 01655-0115
508-856-2323

People who meet the Chancellor of the University of Massachusetts and the Dean of the Massachusetts Medical School for the first time might be taken aback to hear him introduce himself as a state employee, as he occasionally does. He does this to emphasize the fact that he's the head of the state's only public medical school, which is deeply committed to caring for the health needs of the people of the commonwealth of Massachusetts.

The purpose of the University of Massachusetts Medical School at Worcester (UMW) is to graduate clinical staff members for the state's public and private institutions. As such, UMW is a recognized national leader in preparing generalist physicians who are involved in primary care, education, and research.

Relatively speaking, UMW is a new school. It was founded in 1962, but it has not taken long for it to be placed among the top primary-care medical schools in the nation. However, to take advantage of what UMW offers and to get into one of the 100 seats available each year, a student must be a resident of Massachusetts.

UMW's focus on generalist practice gives students a multitude of opportunities to get hands-on training in a full range of settings, from the renowned University of Massachusetts Memorial Health Care hospitals to community health centers and private practices. UMW has a strong dedication to serving people in the underserved urban and rural areas of Massachusetts.

In keeping with the school's primary-care strengths, the Medical School is one of only fourteen medical schools in the nation to have merited the Robert Wood Johnson Generalist Physician Initiative Grant. This project began in 1994 with the intent of increasing the supply of primary-care physicians by 2,000 and provides $2.5 million in funding. The

benefit for students is that they work with the generalist faculty members throughout the curriculum.

UMW encompasses the Medical School, the Graduate School of Biomedical Sciences, and the Graduate School of Nursing. Included are postgraduate residency programs, allied health education, continuing education, and advanced-degree programs through affiliations with other colleges. The University of Massachusetts Memorial Health Care System in central Massachusetts, which includes more than 700 beds and 7,500 employees, was recently separated from the University, but it remains closely linked as a theater for clinical practice for UMW staff members and students.

Not too long ago, UMW revamped its curriculum to stress interdisciplinary learning and clinical correlation of course work. Because the School recognizes that physicians do not stop learning once they get their degrees, students are encouraged to find and use new knowledge as well as to learn the basics. In this age of communication, it is recognized that doctors need excellent written and communication skills, so this is emphasized throughout the curriculum. Students acquire these skills and outlook in a variety of ways—from lectures, small-group sessions, textual sources, and computer-aided instruction to self-instruction. The Lamar Soutter Library has a new Web-based integrated library system for those who are interested in the Internet.

Admissions/Financial Aid

UMW offers advanced standing for any Medical School course. Students have to get the approval of the department.

Students should apply early for financial aid. Latecomers are not likely to receive institutional funding. However, the Financial Aid Office does offer a Learning Contract that students can take regardless of financial need; in it, students who pay full tuition can defer a part of the tuition until after residency training or by giving four years of service to the commonwealth of Massachusetts.

Grading reflects UMW's emphasis on self-motivation, and professors offer periodic evaluations that are used to point out strengths and weaknesses in any given area. If tutoring is necessary, it is available for students in small-group or individual sessions. In addition to specific class work, tutors also help in learning skills, time management, and test taking, among other skills.

Preclinical Years

First-year students are taught the basics of structure and function, but students must participate in a three-week clerkship in family, community, and preventative medicine and a course in human genetics. Twice-weekly sessions, called the Patient, Physician, and Society (PPS) and the Longitudinal Preceptorship Program (LPP), begin the process of learning medical interviewing, physician-patient relationships, physical diagnosis, medical reasoning, and decision analysis. Population-based medicine, epidemiology, ethics, medical informatics, and preventive medicine round out the course work.

Second-year students learn the etiology of disease pathophysiology, pharmacology, and clinical diagnosis. They also begin to explore epidemiology, biostatistics, and psychiatry. In keeping with the multidisciplinary theme, second-year students continue with the Physician, Patient, and Society course within the context of actual patient interviews and small groups led by senior faculty members who explore with the students the societal and cultural aspects of patient health and sickness.

Clinical Years

The same themes are taken into the third year, when students begin a clinical curriculum interspersed with one-week interclerkship courses between their required clinical clerkships and electives.

UMW medical students at the fifteen University of Massachusetts Memorial Health Care System hospitals come into contact with a wide variety of patients from all over the New England area. The University of Massachusetts Memorial Healthcare–Memorial Campus 319-bed hospital offers specialized patient care and research as well as an advanced tertiary-care teaching hospital and clinics. In addition, it serves as a center for high-risk pregnancies, is the regional intensive care center for newborns, and is a center for cancer treatment and care.

UMW students can also connect with other hospitals in the Worcester area. Saint Vincent Hospital is an acute-care general hospital with a wide range of teaching, research, and patient-care facilities. The Berkshire Medical Center is an acute-care community teaching hospital with an active emergency medicine department and a trauma center with coronary, intensive, and respiratory care units. There are many other opportunities for clerkships and electives at other hospitals in the region.

The School has an interclerkship experience in year three that offers interdisciplinary seminars and discussions. During the two- and three-day courses, students are guided by social, clinical, and biomedical science experts on subjects as varied as domestic violence and environmental medicine.

Clerkships, which are usually taken in the third year, require clinical rotations in internal medicine, family practice, pediatrics, obstetrics and gynecology, psychiatry, neurology, and surgery. Clinical practice is particularly important in the clerkships, since it is recognized that UMW graduates are likely to practice medicine outside of a hospital setting.

In addition to twenty-four weeks of electives, fourth-year students take a required four-week clerkship in neurology and a four-week subinternship in medicine. For select students who have demonstrated a special interest or research focus, the Senior Scholars Program provides an opportunity to combine both basic science and clinical experience in a three-month program under the guidance of a faculty member.

One of UMW's other major strengths is research. The adjacent Massachusetts Biotechnology Research Park houses the Medical School's Program in Molecular Medicine. The synergy between the Medical School and the research park provides new ideas, new businesses, and funding. The Medical School and Memorial Health Care attract more than $83 million in research funding annually, with 80 percent from federal sources. The biologic laboratories that are now part of UMW make the University a leader in immunization. Cutting-edge breast cancer research is conducted at the Susan G. Koman Breast Cancer Foundation.

Because primary clinical care for the citizens of Massachusetts is at the center of UMW's curriculum, public service is stressed. The Chancellor is the chair of the Citizen Task Force on Adoption. Medical students participate in public service by working with state agencies to provide health-care and mental health services. Students are not confined to Massachusetts to practice medicine; an International Healthcare Clearinghouse has about 100 organizations all over the world in which professionals and students can volunteer.

Social Life

Medical school is notoriously stressful, and central Massachusetts gives students a number of extracur- ricular outlets. Fishing is a popular pastime. Students can visit Old Sturbridge Village, where the everyday life of a rural New England village in the 1830s is relived, or the National Plastics Center. Hikers can use the Audubon Sanctuaries' five areas. Worcester's Centrum Centre supplies entertainment, from rock concerts to stage shows and sports. The American Hockey League's Ice Cats play in Worcester.

The Bottom Line

As the only public medical school in Massachusetts, UMW students come into contact with a full range of opportunities to work for the public good at an institution that stresses affordable medical education at a top academic health science campus.

UNIVERSITY OF MEDICINE AND DENTISTRY OF NEW JERSEY, NEW JERSEY MEDICAL SCHOOL

Newark, New Jersey

Tuition 1996–97: $24,270 per year
Applications: 3,570
Size of Entering Class: 171
Total Number of Women Students: 246 (35%)
Total Number of Men Students: 453 (65%)

World Wide Web: www.umdnj.edu
Contact: Betty Taylor, Director of Admissions
65 Bergen Street
Newark, NJ 07107-3001
973-972-4631

The oldest medical school in the state, New Jersey Medical School (NJMS) is a relative newcomer to academe. Founded in 1954 as Seton Hall College of Medicine and Dentistry in Jersey City, it fully developed its character after moving to its current site in Newark in 1970. NJMS and its 700 students have a strong belief in improving the quality of life in the community and earned the prestigious Association of American Colleges 1994 Outstanding Community Service Award.

Admissions/Financial Aid

New Jersey Medical School costs $15,509 per year and attracts the majority of its more than 3,000 applicants from within the state. Of those 3,000, approximately 800 are invited to on-site, one-on-one interviews, and 170 are accepted. A variety of students comprise each year's class, including people of all ages. As a result, the mean age of incoming students is approximately 23, but the variance is wide. Also noteworthy is a special program geared toward encouraging students who are members of minority groups to succeed in medical school. Financial aid is offered only to students with demonstrated need. Most students rely on Federal Stafford Student Loans and Federal Perkins Loans. A few scholarships offered by alumni, medical societies, or community organizations exist for students who fit particular criteria, but generally this only provides a few thousand dollars. Another option is the series of primary-care loans that are available for students who commit to a variety of stipulations, including a primary-care residency, often in an area with poor access to health care.

Preclinical Years

A very traditional education at NJMS begins with a strong emphasis on the basic sciences, with lectures in biochemistry and cell and tissue biology followed by genetics, gross anatomy, and physiology, with weekly token cases that attempt to create clinical correlations. Many students study the text book directly and rely on the generally intricate class notes put together by the "scribe," a paid student who organizes and transcribes the lectures. Despite a few dedicated teachers, the first year generally feels like a lost year. The second year, in sharp contrast, embodies the beginning of an academic camaraderie between professors and students, with vastly improved lecture content and stronger clinical relevance. The core curriculum revolves around immunology, pharmacology, pathology, and Introduction to Clinical Sciences (a class that synthesizes the information to date). Interspersed throughout the first and second year are a variety of classes in statistics, psychiatry, and the art of medicine. Also during the first two years, each student is paired with a community preceptor to observe the clinical practice of medicine, and focus shifts away from the competition engendered by the letter-grade system. A variety of electives organized by students are available in topics spanning medical Spanish and violence prevention strategies.

During the approximately twelve-week break between the first and second year, most students take advantage of research opportunities offered by the School, others apply for grants through societies such as AMSA, and others take vacations.

Clinical Years

Clinical education at NJMS is excellent. Third-year students enter the hospital as invaluable members of the health-care team. The third year consists of core rotations in internal medicine, surgery, obstetrics/gynecology, pediatrics, psychiatry, and family medicine, during which students have the opportunity to rotate between the main University Hospital, the Veterans Administration Hospital, and various suburban hospitals. The level of responsibility is dictated by student desire. Because of generally poor ancillary services in the University Hospital, students become facile in the basic procedures of drawing blood, placing IVs, and drawing blood gases. The urban Newark environment provides a patient population unrivaled by many other institutions; few patients have private physicians at University Hospital. Students see rare entities such as tertiary syphilis and advanced tuberculosis. Standardized board exams follow each rotation and combine with house staff and attending evaluations to provide a final grade. Following a two week break, the fourth year begins with a set of mandatory rotations and approximately five months of elective time, during which students often select electives at the site of desired residencies and take time off for interviews or applications. Students generally place very well because of strong support from academic officials and a growing reputation (especially along the East Coast) of the superior, hands-on training, especially in trauma, multiple sclerosis, and physical medicine and rehabilitation.

Social Life

The School is located off of Route 280. Many attempts are being made to revitalize Newark. The newly opened New Jersey Performing Arts Center has begun to attract big-name musical entertainers, and the ever-popular Portuguese sector continues to lure hungry visitors into its restaurants. Most medical students tend to spend much of their time in the NJMS complex with both medical and nonmedical activities. In the spirit of community development, model programs such as Students Teaching AIDS to Students (STATS), in which medical students visit area elementary and junior high schools to dispel myths and teach facts about HIV/AIDS, and Student Family Health Care Center (SFHCC), where medical students form teams that provide free medical care to community members under attending supervision, coexist with traditional activities such as Operation Smile and AMSA. Intramural basketball, tae kwon do, and the Outdoors Club (which participates in such activities as skydiving and white-water rafting) help keep students busy. Annually, students attend the black-tie Golden Apple Awards banquet to honor the outstanding teachers of the year. The rest of the year has few school-sponsored events, and classmates generally band together to travel the ½ hour into New York City. The majority of students move to nearby towns just north and west of Newark.

The Bottom Line

New Jersey Medical School, much like the state's Great Adventure Scream Machine roller coaster, is not for those faint at heart, but at the end of the ride it provides a valuable experience.

UNIVERSITY OF MEDICINE AND DENTISTRY OF NEW JERSEY ROBERT WOOD JOHNSON MEDICAL SCHOOL

Newark, New Jersey

Tuition 1996–97: $24,270 per year
Size of Entering Class: 138
Total Number of Women Students: 396 (47%)
Total Number of Men Students: 448 (53%)
World Wide Web: www2.umdnj.edu/admrweb/

Contact: Dr. David Seiden, Associate Dean for Admissions and Student Affairs
65 Bergen Street
Newark, NJ 07107-3001
732-235-4576

Robert Wood Johnson Medical School (RWJMS) is one of the two allopathic medical schools in New Jersey and is part of the University of Medicine and Dentistry of New Jersey (UMDNJ). UMDNJ claims to be the largest health sciences university in the country, which is true only because Harvard and Johns Hopkins are not solely in the health sciences business. The Medical School began as Rutgers Medical School in the 1960s and changed its name in the 1980s to honor the former chairman of Johnson & Johnson and benefactor of the Robert Wood Johnson Foundation (a $7-billion giant and the nation's largest foundation devoted to health-care issues). However young the Medical School, the preclinical and clinical education provides a solid foundation for the training of clinicians, with an emphasis on primary care.

Admissions/Financial Aid

Students come from many backgrounds, but because Robert Wood Johnson Medical School is state supported, preference is given to New Jersey residents (90 percent are state residents on admission). Out-of-state candidates tend to be members of underrepresented groups (22 percent); the Medical School actively targets such students through separate tutoring programs and maintains them at nationally high levels. The Medical School is quite selective, with about 20 to 25 percent of students coming from state institutions and more than 20 percent from the Ivy League. Interviews consist of one or two relaxed interviews with basic science or clinical faculty members.

The vast majority of financial aid consists of student loans. The financial aid counselors are helpful in finding sufficient loan funds for students, though

the scholarship library is antiquated. The Alumni Association offers limited scholarships and loans to third- and fourth-year students, and the Foundation of UMDNJ also offers a few half and full tuition scholarships to top students.

Preclinical Years

Students begin their preclinical studies in Piscataway on the medical school campus adjacent to the Busch campus of Rutgers University. The Medical School overlooks the Rutgers Golf Course, and preclinical studies continue in a quaint, relatively safe suburban setting. The Medical School does not have dormitories, and students live in one of the many town-house complexes within 10 miles of Piscataway. Students should expect to pay $1200 or more for a three-bedroom town house, with a cost of living that is relatively high by New Jersey standards. Vehicles are usually a necessity in New Jersey. Students have the advantage of being in a college town, and there are plenty of nice restaurants in the New Brunswick area. The Medical School is also an hour away from New York, Philadelphia, and the Jersey shore.

The preclinical curriculum was recently changed to include an introduction to the patient experience, but the curriculum still emphasizes the traditional lecture experience. Many top students do not attend class and instead rely on the student-run note-taking service. Many classes do include small groups for discussion and case presentations. Old exams are placed on file for most classes by faculty members. Grading is by honors/high pass/pass/low pass/fail system, which fosters a friendly competitive environment. RWJ faculty members produce the top-selling review books in biochemistry and pharmacology, but there are few exciting lecture experiences in the first two years. Students regard the preclinical curriculum as a solid foundation to prepare for the Boards. The core of lectures has remained essentially the same for a long time. The Medical School offers a number of student research fellowships for the summer between the first and second years. Research guidance is limited, and finding a research opportunity among the many labs at the Medical School, the affiliated Cancer Institute of New Jersey, and Rutgers University (among others) depends upon student motivation rather than an encouraging dean or faculty member.

Clinical Years

To continue on to the third year, students must pass the USMLE Part I. The core third-year curriculum includes eight weeks each of medicine, surgery, pediatrics, obstetrics/gynecology, family practice, and psychiatry. The rigidity of this curriculum, though well-grounded in primary care, can be stifling. Students do not have the opportunity to take electives until their fourth year, which creates a competitive disadvantage for students interested in specialties with early matching programs.

For the clinical years, Robert Wood Johnson becomes two separate medical schools, each with its own set of deans and faculty members. Students affiliate with either UMDNJ/RWJMS at Camden or at New Brunswick prior to matriculation, though the distinction does not become obvious until after the Boards Part I, when one third of the class moves to southern New Jersey or Philadelphia. Students may petition to change campuses late in their second year, though there is no guarantee that they will get to attend the desired campus. The rivalry between the Camden and New Brunswick faculty members and students is healthy and fierce, with different grading standards, criteria for AOA election, and student award presentations. There are two yearbooks, and students from the two campuses sit separately at the UMDNJ graduation.

The flavors of both campuses are distinct, and the clinical experience diverse. The fifty Camden students spend their third and fourth years at one core hospital (Cooper) and benefit from a close-knit student-faculty relationship. Cooper serves as the primary and tertiary center for all of South Jersey and the heart of an underserved, inner-city population. Third-year students get their fair share of procedures, and the truly motivated can deliver more babies than obstetrics/gynecology interns at community programs. A number of Camden students live in Philadelphia, which is easily accessible to the hospital by subway.

What New Brunswick loses in closeness it gains in the diversity of its faculty and different clinical settings. The 100 New Brunswick students rotate at a number of core teaching hospitals, including Robert Wood Johnson, St. Peter's, Princeton Medical Center, and Jersey Shore. Rotations are chosen by lottery, and with so many hospitals, it is not unusual to see a classmate at graduation for the first time since Boards Part I. Students live in the same Piscataway/New Brunswick area as during their preclinical years and still benefit from the college-town ambiance of Rutgers.

In general, the Camden faculty has stronger affiliations with the Philadelphia hospitals, and the New Brunswick faculty to the New York programs, an important issue at residency application time. Some specialties are stronger at one campus than the other, and students need to be aware of which campus is best suited to their needs. Overall, having two separate medical schools under one umbrella is positive.

The Bottom Line

Robert Wood Johnson Medical School offers a high-quality, affordable state medical school education. Students interested in primary care should consider RWJ over almost any private non-Ivy League medical school. Students do just as well in residency placement in primary care with an RWJ education as with an expensive private one. RWJ students are beginning to break the glass ceiling at some of the top hospitals and in the top specialties. This trend is likely to increase in the coming years, despite the state school connection, with more name recognition. Students interested in highly competitive specialties have plenty of resources and opportunities available within the UMDNJ system to match at great programs and with effort and luck can easily outshine average students at well-connected private medical schools.

UNIVERSITY OF MEDICINE AND DENTISTRY OF NEW JERSEY SCHOOL OF OSTEOPATHIC MEDICINE

Newark, New Jersey

Tuition 1996–97: $23,359 per year
Applications: 3,106
Total Number of Women Students: 148 (49%)
Total Number of Men Students: 154 (51%)
World Wide Web: www3.umdnj.edu/som/index. html

Contact: Dr. Warren Wallace, Director of Admissions/Recruitment
65 Bergen Street
Newark, NJ 07107-3001
609-566-7052

The University of Medicine and Dentistry of New Jersey (UMDNJ) is the largest health-care university in the world, consisting of eight schools. The UMDNJ–School of Osteopathic Medicine's (UMDNJ-SOMs) mission statement reflects the careers of its graduates, many of whom work in primary care: "The School is committed to developing compassionate physicians from the broadest spectrum of backgrounds, themselves dedicated to becoming leaders in their communities and in clinical and academic medicine."

Preclinical Years

The quality of the preclinical education at UMDNJ-SOM is reflected in the 100 percent pass rate students have enjoyed on Step I of the USMLE for the past three years. Basic science faculty members, who conduct their research in the Science Center next door to the Medical School, are always available without an appointment. A student-run note-taking service complements strong, detailed lecture handouts.

During the second year, the major courses—medicine, pathology, and pharmacology—are organized into modules. Although problem-based learning is incorporated into both years, students in the exclusive problem-based learning track work in groups of six with individual faculty members, then rejoin their classmates for the third and fourth years.

Throughout the first and second years, many hours are devoted to nontraditional courses, such as health promotion/disease prevention, biopsychosocial, primary care problem solving, history of osteopathic medicine, and community medicine. Because the material is not tested on Step I of the USMLE, these

courses seem extraneous, but they probably mean more to a student's success as a physician than anatomy or histology. A weekly lab in osteopathic manipulative therapy offers the opportunity to learn a hands-on approach to evaluating and treating patients.

There is considerable exposure to clinical medicine in the first and second years. From the first day, students are assigned to a primary-care preceptor, with whom they work once a month developing physical diagnosis and interpersonal skills. Biochemistry, physiology, and genetics all include clinical correlation involving real patients. In community medicine, students have the opportunity to design and implement health programs. If motivated, students can spend time with any doctor in the hospital or in the free clinic.

The grading system is honors/high pass/pass/low pass/fail, calculated according to numerical exam grades, which are for the transcript only and are not used to calculate class rank. Grades tend to be inflated, with test averages in the high 70s. In general, a sense of camaraderie is strong among each class of approximately 75 students.

The academic center is relatively new and has excellent facilities. Some complain, however, that there is not enough study space, that there are too many hours of course work, and that classrooms are too small. Four 24-hour computer labs provide a variety of educational and noneducational software. A small library contains enough materials, and unavailable resources can be obtained within one day. A cognitive skills coordinator is on staff to help with national

Board preparation and to assist students having academic difficulty.

Clinical Years

The core teaching affiliate is the three-hospital Kennedy Health Systems. Although the three are not far from each other, each is located in a different socioeconomic setting. Students also spend a good amount of time in Our Lady of Lourdes Medical Center, an outstanding facility in Camden, New Jersey. The result is a very diverse clinical education.

The third- and fourth-year curriculum reflects the School's commitment to training primary-care physicians. Students spend three months each year working in family medicine and its related disciplines, such as dermatology and ophthalmology. Students rate these rotations highly and say that the improvement in their interpersonal skills allows them to stand out during outside rotations.

Other excellent rotations include obstetrics and gynecology, pediatrics, surgery, and geriatrics, all of which are well organized and combine variety with structure. For example, on the geriatrics rotation, students spend two weeks in the hospital on a geriatrics internal medicine service, then one week in a geriatrician's office, followed by one week visiting several nursing homes. Throughout the month, there are morning lectures, and in the afternoon, there are ethics lectures, case conferences, or multidisciplinary team meetings.

Students are provided with five months of electives, in which they can train at outside hospitals. Many use this opportunity to study medicine abroad, rotate at a medical facility on a Native American reservation, or perform audition rotations at hospitals in which they may want to train. Because the Kennedy Health Systems have the largest residency and fellowship programs in osteopathic graduate medical education, many students choose to stay.

Social Life

Students are active in a number of clubs, including the roller hockey team, the running club, and the golf team. Other clubs explore issues of religion, gender, and politics. The School's active student council plays a role in nearly every important decision.

Apartments close to campus rent for $250 to $400 per month. Stratford is 15 minutes from Philadelphia, 45 minutes from Atlantic City, and 2 hours from New York City. Philadelphia is a culturally vibrant city whose many young residents support a diverse nightlife.

The Bottom Line

UMDNJ-SOM is the right school for those who want to study osteopathic medicine in a close-knit, student-friendly atmosphere that emphasizes personal and academic development.

UNIVERSITY OF MIAMI SCHOOL OF MEDICINE

Coral Gables, Florida

Size of Entering Class: 142
World Wide Web: www.med.miami.edu/
Contact: Admissions Office

University of Miami Branch
Coral Gables, FL 33124
305-243-6791

Anchoring the city of Miami, the University of Miami School of Medicine (UMSM) campus is larger than the University of Miami's entire undergraduate campus. The medical center complex is situated in an eclectic and diverse city of more than 2 million that serves as the gateway to Central and South America as well as the Caribbean.

For 1998, UMSM received more than 2,400 applications for admission and interviewed about 300 applicants. A well-planned admissions session greets applicants with a one-on-one faculty interview scheduled during the day. Applicants have a chance to interact with current students throughout the day, including a candid, unchaperoned admissions luncheon. About 140 students enroll each year, a percentage of those being from Miami's six- and seven-year Honors Programs in Medical Education. Preference is openly given to Florida residents, even though the University of Miami is a private institution.

The diversity of matriculating students is part of UMSM's character. Classes include former fighter pilots, college mascots, and pairs of students already married to each other. The average age is in the mid-20s but every class includes students of other ages. In 1998, the entering class had an average GPA of 3.71 and MCAT total of 30. In recent classes, students who are members of minority groups have made up more than 40 percent of the class, and some classes are made up of more women than men. Most students majored in either biology or chemistry in college, while about 10 percent were nonscience majors.

Preclinical Years

The first two years of UMSM are extremely structured, and students receive specific schedules. The first semester includes classes on embryology, clinical skills, genetics, biochemistry, and gross anatomy. Students don white coats and interact meaningfully

with patients in the Clinical Skill Program during the first week. Every attempt is made by the faculty, the administration, other first-year students, and upperclassmen to assist new students during the first semester. One of the most important thing that happens during this time is the development of supportive bonds between classmates.

The middle semesters of the preclinical years provide for a much more relaxed and manageable experience. Students generally begin to explore the city of Miami and take on more outside interests. Throughout the preclinical years, lecture hours tend to be well above the national average. A block system of classes begins, in which one class goes on by itself for several weeks at a time, with one final exam. Throughout these classes, the clinical and practical application of the topics is stressed through clinical correlations and problem-based small groups. The summer break between the first and second years is about six weeks, and opportunities for research abound for those willing to look for them. Most students opt for travel and leisure during the off weeks in preparation for a long second year.

The second year revolves around the Mechanisms of Disease course, several months of comprehensive and intense instruction in pathophysiology. There is a strong emphasis on the clinical application of the concepts provided. Students have routinely had four weeks off to study for the USMLE Step I, and the class average is usually in line with the national mean, with several students performing superlatively.

Clinical Years

Most students at the University of Miami consider the clinical years the payoff after two years of seemingly endless lectures and testing. The overwhelming percentage of third-year time is spent at Miami's Jackson Memorial Hospital (JMH), one of the largest hospitals in the country and still growing. Students also rotate to the adjacent Veterans Administration Hospital or Mt. Sinai, a private hospital on Miami Beach. Miami's Bascom Palmer Eye Institute is consistently rated one of the best centers for ophthalmology in the country.

The third year is divided into two blocks, one consisting of six-week rotations in obstetrics/gynecology, pediatrics, psychiatry, and family practice and the other of eight-week rotations in internal medicine, general surgery, and generalist/primary care, a relatively new and somewhat evolving rotation. The pediatrics rotation is felt to be overly lecture- and conference-oriented, but it still provides significant time for meaningful patient care. Opinions of the obstetrics/gynecology rotation are mixed. Family practice offers the opportunity to spend time in Key West practicing rural medicine under the practically complete sponsorship of the University. Internal medicine and general surgery both provide the student with difficult schedules but the greatest health-care team. The generalist/primary-care clerkship focuses on complete wellness; exercise, medicine, and nutrition are considered cohesively.

The UMSM/JMH Medical Complex provides the most complete medical learning environments of which any student could conceive. With multiple organ transplants, a bustling trauma center, and subspecialties that are commonly regarded as among the best in the world, the limit of a student's medical experience begins and ends with his or her imagination. Patient care by medical students in almost every service is not a privilege but a necessity. With the sheer volume that JMH handles daily, it often falls upon students to perform history checks and physicals and present directly to the attending physician.

A large percentage of Jackson's patients speak Spanish or Creole, and students who speak either of these find their skills to be of use. The house staff often includes several alumni of UMSM and is considered to be competent and knowledgeable and inclined to teach. Attendings have an amiable relationship and an overwhelming amount of direct contact with students; most ask questions in order to teach, not intimidate.

During the fourth year, externships and away electives are actively encouraged. Most students do at least one outside rotation, and many do more than one. Given the amount of hands-on clinical experience they receive, Miami students function very well in subinternships.

Social Life

Few cities can compare to Miami in the scope and range of activities and pastimes available at any given moment. Miami is prototypical urban sprawl. With Miami and adjacent areas extending for dozens of miles in any direction, a car is essential. Nightclubs and bars are in no shortage, with South Beach and Coconut Grove both less than 10 minutes from the medical campus. Miami is known for its beaches and weather that routinely reaches 80 degrees at Christmas. Outdoor sports become incredibly attractive whenever free time is available. The cultural diversity of Miami is apparent the moment one arrives, and most students develop a taste for Cuban coffee and other Spanish foods while in the city. Miami is also home to a franchise of each of the major sports as well as the University of Miami Hurricanes, a favorite student attraction. Museums, theater, and concerts can be found easily.

Miami harbors many of the problems associated with any major city. Crime can be a problem, but the campus itself is extremely safe. No violent crimes have been recorded on the JMH campus in more than twenty years. Traffic is a problem for most Miami residents, but given the typical medical student's schedule, rush hour can usually be avoided. The cost of living in Miami is high. Apartments adjacent to the medical campus can be had reasonably. Most students live in the areas immediately surrounding the campus, South Beach, and the upscale Brickell high-rises, although some students live up to 40 miles away.

The Bottom Line

UMSM is a medical school for students with initiative. The first two years are lecture intensive. The clinical years are extremely hands-on and thereby rewarding. The combination of the School itself with the city of Miami, the attached research facilities, and patients arriving from all over the world seeking medical attention specifically from JMH illustrates that there is nothing that cannot be done at Miami.

UNIVERSITY OF MICHIGAN MEDICAL SCHOOL

Ann Arbor, Michigan

Tuition 1996–97: $27,216 per year
Size of Entering Class: 170
World Wide Web: www.med.umich.edu/
  medschool/grad/

Contact: Cheryl J. Grostic, Staff Assistant
  Ann Arbor, MI 48109
  734-936-1508

Admissions/Financial Aid

The University of Michigan is widely regarded as one of the finest medical schools in the nation. It is a public institution, and approximately 55 percent of the students are residents of Michigan. Admission is highly competitive, particularly for those students from out of state. There are approximately 160 students per class, approximately thirty of whom are in Inteflex, which is an eight-year combined B.S./M.D program. There are a few more men than women in the program, but this gap has steadily closed in the last several years. Most students are in their 20s, and enter the School straight from college, other graduate programs, or the work world. However, there are also a number of older students who have taken time to pursue other careers or fields of study. Some students are married and have children. There is no student dorm, but many students live in apartments within walking distance to the medical center.

Preclinical Years

The curriculum is fairly traditional and evolves through small changes made each year. In 1991, the School introduced its "MD 21" curriculum. The first two years of the program remain largely lecture-based, although there has been an increase in other forms of learning, including patient-contact, small-groups, and interactive computer programs. The last two years are spent on clinical rotations, with the M3 year filled with required rotations, and the M4 year largely filled with electives.

Michigan has had a reputation of being a competitive, even cutthroat place. The curriculum is challenging. There are multiple-choice quizzes on most Mondays, which can be a frustrating way to start the week, especially after trying to enjoy the weekend away from classes. However, the first year is entirely pass-fail to reduce emphasis on grades, and the mutual commitment to medicine within the class fosters a strong sense of camaraderie.

The first year begins with the "White Coat Ceremony," in which faculty members present each student with a white lab coat that is symbolic of the entrance into the world of medicine. Many of the administrators and professors give speeches, and family members proudly cheer their new doctors.

Introduction to Pathology is a highlight of the first semester. Dr. Gerry Abrams, always one of the most beloved professors at the School, leads the group through the study of the interesting and unusual. Most of the first-year curriculum consists of the traditional fare, including gross anatomy, biochemistry, physiology, and histology.

The curriculum includes a four-year-long course titled Introduction to the Patient (ITTP), which encompasses many fields of study, including medical ethics, biostatistics, and cultural awareness. Unfortunately, some of these lectures fall short of truly educating students about these issues. The course also serves as the introduction to the patient history and physical. In the first semester, the students learn how to take a thorough medical history, and try out their newfound skills at local nursing homes. In the second semester, the course introduces the physical exam. Class bonding continues as students practice their exam skills on each other.

The second year is more challenging than the first, and is also more interesting. Students learn about all of the diseases and medications that are relevant for the clinical years. The new curriculum introduces an organ system-based course of study that lasts year-long.

For the respiratory sequence, for example, lectures are given on the pathophysiology (how the body goes wrong) of diseases such as asthma and cystic fibrosis. The medications are covered in separate lectures, such as the various inhalers used in the treatment of asthma. This sequence also features medical history tidbits from Dr. Bartlett, and a trip to the hospital to try out pulmonary function to learn about mechanical ventilation. The sequences are complemented by afternoons in the pathology lab during which the students examine the effects of various diseases on tissues under the microscope.

ITTP continues as well. During the year, the students must perform five complete history and physicals on hospitalized patients. They also come across several SPIs—Simulated Patient Instructors. These are people who are paid to be examined by medical students and to offer feedback. As an M2, students learn to perform the female pelvic exam and the male prostate exam on the SPIs. Later, SPIs appear again, for sessions on smoking cessation and HIV risks.

At the end of second year looms the specter of Step I of the Boards. All students take in June, and the School gives students a four-week break to prepare for the boards. The month before the test is long and hard. The U of M exam average is always near the top in the country.

Clinical Years

The transition to the clinical years can be difficult. Interpersonal skills become far more important, and the time commitment to school grows. The School has made a concerted effort in the 1990s to increase student exposure to primary-care and to out-patient medicine. While the overall focus on specialty medicine remains, the administration has been successful in substantially increasing time students spend in clinics.

Michigan students rotate at several hospitals. The majority of rotations are at the U of M Hospital, a large, tertiary-care health center, where many uncommon conditions are seen. Many students spend their time there for rotations in general and subspecialty medicine, surgery, pediatrics, and obstetrics/gynecology.

There is a Veterans Hospital nearby. Students spend several months there, and can get more hands-on experience than at the other hospitals. There are also several community hospitals that are affiliated with U of M, including St. Joseph's Hospital, where almost all of the required rotations are offered. Fewer selections are available at Oakwood Hospital and Beaumont. Students rotate through one month of Family Medicine and a thirteen-week longitudinal primary-care experience at local clinics.

The fourth year is all electives. Everyone must do two months of subinternships, where they act as interns. A month of Science in the Clinics" is also required, in which the basic sciences are integrated in the first two years with clinical medicine. Offerings range from a medicine and law class to learning how to better understand the medical literature. Otherwise, plenty of time is available for residency interviewing and to do rotations away from Michigan (often outside of the U.S.). Another favorite of students is acting as a camp counselor for children with Hemophilia.

Social Life

Outside of medical school, there is no shortage of activities. The School's student life is rich and varied, with many heavily attended community service projects available through groups such as AMSA. The weekends bring nightlife in Ann Arbor, which is a college town of approximately 100,000 people. There are several bars frequented by medical students. The medical fraternities can also be counted on to throw several popular parties each year. Ann Arbor has a remarkable number of excellent restaurants for a city of its size.

Galens is a unique student group at Michigan, which has been around for at least seventy years. This group has monthly meetings, which feature well-known professors telling jokes, and sponsors the Galens Smoker, a yearly medical student musical, which must be seen to be believed. The heart of Galens is "Tag Days," two days in December when students canvas virtually every corner in Ann Arbor to raise money for children's charities in the area—up to $70,000 is raised yearly.

The University of Michigan has a terrific reputation with residency coordinators. The students are well received at interviews. Approximately 90 percent of the students match to one of their top three choices of residency. While many choose to remain within the state for their postgraduate training, others choose to look elsewhere and match successfully all over the country, from New England to California.

The residency match itself is the culmination of the class bonding experience. The students gather for lunch, anxiously awaiting their fates. They are called up to a microphone individually, to share their future destination with their classmates just as they find out themselves.

Choice of specialty varies widely year-to-year. There is an increasing number of students who choose to enter the primary-care specialties.

Michigan has a strong tradition in sending students into surgery and the surgical subspecialties; these represent some of the strongest programs at the U of M itself.

The Bottom Line

Whatever their choice may be for a medical career, alumni feel that they have been extraordinarily well prepared at the University of Michigan.

UNIVERSITY OF MINNESOTA–DULUTH SCHOOL OF MEDICINE

Duluth, Minnesota

Students Receiving Financial Aid: 76%
Applications: 1,142
Size of Entering Class: 53
Total Number of Women Students: 70 (57%)
Total Number of Men Students: 52 (43%)
World Wide Web: www.d.umn.edu/medweb/

Contact: Lillian A. Repesh, Associate Dean for Admissions and Student Affairs
10 University Drive
Duluth, MN 55812-2496
218-726-8511

University of Minnesota–Duluth (UMD) School of Medicine is a two-year preclinical school that emphasizes family practice in rural communities. Students complete two years in Duluth and then transfer to the Twin Cities for their clinical years. The School's focus on rural family practice influences the admission process; the School favors students from small towns who are interested in primary care.

Preclinical Years

The faculty implemented a new, more closely integrated curriculum in 1997. The School's goal with the new curriculum is twofold. First, students learn the complexity of each organ system by studying multiple disciplines at the same time and learning how they interact together. Second, students are encouraged to work together as a team, and competition is discouraged. Some of the courses, such as anatomy and the behavioral sciences, are still taught in the traditional manner. A few of the courses, mostly in the second year, offer some problem-based learning cases in addition to lectures. Though there are still minor problems to work out and the effects on USMLE scores are yet to be seen, students have been happy with the changes.

Throughout the first year, students undertake clinical experiences. Each student is assigned a family practice doctor as a preceptor and shadows the doctor an average of 4 hours a month. Most students find this a welcome break from the typical 8 a.m. to 3 p.m. daily schedule in lecture. In the second year, the monthly preceptorship is replaced with three 3-day preceptorships in a rural community somewhere within Minnesota. During this time, students live with

physicians and their families to observe what work and family are like in a small town. In addition, second-year students participate in minirotations at the local hospitals.

UMD does not have a note-taking service, but one is not needed. Since the class sizes are small, averaging around 50 people, the professors are able to make lecture handouts available to every student. With the exception of biochemistry, in which the book is used for the many diagrams, many handouts are so well done that extensive outside reading is not needed.

For the most part, the teaching is excellent. Because the School is so small, students get to know their professors. It is common for all members of the community to socialize at School functions and play together on intramural sport teams. The support system offered by the School is also quite good. The assistant dean of student affairs goes out of her way to help students, whether a matter is School related or personal.

Between the first and second years, students have several opportunities, including funded, independent summer research projects and teaching opportunities at a summer science program for Native American high school students.

Clinical Years

Students transfer to the Twin Cities campus for years three and four and merge with their counterparts from the University of Minnesota. One of the negative aspects to the transfer is that UMD students are unfamiliar with the hospitals in Minneapolis and St. Paul, and it takes some extra time to adjust to the new setting. Another drawback is that housing is more expensive and more difficult to find than in Duluth. Many of the housing opportunities are through word of mouth and the use of apartment search companies. However, UMD students feel that their education at UMD has left them well prepared for their clinical experiences.

Social Life

Most students at UMD are from Minnesota. In addition to recruiting students interested in primary care, the School actively recruits Native Americans from around the country through its Center of American Indian and Minority Affairs. Last year, 945 people applied, 166 were interviewed, and 53 matriculated. Five of those accepted are members of minority groups, and one half are women. The majority of students are recent college graduates (within two years), but a growing number of students are nontraditional.

The interviews consist of two 1-hour, one-on-one interviews with a member of the admissions committee (members include faculty members and physicians from the community). An optional tour of the School (a short tour, since each class has its own classroom where all lectures are given) and lunch with a medical student are also included.

With such small class sizes, classmates get to know each other well. Several activities are planned throughout the year, such as a welcome picnic, skit/talent night, and a winter social. In addition, there are several student organizations that sponsor activities. Some of the ongoing events include teaching health topics to elementary students, answering phones for a call-in television program on health, and volunteering to take blood pressures at a homeless center.

From the moment students first see the city of Duluth hugging the rocky shores of Lake Superior, they know that this is a unique city. Known for its cold and snow, this town of 65,000 people is home to two colleges, UMD and St. Scholastica. In the summer months, Duluth attracts many vacationers. Grandma's marathon starts the season and draws a few medical students each year, some as runners and others as staff members for the medical tent. Duluth has an abundance of trails and bike paths for the outdoor enthusiast. In the winter months, there are downhill and cross-country skiing, snowshoeing, snowmobiling, and ice fishing. There is even the opportunity for students to get involved in the John Beargrease Dogsled Marathon. Aside from all of the outdoor activities, Duluth also has its own symphony, a playhouse, and a collection of coffeehouses, restaurants, and bars.

Housing is plentiful and affordable. There are many apartment buildings as well as homes to rent. A housing file has been set up for incoming students, as has a list for those students looking for roommates.

The Bottom Line

The University of Minnesota–Duluth School of Medicine is a school for students who love snow and are interested in rural family practice. The class size is small, the professors accessible, and the student support services superb.

UNIVERSITY OF MINNESOTA–TWIN CITIES SCHOOL OF MEDICINE

Minneapolis, Minnesota

Tuition 1996–97: $23,051 per year
Size of Entering Class: 185
World Wide Web: www.med.umn.edu

Contact: Alfred F. Michael, Dean
100 Church Street, SE
Minneapolis, MN 55455-0213

Minnesota is the state with some of the coldest winters imaginable. The governor has, on occasion, canceled all school in the state because the temperature is too low. In spite of the subzero freeze that comes yearly, medical school in Minnesota has much to offer, both educationally and socially.

Preclinical Years

The first and second years consist mainly of lectures in the mornings, followed by labs and clinical experiences in the afternoons. The first year is primarily basic science, and the most difficult classes are biochemistry (grouped with molecular and cell biology and called BMCB) and neuroscience. The perennial favorites are anatomy and microbiology. The first year continues through the end of July, with August allotted for vacation. The entire preclinical curriculum is pass/fail, but there has been a movement recently to increase student motivation by changing to a letter-grading system.

The second year consists of pathophysiology, pathology, and pharmacology. These run for the whole year and are divided into sections based on body systems. There are also small-group sessions, which are case-based didactics. There are many excellent lectures during this year given by the clinicians who act as preceptors during the third and fourth years. The second year ends in early May, which gives students six weeks to study for USMLE Step I.

Students get early exposure to clinical medicine. The first year is spent learning the medical interview and the physical exam through practice on fellow classmates and real patients. The second year consists of minirotations two half days or one full day per week in pediatrics, neurology, medicine, and family practice. At the end of the second year, the clinical medicine class culminates in a 4-hour Saturday exam.

In this session, second years are the "doctors," and they are required to examine third and fourth year students who are acting as patients with specific diseases. This is a good way to receive feedback in a nonthreatening setting prior to beginning the clinical years.

Clinical Years

The University of Minnesota–Twin Cities Campus Medical School differs from many other medical schools in that the third and fourth years are lumped together. The School requires a certain number of core rotations for graduation, but these can be done at any time during the two years. The main reason for this system is that there is not enough room for so many students to do all their core rotations during the third year. The class (already about 180 people) swells with students from the Duluth program and various other students who have taken time off for research or personal reasons. These two years are very flexible. It is possible for students to tailor their rotation schedules so that they have some experience before entering the rotation in a chosen field. It also makes scheduling for vacation, rotations away, or parenting significantly easier. Students are guaranteed one week off at the beginning of December for interviews and one week between Christmas and New Year's for vacation. Many people take extra vacation between those two weeks in order to have a month or more for interviews. Many people also save the last month of the fourth year for one last vacation or for moving to their new home before residency.

The rotations in the third and fourth years are quite good. Hennepin County Medical Center is the Minneapolis County hospital, and it offers several strong rotations. Since it is also close to the Metrodome and the Target Center, it is possible to treat professional athletes in the emergency room as well. Regions Hospital is the St. Paul County hospital and the site of one of the best clinical rotations available: emergency medicine. This is a busy emergency room with great teaching and substantial independence, where medical students work closely with attendings. The University Hospital is good for specialty medicine. The VA is great for the second six weeks of medicine, as everyone serves as a subintern and, therefore, gets a lot of experience with procedures and patient assessment. Several other private hospitals and the Health Partners HMO contribute to the educational experience as well.

Social Life

The Minneapolis/St. Paul Twin Cities area offers many different subcultures for both night life and living experiences. There is not much on-campus housing available for students, but the cost of living in the Twin Cities is manageable. There are three medical school fraternities near campus, which consist of single or double rooms in a fraternity house with cooperative-style dining available. These houses are also the sites of many great parties, especially following a day of exams. There are also many affordable apartment buildings near campus. On the east side of the Mississippi River sits St. Paul, the older of the two cities and the state capital. St. Paul has more stately apartments and large Victorian-style houses than in Minneapolis. Many people also choose to live in any of the surrounding suburbs, which feature chain restaurants and malls, including the Mall of America.

Downtown Minneapolis is a busy social scene. It is full of popular bars and clubs. First Avenue, one of the music clubs downtown, has been the starting point for many big musical names, including Prince. The Metrodome and the Target Center are also in Minneapolis and are the home of the Minnesota Vikings, Twins, and Timberwolves. The uptown area is a subset of Minneapolis and features three lakes in its center, all of which have paths for running, biking, walking, and in-line skating. This is a fairly popular area. The area surrounding the University campus has many college bars.

Students have access to a relatively new athletic facility located across from the medical school buildings. Since the campus is located along the Mississippi River, there are also plenty of trails to explore during the generous lunch hours of the first two years. Students participate in various extracurricular activities, from intramural sports to public health education. In the Doctors Ought to Care (DOC) program, students educate teenagers about various health-related topics, and in the Healthy Moms/Happy Babies program, students pair up with high-risk mothers, helping them with appointments and seeing them all the way through to their delivery.

Financial aid is available in many forms, including federal government, state, University, Minnesota Medical Foundation, and private family scholarships. The financial aid office is excellent at creating a package to cover tuition and cost of living. There are also some programs that can incorporate research or work programs within the financial aid package.

Summer is beautiful and lasts about 2½ months. Spring and fall are equally beautiful and last about one month. Winter is long, snowy, and very cold. People find plenty of activities to participate in despite the temperature. Moreover, the deep freeze creates camaraderie, thickens the skin, and increases the desire to stay inside and study.

The Bottom Line

The medical school is well respected and offers a broad clinical experience. The area offers beautiful summers, with more than 10,000 lakes on which to enjoy them. Students have a chance to experience the night life of the Twin Cities. Tuition is reasonable. All of this is offered to students who have the heart, soul, and unbreakable spirit required to survive the subzero winters.

UNIVERSITY OF MISSISSIPPI MEDICAL CENTER SCHOOL OF MEDICINE

Jackson, Mississippi

Tuition 1996–97: $13,198 per year
Students Receiving Financial Aid: 99%
Applications: 607
Size of Entering Class: 100
Total Number of Women Students: 122 (31%)
Total Number of Men Students: 268 (69%)

World Wide Web: umc.edu/
Contact: Dr. Billy M. Bishop, Director, Student
Services and Records
2500 North State Street
Jackson, MS 39216
601-984-1080

Blue skies, magnolia blossoms, sunny weather, and a healthy dose of smiling Southern hospitality surround the medical campus of the University of Mississippi (Ole Miss). The relaxed atmosphere and friendly faces that permeate Jackson, the state capital and home to the medical campus, belie the aggressive expansion that the medical center has experienced during recent years and continues to undergo. Nestled in the heart of the deep South, the Medical School might best be described as a sleeper program that is content to stay that way.

Preclinical Years

Ole Miss has its fair share of uninteresting courses in the first two years, despite recent initiatives to incorporate clinical medicine. The situation has improved, however, as problem-based learning has worked its way into many classes, effectively improving the School's traditionally dreary, lecture-based, didactic format. Almost all of the lectures take place in one of two lecture halls.

The first year begins with gross anatomy, which, despite its reputation as a difficult course, proves to be quite benign. The anatomy lab sits on the seventh floor of one of the School's research towers and offers a panoramic view of northeast Jackson. The course goes quickly and leads to histology. Physiology stands out, as it is directed by one of the coeditors of Dr. Arthur C. Guyton's venerable Textbook of Medical Physiology.

The second-year exam schedule is somewhat tiresome, with a protected block of time each Monday morning designated as test time. Professors are required to schedule their examinations during this time. This guarantees at least two days of solid study time, but weekends are forsaken. Pathology dominates the second year. The course is extremely well taught and provides students with a solid foundation for USMLE Step I. A comprehensive, well-organized, student-run note service makes the endless number of lectures during the first two years almost tolerable, as it virtually eliminates the need to take notes during class.

Students get their first clinical experience in the second year during Introduction to Clinical Medicine, a somewhat haphazard course that attempts to combine mentorship by a clinical faculty member with lectures on basic and clinical science. Although there is much room for improvement, the course is reasonably successful at preparing students for the wards. There are also ample opportunities during the first two years to volunteer in the Emergency Department and gain early experience suturing and seeing patients.

Research opportunities for medical students are somewhat difficult, but not impossible, to find. The research landscape around Ole Miss seems to be improving, however, with many new opportunities on the horizon. For example, Ole Miss recently received a massive NIH grant to fund an ambitious study that will track and explore the natural history of cardiovascular disease in African Americans.

Clinical Years

The clinical training is excellent, and the third and fourth years prove to be the highlight. The third year consists of an exhausting forty-eight weeks of core clinical clerkships, including ten weeks of internal medicine, two weeks of neurology, twelve weeks of surgery (divided among the various specialties, including general, orthopedics, and neurosurgery), and six weeks each of pediatrics, obstetrics/gynecology, family medicine, and psychiatry. The clinical faculty consists of professors who are devoted to teaching medical students. Of the remaining four weeks, two are allocated to vacation and one to study time. The fourth week of this block consists of six exams in five days that cover each of the six clinical subject areas. This seems like a lot to do in a week, but four weeks later, students face USMLE Step II without much effort and do well.

Clinical rotations are divided between two hospitals that are within easy walking distance of each other: the Jackson Veterans Administration Medical Center and the University of Mississippi Medical Center (UMMC). Rotations at the former provide experience with managing routine Veterans Administration cases: diabetes, cardiovascular pathology, and a wide variety of cancers. The latter offers experience in trauma, infectious disease, oncology, and an array of other pathology. Furthermore, the high patient volume and insistence that students fend for themselves ensures abundant opportunity for procedures ranging from blood draws to central lines and chest tubes to deliveries. With a bit of interest and determination, there is not much that an energetic medical student cannot get his or her hands into at UMMC.

New clinical facilities seem to be sprouting up everywhere, with more than $211 million worth of construction to be either completed or planned over the next five years. Projects include the recently completed 130-bed Batson Children's Hospital, a women's hospital, and a student union, which will include a basketball court, workout facilities, and a food court. Also in the works are an adult inpatient tower and a critical-care tower.

Social Life

Students, for the most part, come to Ole Miss from other Mississippi and Southeastern schools. They are friendly and not overly competitive. Many are married and family oriented.

Jackson offers restaurants to suit almost anyone's tastes, particularly if one is a fan of down-home Southern cooking and barbecue. The town also has sushi bars that are remarkably good and several solid Italian and California cuisine restaurants. While the nightlife is not for everyone, those interested can go to one of several line-dancing clubs or honky-tonks. The Medical School sponsors several well-catered formals over the course of the year, which are particularly well attended by first- and fourth-year students.

The cost of living is low, and some medical students choose to purchase homes during their four-year stint, typically coming out ahead when the time comes to sell. Several old picturesque neighborhoods, complete with arboreal canopies over streets, which are replete with joggers and dogs, are within 5 minutes of the medical center. Rent is very reasonable in town, and UMMC even offers low-cost, bare-bones housing on campus. The suburbs in Madison County, north of Jackson, lie within 20 minutes and offer a nice alternative to living in the city. Although certain national statistics make Jackson seem a dangerous place to live, crime is centered in several easily avoidable parts of the city.

The year-round warm weather and sunshine are a wonderful combination for anyone who enjoys outdoor sports, including golf and tennis, as well as waterskiing and sailing. Mississippi is a rural state and offers outstanding hunting and freshwater fishing. Moreover, Jackson lies only a short drive from New Orleans and the Florida panhandle beaches.

The Bottom Line

Ole Miss offers an excellent clinical, above-average preclinical, and solidly mediocre research experience and is an overall good deal for those paying in-state tuition. For someone interested in practicing in the Southeast, it is difficult to beat in terms of the quality of clinical training, cost of living, weather and friendly atmosphere. The cost is much higher for nonresidents.

UNIVERSITY OF MISSOURI–COLUMBIA SCHOOL OF MEDICINE

Columbia, Missouri

Tuition 1996–97: $28,224 per year
Size of Entering Class: 95
Total Number of Women Students: 219 (45%)
Total Number of Men Students: 266 (55%)
World Wide Web: www.muhealth.org

Contact: Dr. Judy Nolke, Coordinator of
Admissions and Recruitment
305 Jesse Hall
Columbia, MO 65211
573-882-2923

Located in the small town of Columbia, the University of Missouri (MU or Mizzou) has been a leader in health care in the Midwest for many years. The School of Medicine is part of the MU Health Sciences Center, which includes University Hospital and Clinics, Children's Hospital, the Ellis Fischel Cancer Center, and the Missouri Rehabilitation Center. These hospitals make up the largest health-care network in mid-Missouri and, through the University, are also affiliated with Mid-Missouri Mental Health Center and Truman Veterans Hospital. The School has recently made many changes to update its curriculum, becoming a national pioneer in problem-based learning.

Admissions/Financial Aid

In 1997, Mizzou had 988 applicants (452 in-state). Of the 265 applicants interviewed (250 in-state), 95 were accepted. That class had an average undergraduate GPA of 3.6 and MCAT score of 29.2. The average age of the class was 23.5, and 43 percent are women. Seventy-five percent majored in sciences. The tuition for the 1997–98 school year was $14,254. Most students were from St. Louis, Kansas City, or somewhere in between.

Preclinical Years

Mizzou's curriculum is constantly updating itself. Over the past several years, the School has dramatically reduced the number of lecture hours and replaced traditional didactics with problem-based learning (PBL). The class is divided into groups of eight, which alternate every two months. Through self-directed learning and group teaching, each group focuses on a

different clinical case each week. The goal is to master the basic sciences by learning from classmates. This approach has helped reduce the level of competition and stress among students, and most students value the free time away from the lecture hall. Some complain, however, that students are left with too much uncertainty and that the depth and structure of material covered is sometimes insufficient. One example is anatomy. Traditionally taught as a course unto itself, anatomy is broken into pieces and integrated into lectures and PBL. The School has not made it clear yet how much anatomy it expects students to know or how it intends to incorporate the material into the new curriculum.

The first two years are organized into two-month blocks, with a week of exams followed by a week off (a rarity in medical school). The blocks for the first year are biochemistry, physiology, neuroanatomy, and microbiology/immunology. Class time is limited to 8 a.m. to noon In the second year, class starts at 1 p.m. and covers pathology and pharmacology as well as more physiology and microbiology. The lectures vary tremendously in quality, but there are usually more good than bad. There are usually only six or seven lectures a week; the rest of the class time is devoted to PBL and Introduction to Patient Care (IPC). IPC begins during the first block of medical school, and by the second block, students begin shadowing doctors in the hospital.

Examinations are held at the end of each block. Usually consisting of four separate exams, the tests tend to be quite fair, though the variation in PBL experiences leaves some students unprepared. Nevertheless, the quality of the curriculum appears secure; last year, 99 percent of students passed USMLE Step I, and ten people scored in the 99th percentile.

Clinical Years

All third-year clerkships, except family practice, must be done in Columbia. The third year is divided into six 2-month rotations. The third year is quite grueling, with the easier rotations in family practice and obstetrics/gynecology and the harder in surgery and internal medicine. The fourth year is quite flexible and leaves plenty of time for interviews and electives. The School's strongest rotations are in primary care. Most students enjoy their family practice rotation, where they rotate for four weeks at a rural clinical site. Mizzou is ranked consistently by *U.S. News & World Report* as one of the top schools in the nation oriented toward primary care, and the family medicine program has been ranked among the best in the country.

Students tend to do quite well in the residency match. Eighty-five percent or more receive their first or second choice of residency programs, with 70 percent matching at their top choice.

Social Life

Largely, a consequence of the PBL curriculum, the class tends to be close. Class social activities are abundant, including hayrides, mixers with law students, and monthly birthday celebrations. In addition, there is always a Halloween party, a Spring Formal, or A-Review (an opportunity to make fun of friends and classmates) to attend.

With a population of 71,000, Columbia is the consummate college town, and most activities are geared toward its 25,000 students. Many professional students intermingle with medical students. The School has Schools of Nursing and Health-Related Professions, a master's program in public health, and Law and Veterinary Schools. Downtown Columbia is quaint, with many restaurants and bars, a symphony theater, and stores. Even though it is improving, Columbia is not diverse. Thankfully, St. Louis and Kansas City are each about 2 hours away. The cost of living is reasonable. Most people live within 5 or 10 minutes of school and usually rent apartments for $250 to $300 per month.

The Bottom Line

Mizzou is a university with an old tradition and a new approach to learning. Located in an affordable, fun college town, the School offers students a solid education, with a particular emphasis on primary care.

UNIVERSITY OF MISSOURI–KANSAS CITY SCHOOL OF MEDICINE

Kansas City, Missouri

Size of Entering Class: 113
World Wide Web: www.med.umkc.edu

Contact: Kansas City, MO 64108

At the University of Missouri–Kansas City School of Medicine (UMKC SOM), students must be self-motivated learners. UMKC SOM is a six-year combined B.A./M.D. program. When the School of Medicine accepted its first class in 1971, it drafted a new blueprint for medical education, which many schools around the nation have studied and adopted. The School's innovation has proven to be a viable alternative to the traditional four years of college followed by four years of medical school.

By design, most students are recruited from Missouri. The School seeks people who are intelligent, compassionate, and dedicated to studying medicine. Since most of the class is accepted from Missouri, many (40 percent) also choose to stay in the state after they graduate. This is actually a goal the UMKC Board of Curators and state legislature have set to satisfy the health-care needs of Missourians. The School is also sensitive to the need for primary-care physicians. As a result, 45 to 55 percent of graduates eventually become generalists.

Admissions/Financial Aid

Roughly 100 students (ninety in-state, ten out-of-state) are selected directly from high school to enter the six-year combined B.A./M.D. program. Besides a high GPA and ACT score (recommended above 27 out of 36), the interview is a major part of admission into UMKC. Interviewers (one physician and one nonphysician) look for personal characteristics such as maturity, leadership, reliability, motivation for medicine, a range of interests, and interpersonal skills. Another possible route of admission is advanced standing. These positions are created when students drop out between years. Candidates who fill the vacancies must be from Missouri and must have at least a baccalaureate degree. This past year, only one advanced standing student was accepted.

Long-term financial planning is essential. Tuition, supply costs, and room and board are likely to increase over the six years in school. Already, tuition for in-state students begins at $19,323 per year ($38,995 out-of-state) for years one and two and rises to $22,093 per year ($43,929 out-of-state) during years three through six. UMKC participates in numerous grant and loan programs, and several need-based and academic scholarships are available for qualified individuals.

The best part of year one is that students have practicing physician counselors (Year One Docents) with whom they meet their first patients at local hospitals. Once a week, at the hospitals, students are exposed to the various wards and pick up their first bits of medical vocabulary. One of the most tedious courses is the mandatory Learning Basic Medical Science, taken to develop study skills. During the academic year, students take their regular B.A. classes as well as Introduction to Anatomy and Microbiology. Classes are usually manageable and, for those having difficulty, study groups are available. In year two, courses such as biochemistry and physiology are more challenging.

Clinical exposure is focused on Introduction to Pediatrics and Obstetrics/Gynecology. Some assigned physician groups visit the wards every week, while others read journal articles for a semester. During the second year, the number of students decreases. Whether due to low GPAs, poor clinical evaluations, or personal reasons, about twenty-five students from each class are expelled or extended (graduate in seven years). On average, 82 percent of first-time freshmen who enter the B.A./M.D. program graduate from it.

The beginning of the third year is known as "making it to the Hill" (Hospital Hill). During years three through six, the curriculum lasts forty-eight weeks and consists primarily of health sciences and clinical rotations. The basic sciences are taught in years three and four. One complaint students have perennially is that gross anatomy is taught without cadavers. The School has recently formed a Basic Medical Science Department to restructure the curriculum.

The strength of the School lies in its clinical training, which revolves around the docent unit. Students join a unit of twelve students during years three through six and stay on the same unit for four years under the supervision of a docent. Docents fulfill many roles: teachers, curriculum advisers, career counselors, evaluators, and role models. The design of the docent group, with offices located together in pods in the medical school, helps build small-group teamwork. The quality and quantity of teaching by docents is highly variable. With their unit and docent, students participate in the care of inpatients for a two-month period during the last three years of school at the Truman Medical Center West.

Truman is an inner-city hospital and Level I trauma center, so exposure to a wide variety of cases is possible. Students have a large amount of responsibility in the care of the patients. Students take overnight call, attend outpatient clinics weekly, care for ICU patients, and may be responsible for up to ten patients per day. Sometimes, the clinical schedule is so heavy that little time is left for reading and studying. To succeed, students must be highly motivated to sneak reading into their free time.

Other hospitals include St. Luke's Hospital, Children's Mercy Hospital, Western Missouri Mental Health Center, and Truman Medical Center East. Many students take as many core rotations and electives as possible at St. Luke's Hospital because it is a private hospital with pleasant facilities—a definite contrast to the inner-city population and bare-necessities wards of Truman.

Social Life

Kansas City's (KC's) suburbs (i.e., Overland Park) is one of the best places in the nation to raise children; thus, most of its attractions are family oriented. Shopping is superb in KC and the metropolitan area, especially the Plaza, with its high-end retail shops near the undergraduate campus. There are art museums, a zoo, and several good theaters. A strip of bars called Westport is one of the few places where college students gather. Crime deters most students from living within a 5-mile radius of the School. Rather, most students move into apartments in Mission, Kansas, a suburb about 15 minutes away by highway. Housing is reasonable (approximately $500–$800 per month for a two-bedroom apartment), especially when rent is split with roommates.

The Bottom Line

UMKC offers students an opportunity to get excellent clinical training at an accelerated pace. This program works for students who are willing to commit themselves to medicine at an early age and are able to learn through independent study.

UNIVERSITY OF NEBRASKA MEDICAL CENTER COLLEGE OF MEDICINE

Omaha, Nebraska

Tuition 1996–97: $23,051 per year
Students Receiving Financial Aid: 92%
Size of Entering Class: 120
Total Number of Women Students: 216 (44%)
Total Number of Men Students: 270 (56%)
World Wide Web: www.unmc.edu

Contact: Cheryl E. Scruggs, Director of Admissions
Nebraska Medical Center
Omaha, NE 68198
402-559-2259

Nestled in the heart of Omaha, the University of Nebraska Medical Center (UNMC) is one of the state's two medical schools. More than a century old and the provider of many of Nebraska's clinicians, the College of Medicine draws students primarily from the Midwest. It has a special mission to train physicians to meet the health-care needs of Nebraska citizens, but it is also an established research institution. The M.D./Ph.D. program is very competitive and well-known for its graduates. The Eppley Institute provides students with the opportunity to experience innovative cancer research, and the University Hospital is internationally known for its organ transplant program.

Admissions/Financial Aid

Applications for matriculation have been slowly decreasing over the past several years. Last year, excluding international applicants, 857 people applied, 323 were interviewed, and 123 matriculated. Applicants are competitive and have above-average MCAT scores and GPAs. The ratio of men to women is nearly equal, and members of minority groups comprise 5 to 6 percent of the newly admitted class. The tuition is somewhat high, considering UNMC is a state-funded school. Compared to other schools in Nebraska, the School is inexpensive, at about $13,000 per year. Out-of-state tuition is double this amount. The average debt upon graduation is usually $80,000.

The interview process for UNMC is fairly relaxed. The applicant meets with a member of the admissions committee to discuss anything from career choices to leisure activities. After the interview, the applicant goes on a tour with either a first- or second-

year medical student. This is the best time for the applicant to learn more about the School.

Preclinical Years

The curriculum is based on a core system, with the first two years divided into four cores each. For example, the first-year student starts out with anatomy, embryology, and living anatomy for ten weeks. The School complements the lectures with problem-based learning, labs, audiovisual materials, and small groups, though the pace is sometimes too frenzied to appreciate each of the experiences. The testing system consists of conjoints on Saturday mornings that cover all the material from the previous several weeks. After core one, the student experiences biochemistry; the material is dry and the class is poorly taught. The next two cores of neuroscience and physiology are significantly more palatable.

In the second year, the material gets better. Pathology is the most difficult class. The large pathology text sometimes seems to be an abbreviated version of what students are expected to know. The quality of the lectures varies from core to core, but overall, there is a fair number of entertaining and dedicated professors. By the end of the year, students often seem overwhelmed by class work and the anticipation of USMLE I. Nevertheless, the school is above the national average in the percent of students passing.

Students develop their experience with patients in Integrated Clinical Experience (ICE). This program combines ethics, behavioral science, preventive medicine, and psychosocial dimensions of medicine. The student learns how to perform a history and physical. Students practice on simulated patients as well as on each other. Students also spend five half days per semester with a local preceptor. In the second year, students can also precept in an indigent care clinic or in a geriatric center. Between the first and second years, the student spends three weeks in a rural family medicine clinic. This experience is often highly rated because the preceptor often allows the student to suture, assist with deliveries, watch surgeries, and take histories. Students learn to appreciate their instruction in ethics, physical exams, and patient communication when they reach the third year.

Clinical Years

During the third year, most rotations are done either at UNMC or the VA hospital. The student rotates through family practice, pediatrics, surgery, internal medicine, obstetrics/gynecology, and psychiatry. Family practice and pediatrics rotations can be done away from Omaha. There are nearly six other hospitals in town for the student to rotate through, depending on the service and the attending physician. In the fourth year, all rotations are monthlong electives.

Medical students at UNMC get a large amount of patient-focused care and, depending upon the rotation, considerable input on patient management. Third-year students can expect prerounding, holding retractors, doing scut work, and occasionally performing procedures (blood draws, IV starts, and chest tube placement). Because they are in an urban medical center in a largely rural state, students get exposed to a wide variety of small-town and big-town problems, as well as considerable experience with outpatient, real-world medicine.

The best third-year rotation for most people is surgery, which, despite its long hours, lets people participate in exciting emergency procedures and the occasional organ transplant. The other highlight is family practice, in which students probably get even more experience in procedures than in other rotations. Students spend two months in a rural Nebraska town working closely with attending physicians. With no house staff to compete with, students get to cover the emergency room, first assist in surgeries, and deliver babies. The fourth year gives students a number of elective months. The most highly ranked rotations are those in which students are given a lot of responsibil-

ity to manage emergency situations (the emergency room, trauma, and critical care).

Social Life

The lifestyle is slow paced, considering that nearly 520,000 people live in the two surrounding counties. Housing is affordable, with apartments renting for $300 to $575, depending on location and desired amenities. Sharing a house with other students minimizes costs considerably. In addition, the local chapter of Phi Chi medical fraternity offers cheap housing for students. Campus housing is available, affordable, and within a few minutes' walking distance of campus.

Omaha has a large number of attractions for students and families alike. The Old Market area in downtown Omaha is stocked with quaint shops, coffeehouses, old-fashioned ice-cream parlors, thrift stores, antique stores, and a great selection of pubs, bars, clubs, and restaurants. There are a variety of operas, plays, and symphony performances, and the city is a destination for big-name popular music performers. The Joslyn Art Museum is truly an architectural masterpiece and houses a fine collection of artwork. The Henry Dorly Zoo is world renowned for having the largest indoor rainforest, an aquarium, and the newly added Lied IMAX theater.

For sports fans, the College World Series is held yearly at Rosenblatt Stadium, home of the Omaha Royals, a Triple A baseball team. There are two universities in town that provide exciting sporting events—Creighton University and the University of Nebraska at Omaha, with many events free to UNMC students. Lincoln, home of the Cornhuskers football team, is 50 miles away. Omaha has a large number of inexpensive public golf courses, trails for hiking and biking, and several road races. Every year, many medical students organize skiing trips to the Rocky Mountains or spring break trips to Jamaica.

The Bottom Line

Located in a small but exciting midwestern city, UNMC provides an above-average preclinical experience and a superb clinical experience. There is an emphasis on primary care, with a goal of graduating clinicians who will work in rural Nebraska.

UNIVERSITY OF NEVADA SCHOOL OF MEDICINE

Reno, Nevada

Tuition 1996–97: $21,931 per year
Applications: 128
Size of Entering Class: 52

World Wide Web: www.unr.edu/med/index.html
Contact: Dr. Robert Daugherty, Jr., Dean
Reno, NV 89557

Nevada often conjures up images of bright lights, gambling, and 24-hour entertainment. Part of its image is based upon reality, but there is much more to Nevada than that. The University of Nevada School of Medicine (UNSOM) provides many student options and good clinical training. The Medical School is statewide, with the preclinical years based in Reno and the clinical years located in Las Vegas or Reno. Students have the option of living 40 minutes from world-class skiing in Lake Tahoe or enjoying the sun and fast-paced lifestyle of Las Vegas. As Las Vegas is the fastest growing city in the United States, Nevada's clinical opportunities are excellent and expanding every year.

Admissions/Financial Aid

The University of Nevada School of Medicine receives about 2,500 applications each year, but only offers about 250 interviews. The School puts a strong emphasis on accepting Nevada residents, with only a few spots available each year for out-of-state applicants. Of these, a majority are from Wyoming, Alaska, Montana, and Idaho—states that don't have a medical school. The class is typically 60 percent men and 6 percent members of minority groups. The average age for the entering class is usually 24, with a range from 21 to 36.

The interviews consist of one interview with a faculty member or a practitioner from the local community and another interview with a second- or third-year medical student. Both interviews have equal weight. The interviews are closed (the interviewer knows nothing about applicants except their names). This seems to be popular with applicants because it gives everyone an equal chance based upon their interviewing skills.

The school is affordable for Nevada residents, with tuition averaging $9,000 per year. Financial aid is generous, with most students receiving some form of scholarships or loans.

Preclinical Years

The School is one of the smallest in the country (52 students per class) and offers a unique environment. The students know each other and become quite close in their two years together in the classroom. This is great for fostering lifelong friendships, but everyone knows others' personal business. In addition, because it is such a small school, students have ample opportunity to interact with faculty members and the administration. Every major committee at the School has at least one student representative, including the admissions committee, curriculum committee, and a committee to assist students in need.

The first year of medical school begins with an orientation week, where students are assigned a Senior Colleague to help them through their first year. Senior Colleagues are a resource for used books and advice about how to study. Highlights of the week are several parties thrown by the second-year class so that everyone gets to know each other, and a first-year versus second-year student softball game takes place.

The curriculum at UNSOM is a combination of the traditional format of semester-based basic sciences (anatomy, biochemistry, physiology, histology, and others) and problem-based learning. Students tend learn well from this mix of methods. Nevada has a 100 percent pass rate for Step I in the past three years, and many students score in the top tenth to twentieth percentile every year. The only negative aspect of Nevada's integrated curriculum is that students spend a lot of time in class. The grading system is a combination of letter grades for the traditional science courses and honors/pass/fail for the clinical experiences.

One of Nevada's strong points is the early clinical experiences for first and second-year students.

Students spend one afternoon per week with a primary-care physician in an outpatient setting, which gives them the chance to practice the concepts and skills that they learn in the clinical medicine class. Students also have the chance to see patients in a new Student Outreach Clinic. Created by students three years ago to help underserved people in Reno, the clinic is a great opportunity for students to learn clinical medicine before their third-year clerkships.

Students are active in biomedical research. Last year, about one half of the second-year class participated in a research project. Students have the option of conducting research in Reno, Las Vegas, or other institutions, including the Mayo Clinic; Harvard; the University of Southern California; the University of California, Los Angeles; Vanderbilt; and McGill. The medical school is extremely supportive of students traveling to other schools or other countries for research or training. Some students elect to go to South America to hone their foreign language skills.

Clinical Years

About half of the class spends its clinical years in Reno, the other half in Las Vegas. This allows for a diverse clinical experience. Las Vegas's burgeoning population has increased the number of trauma cases seen at the University Medical Center, one of UNSOM's major teaching hospitals. The medical center is one of the top-ten trauma centers in the U.S., and students get to play an active role in caring for patients in emergency situations.

One of the highlights of the third year is the Practice of Medicine Clerkship. One of the goals of the School is to increase the number of primary-care physicians in Nevada, and the Practice of Medicine Clerkship is an intense outpatient primary-care experience that gives students a strong base of real-world experience. Many of the School's graduates feel that the strong hands-on experience that they gained during medical school really gave them an advantage during residency.

UNSOM graduates match very well, with 90 percent typically matching in their first or second

choice. Even though the focus of the School is to produce primary-care physicians, students find that they are well prepared to enter any specialty of medicine they desire. The only negative aspect to clinical training is that the School does not offer residency programs in certain areas, including ENT and orthopedics, so students who wish to enter these fields do not get much exposure to the life of a resident or to a residency director who will direct them through the application process. The School recognizes this limitation and actively encourages students to perform subinternships at other institutions to increase their chance of matching in their specialty.

Social Life

One of Nevada's greatest strengths is the choice of location that students have for their clinical years. Reno provides good skiing, hiking, and anything related to snow. Many ski resorts, such as Mount Rose, offer special student rates on certain days. Many first- and second-year students can be found skiing on a Wednesday for half price. Despite the great skiing, the weather is surprising mild, and in the summer, Lake Tahoe offers abundant water sports and hiking.

Life in Las Vegas offers all the advantages of living in a big city. Because so many tourists come in each weekend, there are always concerts, shows, and sporting events, and Las Vegas is one of the best sites in the world to celebrate the new year. Almost all students live off campus, and housing is relatively inexpensive and abundant. Some students decide to share a house to reduce the costs. Most students find that their financial aid package allow them to live comfortably.

The Bottom Line

UNSOM is a great medical school for those who want an intimate education at an inexpensive price in two unique cities. Nevada provides both world-class skiing and fun in the sun.

UNIVERSITY OF NEW ENGLAND COLLEGE OF OSTEOPATHIC MEDICINE

Biddeford, Maine

Tuition 1996–97: $23,850 per year
Applications: 2,976
Total Number of Women Students: 171 (43%)
Total Number of Men Students: 225 (57%)
World Wide Web: www.une.edu/COM/compage1. html

Contact: Patricia T. Cribby, Dean of Admissions and Enrollment Management
Hills Beach Road
Biddeford, ME 04005-9526

The University of New England College of Osteopathic Medicine (UNECOM) is situated in an idyllic setting, a short walk from the beach, where the Saco River empties into the Atlantic Ocean.

The focal point of the College is the new multimillion-dollar Alfond Center for Health Sciences, which was completed in 1996. The building is equipped with amphitheater-style lecture halls, laboratories, and study areas. Recognizing the need for future physicians to be computer literate, UNECOM has instituted a mandatory laptop computer requirement. Each seat in the lecture halls is wired to accommodate computer and modem access.

UNECOM opened in 1978 and is young compared to many medical schools, yet it attracts a varied student body. Predominantly, students are nontraditional and have often spent time in other careers or pursuing advanced degrees. The average age is almost 30. Many students are married and have families. With a class size of 115 students, the atmosphere is friendly. Faculty members and Deans are accessible. In fact, the Deans meet monthly with the student body in an open forum to discuss student issues and concerns.

Admission has become increasingly more competitive over the past several years. Since UNECOM's mission is to educate high-quality osteopathic physicians who will provide primary care for the people of the New England states, preference is given to New England residents. However, students come from all over the U.S. and other countries. Tuition is currently about $25,000. Financial aid is available in the form of loans, scholarships, and grants.

Preclinical Years

During an orientation week, first-year classes begin with gross anatomy. First-year students take gross anatomy for the entire fall of first year. The state-of-the-art lab provides plenty of space and equipment. Embryology, parasitology, and histology courses run alongside gross anatomy.

A physical exam course teaches students how to use all of the medical equipment that students purchase during the orientation week. Introduction to Clinical Medicine runs throughout the first year and teaches students how to take a medical history and describes physician patient relationships. At the end of the fall, students celebrate the end of gross anatomy with a bonfire held near the river, where students enthusiastically burn their lab clothes, books, and whatever else they can find.

In the winter, histology becomes important as well as courses in microbiology (including immunology, virology, and bacteriology), biochemistry, and cell biology. A course called Physician Skills helps students become proficient at injections, blood draws, and other skills. In January of the first year, the first clinical experiences begin through the preceptor program, in which students spend time with a family physician and are exposed to allied health professionals. Spring brings classes in pathology, pharmacology (traditionally the weakest class at UNECOM, but improvements are being made every year), medical jurisprudence, public health, nutrition, and epidemiology.

A course in Osteopathic Practice and Principles continues throughout the first two years. Through lectures and hands-on laboratory time, the principles of osteopathic medicine and the application of manual techniques of diagnosis and treatment are emphasized and taught.

Following a month or so of vacation, the second year begins. A major part of the fall is spent with neuroanatomy. The rest of the second year is occupied by courses based on organ systems (musculoskeletal, respiratory, cardiovascular, and others). These courses integrate anatomy, physiology, pathology, pharmacology, internal medicine, pediatrics, and family medicine topics. The clinical experience continues with a yearlong geriatrics course and the continuation of the preceptor program.

All classes are graded on a high pass/pass/fail system. Class rank is nonexistent, making competition an individual rather than general feature of the students. Most students tend to be supportive and willing to help each other. Perhaps the most nerve-racking experience of second year is the first part of the osteopathic medicine licensing boards—COMLEX Part I—which students must take before moving on to clinical training in the third and fourth years.

Clinical Years

Clinical experiences at UNECOM are varied. The third year is comprised of core rotations taught at Clerkship Training Centers (CTCs) in internal medicine, pediatrics, surgery, obstetrics/gynecology, family practice, and psychiatry. CTCs consist of a group of several hospitals and clinics in one general geographic location. UNECOM currently utilizes CTCs in Maine, New Jersey, Pennsylvania, New York, and Ohio; students can plan on spending a good deal of time away from Maine and New England in the third and fourth years. Depending on the hospital, student experiences can range from hands-on to purely observational. Most students get to do more than they might expect, including first assisting in surgery and delivering babies with the attending looking over their shoulder.

The fourth year is made up of electives (approximately six months worth) as well as required rotations in internal medicine, surgery, emergency medicine, and rural family practice. Students use the elective time to pursue interests in subspecialties, research, and/or international health.

UNECOM students participate in the military, the American Osteopathic Association (AOA), and the American Medical Association (AMA) matches for internship or residency. Most students match with their first or second choice of residency. COMLEX Part II must be taken in order to graduate. Graduates are awarded the degree of Doctor of Osteopathic Medicine (D.O.).

Social Life

Biddeford is a small community of just under 20,000, and it often seems like there isn't much to do. However, Portland (a small city of 64,500) is only a 20–25-minute drive away and has many cultural activities, sporting events, and shopping areas. The Old Port section of Portland is a particularly popular spot to congregate and has many restaurants, specialty shops, microbreweries, and small clubs. Boston is an easy 90-minute drive away.

Housing is affordable. Although a small number of graduate student apartments are found on campus (quite utilitarian, but convenient), almost everyone lives off campus. One can find almost any type of rental situation in Biddeford or the surrounding towns (Saco, Old Orchard Beach, Kennebunk, and Portland). A large one- or two-bedroom apartment averages $500–$600 per month, which often includes heat and hot water. Traditionally, many medical students have chosen to live on the beach in seasonal housing that is quite affordable through the off-season. An entire house may rent for $1,000 per month and is usually shared by 2 or 3 people.

Numerous school clubs and organizations sponsor activities and events throughout the year that are open to the entire student body. Students can expect plenty of parties, particularly after each big exam. The annual Holiday Party in December is a formal dinner and dance. Intramural sports teams are available, with competition involving the undergraduate college.

The Bottom Line

UNECOM is a great place for students who have an interest in primary-care or holistic medicine, have a strong desire to understand medicine and the human body, or consider themselves nontraditional.

UNIVERSITY OF NEW MEXICO SCHOOL OF MEDICINE

Albuquerque, New Mexico

Tuition 1996–97: $18,572 per year
Applications: 1,422
Size of Entering Class: 73
Total Number of Women Students: 171 (57%)
Total Number of Men Students: 131 (43%)

World Wide Web: hsc.unm.edu/som/index.html
Contact: Diane Klepper, Associate Dean for
Admissions
Albuquerque, NM 87131-2039
505-277-3414

Founded in 1964, the University of New Mexico School of Medicine (UNMSOM) is a recognized leader in primary-care medical education and has been ranked by *U.S. News & World Report* among the top ten medical schools in the area since 1996. Possessing a new curriculum twenty years in the making, UNMSOM is the model for Harvard Medical School's New Pathways program.

UNMSOM is small in size and less burdened by the often-inflexible traditions of older schools. Most interactions are on a first-name basis, even with the Chief of Surgery.

UNMSOM's efforts are aimed at graduating well-educated, conscientious primary-care physicians who may someday choose to practice in New Mexico.

Admissions/Financial Aid

UNMSOM is committed to enrolling students who are residents of the state of New Mexico. Typically, about 5 percent of the incoming class are nonresidents. All out-of-state applicants must apply to the Early Decision Program (with an application deadline of August 1), which requires an exclusive application to UNMSOM.

UNMSOM grants interviews to all applicants who are state residents; moving to New Mexico a year prior to applying can make a large difference by guaranteeing an interview. With an in-state tuition of approximately $6,000 per year, the School is affordable.

The average age of the student body is 26, and Latinos and Native Americans are well represented.

The admissions interview is a critical feature of the application process. Interviewers dress casually and are impressed by candidates with proven track records in community involvement, knowledge of the Spanish

language, and an expressed desire to practice in underserved areas of New Mexico.

Preclinical Years

The basic science years are a mix of lectures, tutorials, and weekly clinical training at various local practices. By the time the formal clinical years begin, students from UNMSOM are quite comfortable and seasoned in interacting with patients, a fact often underscored by interns coming from other universities.

The format of tutorials is based on the new paradigm in primary-care medical education: problem-based learning (PBL). In PBL, relevant areas in medicine (e.g., histology, pathophysiology, and pharmacology) are covered by going over case studies, which are actual patient presentations discussed in the setting of small tutorials that consist of round table groups of six or seven students with one or two physicians as guides. In each block, tutorials are interspersed each week with traditional morning lectures, in which cases relevant to the topics of the block are discussed.

Paper cases, often based on real-life situations, are handed out to all students, along with the relevant history, physical examination, labs, and other information. A sample case may begin, "A 34-year-old diabetic male comes to see you with a one-week history of nausea and vomiting." Like a slowly revealed mystery novel, the cases are given in discrete segments, allowing students time to anticipate and discuss issues with limited amounts of information.

Throughout the discussion, basic science and clinically oriented questions arise. What is the anatomy and physiology of the gastrointestinal tract? How does diabetes effect gastric motility? This exercise is the essence of student-directed teaching, which balances the formal lecture content of the curriculum and prepares each student for the art of effective presentations.

The lectures are limited to 4 hours per day, with no Saturday morning exams. There is no note-taking service, but lecture outlines are beginning to appear on the Web. Basic science blocks are of various lengths, ranging from three to nine weeks. The afternoons are typically free, except for the occasional labs or ethics forums, where students from the first through third years and attendings gather for formal discussions of ethical dilemmas associated with actual clinical experiences.

The grading system at UNMSOM is letter based. Unfortunately, this feature encourages some degree of competition, although it is quite benign relative to some other medical schools. As a counterbalance, direct written evaluations from the tutorial settings provide a more personalized and meaningful evaluation of each student.

Unlike the standard three-month vacation that follows the end of the first year at other medical schools, at UNMSOM most students are involved with the Practical Immersion Program. Those without extenuating circumstances are relocated to various rural sites around New Mexico, provided with room and board, and assigned to a local physician, who precepts them in the daily practice of medicine, a most valuable preparation for the clinical years ahead. There are still about three months of vacation time built into the first two years in smaller segments.

Clinical Years

At UNMSOM, students may delay taking USMLE Step I until after their third-year clerkships. This rule was instituted as a measure to further strengthen each student by postponing this critical exam until after exposure to the clinical sciences.

The clinical years take place at the University Hospital, a 384-bed acute-care facility with New Mexico's only Level I trauma center, the Albuquerque VA, and many satellite clinics.

Traditionally, the third year is the hardest year in medical school because of overnight call every third or fourth night. At UNMSOM, depending on the clerkship, call frequency ranges from every fourth to every tenth night, with only obstetrics/gynecology requiring students to actually stay overnight. While on call, most students on other clerkships are done by 11 p.m.

To some extent, the intensity of clinical training during the third year at UNMSOM is clerkship dependent. Consistent with the primary-care focus at this institution, the clerkships in family practice, internal medicine, and pediatrics are the strongest, with the faculty and senior residents more comfortable with relegating responsibility for patient care to third-year students.

A common complaint of many medical students here is that they do not get as much hands-on exposure to doing medical procedures as they would like. Unfortunately, it is also possible to complete the third year somewhat lacking in the standard technical skills often expected of starting fourth-year students. To gain experience in this area, students have to be disciplined and driven enough to actively pursue opportunities.

The fourth year is quite standard, with monthlong electives and ample time off for board preparation (USMLE Step II).

Social Life

Life in Albuquerque, with a population of more than 800,000, is a slow-paced affair, with outstanding weather, breathtaking sunsets, and great New Mexican food. In addition to the expected array of museums and naturalist venues (a zoo, an aquarium, a natural history museum, and botanical gardens), there are seasonal activities at the surrounding Native American pueblos, including Harvest Festivals, Spiritual Dances, and others. Acoma City, the home of one of the nineteen Pueblo Indian groups in New Mexico, is a mesmerizing cluster of ancient homes, cisterns, and timeless passageways atop a 300-foot flat mesa. Today, a handful of Acomans still live there, and the site is mostly reserved for ceremonials and special occasions. The public is welcome to daily tours and the Corn Festival celebrations.

A 15-minute drive takes students to the nearby Sandia Mountains, a magnificent landmark for hiking and short day trips and the site of the world's longest tram, which carries people to the top effortlessly. Sante Fe is an hour's drive north; renowned artists display their works in expansive galleries in an otherwise quiet town. Taos, 90 minutes from Albuquerque, is the site of the world-famous Taos Ski Valley, the Taos Pueblo, and more galleries in a sleepy hamlet scented by the constant aroma of cedars.

For outdoor enthusiasts, there is plenty of opportunity for activities all around the state, with natural hot springs, Indian ruins, great hiking, and more.

The Bottom Line

UNMSOM and its hospitals are primarily focused on clinical training. The faculty is superb and quite approachable. The lifestyle afforded to medical students here leaves reasonable time for pursuing outside interests and is family friendly. In addition, with a tuition that is the second lowest in the country, these four years do not pin students into the unpleasant spot of having debt decide their chosen discipline.

UNIVERSITY OF NORTH CAROLINA AT CHAPEL HILL SCHOOL OF MEDICINE

Chapel Hill, North Carolina

Tuition 1996–97: $22,984 per year
Size of Entering Class: 160
World Wide Web: www.med.unc.edu/

Contact: Dr. Paul B. Farel,
Chapel Hill, NC 27599
919-962-8831

The University of North Carolina (UNC) is located in Chapel Hill, North Carolina, also known as the Southern Part of Heaven. Chapel Hill is the quintessential college town—one main street with shops and bars, tree-lined quads, brick paths, and basketball. Even students who aren't sports fans or went elsewhere for undergraduate education quickly realize that UNC is fun.

UNC is the oldest state university, founded in 1795. The medical school was founded in 1879. The medical campus is undergoing an extensive renaissance, with a new neurosciences hospital and construction under way for a Women's and Children's Hospital and an additional parking deck. UNC has one of the largest health affairs complexes in the country and offers degrees in nursing, physical therapy, dentistry, pharmacy, speech therapy, occupational therapy, social work, and public health.

The vast majority of students at the University of North Carolina School of Medicine (UNC-SOM) are North Carolina residents. A large percentage of students declare state residence as they complete undergraduate studies to take advantage of the incredibly low tuition ($3,300 per year) and preferential admission of in-state students. Only 10 percent (about 16 students) of each class are admitted as out-of-state applicants. In 1998, the Admissions Office had a major restructuring. The Admissions Committee seems to be accepting younger and more focused students (average age 23) while maintaining their commitment to a diverse student body. The percentage of women medical students hovers between 40 and 50, and members of minority groups comprise almost 20 percent of the student body.

Preclinical Years

A North Carolina legislature mandate to the state medical schools to produce primary-care physicians resulted in the creation of the course Medical Practice and the Community. The course name is being changed to Introduction to Clinical Medicine; it introduces students to physical diagnosis, history and physical exam skills, and clinical problem solving in the first two preclinical years. For five weeks over the first two years, students are sent to work with a community practitioner.

The first-year curriculum is the standard fare for most medical schools. Award winners include neuroanatomy, physiology, and pathology.

Between the first and second years, UNC students are ambitious. Many go abroad for an international medical experience, and the rest do research or community health projects. Students can get credit for these experiences if they are willing to do the paperwork.

The second-year curriculum is organized around organ systems. The quality of these courses varies, but high points are hematology/oncology and cardiovascular and musculoskeletal systems.

All courses are graded honors/pass/fail for the first two years. For each course, the top 15 percent of students are awarded a grade of honors. For the most part, students work with each other and for each other. It is a wonderful environment in which to make lifelong friends.

One of the best features of UNC is the lab system that is used during the preclinical years. Each student is assigned a lab desk, which comes with a microscope, path slides, and a key for nearby cabinets and drawers. In addition, each desk has outlets for the requisite laptop computer. All entering medical students are required to have a laptop computer—financial aid is available for this. The use of PCs is integrated into the curriculum, with course work and syllabi available over the Internet. Electrical outlets are also available for microwaves, refrigerators, toasters, and coffee makers.

Clinical Years

In the early 1970s, the state of North Carolina established the Area Health Education Center (AHEC) system. Regional centers where students do their clinical rotations are located throughout the state. Students typically rate their experiences at AHECs very highly, and the AHECs typically rate the students highly, too. Grades in the clinical years are honors/high pass/pass/low pass/fail. Because grades are higher at AHECs and they provide housing free of charge (except in Raleigh), many students virtually disappear from Chapel Hill during the third year.

Rotations at the UNC Hospitals in Chapel Hill are largely dependent upon the team. Overall, students have little negative feedback about rotations. Attendings and house staff members are generally nice and helpful. This is also true of staff interactions at AHECs; the AHEC hospital staff is more likely to learn students' names and help them than the staff members at the UNC Hospitals.

Fourth-year students have the most flexibility in their schedules. UNC has few requirements for senior students, leaving ample time to study for USMLE Step II, fill out applications and interview for residency, and travel. Extensive time is spent writing the Dean's Letter with the Office of Student Affairs; UNC students are very competitive. Classmates scatter for residency, but a good portion stay in the Southeast.

Social Life

UNC is dedicated to graduating the students it admits. Counseling, academic assistance, and scheduling adaptations are readily available to students in need.

Students tend to have many interests and participate in many activities. Approximately 10–15 medical students per year attend the UNC School of Public Health (one of the country's best), an equal number do research, and several pursue other interests, including travel and personal relationships. There are clubs and organizations for everything, including the American Medical Association, the International Health Forum, a soup kitchen, wilderness medicine, and low-income health clinics. Students are locally, nationally, and internationally active at UNC.

Class parties are held on a regular basis. A winter semiformal is scheduled every year. One of the best parties is the annual 1970s party. Bell-bottoms and gold medallions are de riguer.

UNC dominates Chapel Hill but not the Triangle, a geographic triangle composed of Durham, Chapel Hill, and Raleigh. Durham is only a few miles away, and Raleigh is about 30 miles away. Carrboro, which abuts Chapel Hill, bills itself as the Paris of the Piedmont. It has a bohemian air with a farmer's market and a food co-op, which hosts wine tastings with live music. The music scene in Chapel Hill is quite vibrant, with multiple venues for up-and-coming rock and alternative music acts. For its size, Chapel Hill has excellent restaurants and attracts residents from all corners of the Triangle.

The Bottom Line

As the only school east of the Mississippi that is ranked in the top 20 percent in both research and primary care, UNC is a great place for students with many interests and a desire to pursue them all. In addition, the climate; the opportunity to see medicine in rural, urban, and suburban settings; and the attraction of being a Tarheel are all positive aspects of UNC.

UNIVERSITY OF NORTH DAKOTA SCHOOL OF MEDICINE

Grand Forks, North Dakota

Tuition 1996–97: $27,302 per year
Students Receiving Financial Aid: 13%
Applications: 447
Size of Entering Class: 60
Total Number of Women Students: 166 (48%)

Total Number of Men Students: 179 (52%)
World Wide Web: www.med.und.nodak.edu/
Contact: J. DeMers, Associate Dean
Grand Forks, ND 58202
701-777-4221

The University of North Dakota School of Medicine and Health Sciences (UNDSMHS) has a nearly century-old tradition of preparing medical students, with a strong emphasis on primary care and rural service. The medical school is housed in what was Saint Michael's Hospital. The architecture and function of the old building are immediately and easily appreciated. A flood in 1997 virtually destroyed the lower levels of the building, which had to be entirely refurbished. This results in a wonderful facility that is steeped in history but entirely state of the art.

Admissions/Financial Aid

UNDSMHS admissions are heavily weighted to residents of North Dakota, Minnesota, and the states participating in the Western Interstate Commission for Higher Education (WICHE). Through the federal Indians into Medicine (INMED) program, an additional seven spots are open to Native American students, regardless of their state of residence. UNDSMHS does not participate in AMCAS and does not have rolling admissions. Demographics for the class of 2001 include 53 percent women and 18 percent members of minority groups. Almost half of the class is married, and nearly one quarter of the students have children. The mean age at matriculation was 24.2 years.

The average cost of medical school tuition, room, board, books, and other expenses is about $25,000 per year. Approximately 90 percent of students receive some type of financial aid. The average indebtedness after four years is $81,500.

Preclinical Years

The first two years are divided into eight 10-week blocks. The first eight weeks consist of Patient-

Centered Learning (PCL), which makes up ~about 80 percent of contact hours for the week. In the PCL experience, students are divided into groups of seven or eight students who collaborate to direct their own learning. Students examine a "paper patient" case and determine what they know as a group. Students study the case as if the patient were seen in a physician's office. The process consists of identifying the chief complaint, constructing hypotheses, and identifying a diagnosis. The diagnosis, however, is not the goal of the PCL experience; some cases are presented with the diagnosis given on the first page. The experience is to learn about the physiology, biochemistry, anatomy, and pharmacology involved with the patient and the disease state. Students spend the week teaching and learning from each other. In addition, there are 8–10 hours of didactic lectures each week to supplement and guide student-directed learning. Following the last group session on Friday, there is a 1-hour patient wrap-up session. A physician with expertise in the area covered by the case comes into the classroom to speak to the students about the case. He or she gives insight as to what the thought processes are at various points in the case, in addition to giving advice about why treatments were given and what the patient's prognosis would be. Frequently, actual patients are present to describe their experiences with a particular disease. This has been the most rewarding PCL experience, based on student feedback, because participants can connect a face with their paper case. Patient perspectives give added meaning to this experience. Students like this curriculum because it helps them develop working relationships with colleagues and teaches them how to find answers for themselves. Both of these skills are key to future practice as physicians.

The rest of the week (20 percent) is spent in Introduction to Patient Care (IPC). In these sessions, students learn to take histories and conduct physical exams. Additional lectures and assignments are related to biostatistics, ethics, human behavior, doctor/patient interaction, and family life cycle. IPC provides students with the opportunity to have hands-on exposure to patients, beginning in their very first semester. The emphasis on the art of medicine that this course provides makes it a student favorite.

At the end of eight weeks, during which students have covered eight distinct patient cases in PCL, students enter into assessment week, which consists of passing an exam covering all of the material examined in PCL and IPC in a national Boards-type format. Students also are required to pass necessary history-taking and physical exam–taking exercises with their IPC facilitator. In addition, a patient case is covered, in which each student is required to address specific questions regarding the patient, as they have already done in the block with the PCL patient cases. Following assessment week is a special studies week, during which students are required to remediate if they have failed any component of the block. If they have passed all of the components assessed, this week is unscheduled time. Some students find the length of time between exams a little unsettling, but most enjoy the low-pressure schedule.

Clinical Years

Third-year medical students have three educational models to choose from: a traditional model of third-year clinical rotations, Rural Opportunities in Medical Education (ROME), and a new model that is in development—Practice-Based Medical Education (PBME).

The traditional third-year model includes six 8-week clerkships in internal medicine, obstetrics/gynecology, pediatrics, psychiatry, surgery, and family medicine, which are followed by two acting internships of four weeks each in surgery and internal medicine at the beginning of fourth year. The family medicine rotations are held in rural communities around the state.

ROME is an eight-month experience in a rural primary-care setting. Students live and train, individually or in pairs, in a nonmetropolitan community under the supervision of physician preceptors. ROME's goal is to encourage students to practice in rural areas throughout the state, where access to care is often not readily available. In this model, students enjoy the highest degree of autonomy, which provides them with a great opportunity to really participate in the practice of medicine. Students who apply for this program must be very self-directed, since there are few, if any, lectures and limited contact with other medical students.

PBME is a twelve-month experience in a multispecialty clinic in an urban North Dakota medical education teaching center. PBME students are introduced to patients in the clinic and follow those patients throughout the year in the clinic, at home, and when admitted to the hospital. This program stresses continuity of care, is practice based and patient centered, and emphasizes community health. This model has not yet been implemented.

While the first two years of medical school take place on the Grand Forks campus, third-year students move to either the Fargo or the Bismarck campus. Fourth-year rotations are in Fargo, Bismarck, Grand Forks, or Minot. Site assignment is determined by a lottery system. This means that a few students do not get their first choice of campus, but students have occasionally switched sites. Some students choose to move twice for more variety, but most (especially parents) prefer to stay in one place for both clinical years. Because there are no fellowships and a limited number of residency programs in North Dakota, students in any of the models receive a high degree of individual attention from attending physicians. This also results in more hands-on practice of medicine than may be available in other schools. All three models place a heavy emphasis on primary care, regardless of the student's final career choice.

Social Life

Grand Forks is a community of about 50,000 located on the natural prairie of North Dakota. State parks, lakes, and rivers in the area provide opportunities for mountain biking, hiking, and fishing, and, in good weather, medical students can often be found on area golf courses. Winter sports are also common, such as skiing, snowmobiling, and ice fishing. The winter temperatures can fall below zero for a week at a time, but the medical school is housed entirely in one building, and most students feel that with adequate clothing, the fabled prairie winters are not a problem.

The University of North Dakota fields many sports teams each year. The hockey and women's basketball teams are perennial NCAA division champs, so sports fans can always find a team to support. UND also has good theater and performing arts opportunities, but, in general, major cultural events are limited in Grand Forks, so students travel to Winnipeg (less than 2 hours away) to enjoy the arts, festivals, and restaurants of that beautiful city.

Although student housing is available, students generally live off campus. A nice three-bedroom house in the area costs about $600 per month. Public transportation is limited, so most students find that a car is necessary. Because the crime rate is also quite low, most students feel very safe. There is a very active social committee at UNDSMHS, which plans a number of activities throughout the year. Social events include a welcoming picnic, a Halloween party, a Christmas formal with the faculty, and a Sophomore Sendoff in April. One favorite tradition is the two

Malpractice Bowl games. The law school and the medical school play a game of touch football every fall and, in the winter, a game of volleyball. This grudge match has become an extraordinary opportunity to generate donations to the local food shelf or other charitable organizations.

The Bottom Line

The University of North Dakota School of Medicine and Health Sciences provides a solid foundation in the sciences, which is evidenced by a 100 percent pass rate on the 1997 USMLE Step I. Also, students receive an excellent preparation for future years of study; UND students do very well in the match. Eighty-three percent of 1999 graduates matched in one of their top three choices. This program centers students on patients as people, teaches students to work together, and prepares future doctors for a career of lifelong learning.

UNIVERSITY OF NORTH TEXAS HEALTH SCIENCE CENTER TEXAS COLLEGE OF OSTEOPATHIC MEDICINE

Fort Worth, Texas

Students Receiving Financial Aid: 82%
Applications: 2,194
Size of Entering Class: 449
Total Number of Women Students: 187 (41%)
Total Number of Men Students: 267 (59%)
World Wide Web: www.hsc.unt.edu/

Contact: Dr. T. John Leppi, Associate Dean of Admissions
3500 Camp Bowie Boulevard
Fort Worth, TX 76107
817-735-2204

The University of North Texas (UNT) Health Science Center is comprised of the Graduate School of Biomedical Sciences and the Texas College of Osteopathic Medicine (TCOM). Located in the heart of the Fort Worth Cultural District, the center's mirrored glass buildings rise above the surrounding shops, restaurants, and museums and afford one of the most popular views of downtown Fort Worth. While numerous civic and cultural events are hosted in the area each year, only students with exemplary time management skills are able to participate in many leisure activities.

Preclinical Years

At TCOM, the preclinical years begin at a relatively easy pace. The first semester is viewed as a transition, which allows students to adapt to a new mode of learning. The most time-consuming course is Gross and Developmental Anatomy. The school provides 24-hour access to the gross anatomy lab. It is not uncommon to find groups of students studying at any hour. The faculty and administration are earnestly trying to trim the number of hours students spend in a traditional lecture-based curriculum, electing for a more problem-based and small-group–oriented curriculum instead; however, students still spend a majority of the first eighteen weeks of medical school in the library or the lab.

Exams and classes are graded on a numerical scale, with passing set at 75 or greater. Classes with laboratory sections, such as gross anatomy or manipulative medicine, generally grade lab portions separately and combine the score with the lecture component to arrive at an overall grade. Professors are

readily accessible, and most see students by appointment in their office or lab. Some professors are known to roam the library the night before a big exam looking for groups of students who could benefit from last-minute clarification.

During the summer between the first and second years, students are required to complete a one-week preceptorship in family medicine with a local physician. Also available are paid positions as gross anatomy prosectors and teaching assistants. A number of dual-degree programs and fellowships are offered for qualified students in good academic standing. These include D.O./Ph.D. and D.O./M.S. combinations, which are available in most of the biomedical sciences, such as pharmacology, biochemistry, integrative physiology, or immunology. A Master of Public Health (M.P.H.) degree is also offered.

Students finish their preclinical sciences by the end of the second year and have three or four weeks to prepare for Step I of the USMLE and COMLEX. While students are required to pass the COMLEX to advance to the clinical phase of their training, the USMLE is optional. Still, TCOM students are encouraged to sit for the USMLE examination, especially if they intend to pursue ACGME-approved residencies after graduation.

Clinical Years

Students rotate at several local hospitals and clinical health-are facilities. In addition, the UNT Health Science Center is a member of the North Texas Medical Educational Consortium, whose mission is to demonstrate a community health model of generalist medical education that draws on the strengths of both allopathic and osteopathic traditions of American medicine. This translates into a wide variety of choices for rotations situated in the Dallas-Fort Worth Metroplex. While some placements are determined by lottery, students maintain considerable control in securing their preferred practice setting for a number of rotations. Some students elect for more rural-based experiences, while others prefer exposure to more urban and city-based locations.

There are fifty-six weeks of required core rotations, which, barring unusual circumstances, must be completed at locally approved sites or at American Osteopathic Association–approved clinical education sites elsewhere. This leaves twenty weeks for electives, which may be completed anywhere the student wishes, and one academic month. The academic month is traditionally spent working on individual projects or arranging internship and residency interviews. Sites with consistently strong reviews include obstetrics and gynecology at the Dallas-Fort Worth Medical Center, psychiatry and emergency medicine at John Peter Smith Hospital, and subspecialty internal medicine at the University of Texas Health Science Center at Tyler.

Predoctoral teaching and research fellowships in osteopathic manipulative medicine are available to students on a competitive basis. Fellows rotate into the manipulative medicine department in four 3-month blocks during the third and fourth years. While in the department, teaching fellows concentrate on assisting the faculty in working with first- and second-year students, while research fellows oversee research endeavors.

Social Life

TCOM students have a reputation for being hardworking, serious, and collegial. The state-sponsored school is required by law to draw at least 90 percent of students from Texas. The average age is 25 at matriculation. Most medical students rapidly build friendship networks, and in time, a wider sense of community develops between all students at the Health Science Center.

The roster of campus clubs and student organizations reflects the traditionally diverse student interests. Among the largest are the Internal Medicine Club, Surgery Club, Pediatric Club, and Business and Medicine Club. The Health Science Center is also home to student organizations with a significant national presence, such as the Student Movement of the Medicine/Public Health Initiative, Student Osteopathic Medical Association (SOMA), and American Medical Students Association (AMSA). All student organizations sponsor community outreach projects and provide preclinical students with experiences aimed at familiarizing them with the health needs of the surrounding area.

Fort Worth offers a wide variety of entertainment and nightlife. Its revitalized downtown is a common destination for medical and college students who often socialize in pubs, listen to the latest musical talent, or simply people watch. Dallas is 50 minutes away by car. Students also organize intramural sporting events and go hiking, skiing, and camping.

Plenty of affordable off-campus housing is available, and many students rent small homes near campus. The average rent for an efficiency apartment is $400, which usually includes such amenities as a pool, weight room, and/or spa.

The Bottom Line

TCOM, while dedicated to generalist medical education and primary care, offers something for everyone. Those seeking an exceptional primary-care–focused medical education are as likely to be satisfied as are those who wish to pursue a career in academic medicine or research. It offers all of the resources of a large state-sponsored institution combined with the unique and compassionate approach to patient care for which osteopathic medicine is best known.

UNIVERSITY OF OKLAHOMA HEALTH SCIENCES CENTER COLLEGE OF MEDICINE

Oklahoma City, Oklahoma

Tuition 1996–97: $21,460 per year
Size of Entering Class: 154
Total Number of Women Students: 288 (42%)
Total Number of Men Students: 403 (58%)
World Wide Web: w3.uokhsc.edu/home/college/
  medicine.html

Contact: Dr. Edward N. Brandt, Executive Dean
PO Box 26901
Oklahoma City, OK 73190

In the June 1998 administration of the USMLE Step I, 99 percent of the University of Oklahoma (OU) medical students passed the exam. Few other medical schools can claim that their students were better prepared.

The College of Medicine's main campus is located at the OU Health Sciences Center in Oklahoma City (OKC). Eighty-five to 95 percent of students at OU are residents of Oklahoma. Applicants are screened for minimum academic requirements, and interviews are offered primarily based on MCAT scores. Applicants who find small envelopes in their mailboxes are offered a unique opportunity—a workshop on how to bolster their application and successfully reapply next year.

Among public medical schools, OU ranks as a bargain, with tuition of $9,552 per year and a housing market that is one of the lowest in the country. The average student in the class of 1997 finished with $63,254 of debt.

Preclinical Years

The first year consists of traditional courses in the anatomical sciences: gross anatomy, histology, and embryology. Biochemistry is a more difficult first-year class. Principles of Clinical Medicine uses preceptorships and patient simulators to cultivate history-taking skills, empathy, and bedside manner. A neuroscience course integrates neuroanatomy and neurophysiology and also covers some psychology. Physiology and medical statistics round out the year.

There are no electives in the first two years. Grading at OU is A/B/C/F, and students must pass all courses to continue to the next year.

Attendance at basic science lectures is optional, and a student-run note-taking service transcribes all the lectures. Numerous clinical correlations with real patients are presented to the class in the lecture hall to encourage students. Two years ago, one of the patients, a 10-year-old boy, inspired the class to raise enough money to send him to a Chicago Bulls game. This grew into Foundation 2000, a nonprofit charity project of the class of 2000 that is designed after the Make-a-Wish Foundation. Even with incredibly busy schedules, students at OU also found time to volunteer nearly 2,500 hours working in local free clinics in 1998.

In an effort to create a support network, students are broken up into eight small group modules. Each module has its own laboratory and study space, which is equipped with computers for viewing OU's extensive online curriculum. Labs, case discussions, and studying are done in this environment, which fosters a team outlook that students take with them into the wards. Students tend to be noncompetitive.

During the summer following the first year, about a quarter of the class usually participates in the Future Physicians of Oklahoma program, which pairs students with family practice physicians in rural Oklahoma for a month and offers a stipend. A smaller number of students are selected for the more prestigious and rigorous honors research program, which consists of both basic science and clinical projects with top-notch professors.

Most of the second year is spent in Introduction to Human Illness, which is a yearlong course in pathology and pathophysiology. In the fall comes an excellent course in medical microbiology and immunology. Pharmacology is historically a self-taught course but has been redone as a result of student feedback. In the spring, students take more courses on human behavior and a short medical ethics course that provides for a nice philosophical intermission.

Clinical Years

About one quarter of each class chooses to do the third and fourth years on the smaller community-based Tulsa campus. Tulsa offers a prettier landscape, a faculty composed entirely of private physicians, and four large private hospitals where students train. Those choosing to stay in OKC consider themselves to be working in the trenches. Either way, the clinical education at OU is superb.

In OKC, University and Children's Hospitals are jointly run by the state and Columbia HCA in a recent partnership that infused millions of dollars into the two main teaching hospitals. This unique venture brings the state hospitals face to face with managed care. Columbia also owns Presbyterian Hospital, a private facility located on campus that plays a lesser role in medical education. Students can also gain experience at the VA.

In the third year, students spend eight weeks each with internal medicine and general surgery; six weeks each with obstetrics/gynecology, pediatrics, and psychiatry; four weeks with family medicine; and two weeks with neurology. Surgery requires long hours, but most students enjoy the level of responsibility given to students. Obstetrics/gynecology is a clerkship that is very student friendly. It is also demanding, but students get to deliver babies and continue to develop their skills with even more hands-on training. Pediatrics can be fun, as students work at Children's Hospital with enthusiastic residents and attendings. The two least favorite rotations are psychiatry and neurology. Family medicine is very strong at OU; the Family Medicine Interest Group is the largest student organization on campus. Primary care is emphasized at OU, and family medicine is the flagship of all primary-care clerkships.

The fourth year at OU, like most schools, is not as stressful. Students are busy doing off-campus externships and interviewing for residency slots.

Students are required to do ENT, dermatology, ophthalmology, ambulatory medicine, and a rural preceptorship. This leaves seven electives, three of which can be done off campus. An International Studies Program places several students per year in places such as Zimbabwe and Nepal.

The Dean's Office conducts a daylong workshop in the spring of the third year to help inform and guide students through the Residency Match Program. Last year, the Class of 1998 matched well: 83 percent of students got their first or second choice. About half of each class stays in state, and about half of each class goes into primary care.

Social Life

There is no on-campus housing at OU, and the neighborhood surrounding the Health Sciences Center is not always safe. Instead of living near the school, students commute from nearby historic neighborhoods in OKC or suburbs like Edmond or Norman, which are just 20 minutes away. Housing costs and the cost of living are low, and there is little traffic.

There is a health club located on campus that offers generous hours and inexpensive student rates. The Bricktown area nearby is an old industrial district that is being transformed. A new all-brick ballpark, numerous restaurants, and nightclubs recently opened; a riverwalk with retail shops, loft apartments, and a twenty-four-theater complex are all underway. A second development is centered around a local reservoir, Lake Hefner, and includes jogging and bike paths, parks, two golf courses, and a marina. Soon, there also will be lakeside restaurants, nightlife, and shopping.

At the end of the year, students revel in a long-standing tradition of debauchery known as GridIron. This tradition is running out of venues in town, because every year the College of Medicine is banned from ever returning.

The Bottom Line

Students at OU are known for their solid clinical skills and enjoy some of the lowest tuition and living costs in the country. Value is OU's strongest asset, followed by sensibility among students, faculty members, and the city.

UNIVERSITY OF OSTEOPATHIC MEDICINE AND HEALTH SCIENCES COLLEGE OF OSTEOPATHIC MEDICINE AND SURGERY

Des Moines, Iowa

Students Receiving Financial Aid: 97%
Applications: 4,100
Total Number of Women Students: 255 (32%)
Total Number of Men Students: 547 (68%)
World Wide Web: www.uomhs.edu

Contact: Dr. Dennis L. Bates, Director of
Admissions
3200 Grand Avenue
Des Moines, IA 50312-4104
515-271-1450

The University of Osteopathic Medicine and Health Sciences College of Osteopathic Medicine and Surgery is the second-oldest and second-largest osteopathic medical college in the country. Students and faculty conveniently refer to their school as UOMHS. Established in 1898 as the S. S. Still College, the school has undergone four name changes and many tumultuous years to celebrate its centennial this year. Its primary focus is teaching rather than research, and the school is known for its high-quality instruction in osteopathic manipulative therapy (OMT).

Admissions/Financial Aid

Although competition for the medical school is intense (more than 3,000 applicants for 200 spots), the admissions committee uses more than GPA (average of 3.61) and MCAT scores (average of 27) for selection. Personal experiences play a large role in the committee's evaluation. Many medical students have abandoned other careers to pursue their dream of becoming a physician, and each class has a mix of former physician assistants, pharmacists, nurses, lawyers, chiropractors, engineers, and accountants. Students from nearly all the states and many ethnicities are represented.

UOMHS is expensive, with a yearly tuition of approximately $20,000. Through the Iowa Forgivable Loan Program, Iowa residents get a small discount that totals close to one year's tuition. Many students get assistance through military or public health scholarships. Others receive aid from national and alumni foundations. Primary-care scholarships are available to third- and fourth-year students who are

committed to family practice, general internal medicine, and pediatrics. At the end of the second year, students can apply for an Osteopathic Fellowship. Fellows give lectures, run OMT lab, and see their own patients. This requires an additional year, but years four and five are funded, and fellows receive a stipend. The most popular method of financial assistance, however, continues to be loans.

Preclinical Years

In the first two years, students spend the majority of their time in lectures, labs, and the library. After a quick course on the history and philosophy of osteopathic medicine, students take anatomy, which includes long hours of dissecting, squinting through microscopes, and memorizing minutiae. Every three weeks, students have practical and written exams. Basic sciences continue through the first year, with the material changing but the schedule remaining nearly the same: three weeks of memorization, followed by a day of testing. Comprehensive shelf exams are given after the completion of each course. These exams are modeled after the USMLE and are good practice for Step I.

Throughout the basic science years, there are weekly lectures and labs in osteopathic manipulative therapy. By the end of the first year, students know enough OMT to do a full-body treatment. OMT is a great break from the basic science, which can get tedious, and it greatly enhances physical diagnosis skills. UOMHS is known nationally as one of the best osteopathic medical colleges for OMT. This is due to the administration's commitment to the field and to the department director. Students also have clinical experience through physical diagnosis labs at local hospitals and half-days in University Clinics seeing patients with upperclassmen.

In year two, students begin the systems curriculum, which consists of intensive study of embryology, anatomy, physiology, pathology, and pharmacology specific to each system (e.g., cardiology). Specialist clinicians present specific topics in their field, with emphasis on diagnosis and treatment for specific pathology. This is an excellent foundation for the clinical years.

Opportunities for dual degrees at the University are also available. After the first semester, students can apply for the D.O./M.H.A. or D.O./M.P.H. program. Classes are offered in the evenings and weekends. A few students graduate with these degrees each year.

Clinical Years

UOMHS has affiliations with hospitals and clinics all across the U.S. Students have the opportunity to do their clinical work in central Iowa or to go elsewhere in the state or country for their rotations. Students begin the year by scheduling a core curriculum. This consists of one year of clinical experience in a core hospital, rotating through the required fields, and one elective block. Throughout the year, there is a great emphasis on primary care. Students spend a significant amount of their training in family medicine clinics, especially in underserved rural or urban settings. In the fourth year, students get ample time for subspecialty rotations.

The system of clinical education is one of the school's greatest strengths but also one of its weaknesses. The curriculum works well for self-motivated students who can design a challenging curriculum and take advantage of their given facility to learn as much as they can, but because the curriculum is so loosely structured, those who just want to get by can often do so. The school has responded to this problem by placing tighter controls on students, requiring them to keep patient logs, document clinical experiences, and take examinations on line after rotations. The opportunity for UOMHS students to do many rotations with other training facilities helps with residency selection. Students have the opportunity to experience many different clinical settings and to meet residency directors at other institutions.

Social Life

Though students are hard pressed to find the time, Des Moines offers many opportunities for cultural edification, including concerts, plays, a symphony orchestra, and fine dining. People are genuinely friendly, and housing is inexpensive, easy to find, and crime free. The winters are cold in Des Moines. From late October until mid-April, no one ventures out, except for the dash between the parking lot and the lecture hall. In the spring, however, outdoor activities abound; there are lakes, festivals, trails, and golf courses.

In the fall and spring, the school sponsors parties, not unlike homecoming and the prom, for the students. Other activities include Coffee House, a faculty roast, and the Malpractice Bowl, an annual brutal football tournament against local law students. The school also has an active extracurricular life, including local chapters of national organizations and clubs devoted to various medical fields. Students can also become involved with local health initiatives, including school athletic physicals, wellness exams for indigent children, public health clinics, and medical support at sporting events. Each fall, medical students also participate in Health Fair, a UOMHS-sponsored event designed to educate the public about major health issues.

The Bottom Line

UOMHS is a friendly institution that emphasizes clinical training over research and allows students flexibility in designing their education. It provides an excellent education in a comfortable town with an inexpensive cost of living.

UNIVERSITY OF PENNSYLVANIA SCHOOL OF MEDICINE

Philadelphia, Pennsylvania

Tuition 1996–97: $28,470 per year
Applications: 8,873
Size of Entering Class: 150
Total Number of Women Students: 521 (42%)
Total Number of Men Students: 708 (58%)

World Wide Web: www.med.upenn.edu/
Contact: Dr. William N. Kelley, Dean
34th and Walnut Streets
Philadelphia, PA 19104

From the first day of orientation, when one of the deans shows students his paintings and reminds each of them to "find whatever it is that makes you you" and to keep doing it throughout their lives in medicine, students know that Penn Med is a kinder, gentler medical school. In addition to a commitment to top-notch education and medicine, students find a commitment to collegiality and to life outside of medicine that goes beyond lip service. In fact, the only true stereotype about Penn Med that may be true is that there are not many stereotypically competitive, work-obsessed medical students at the School. Approximately half of the students have worked, and many have had other careers in fields ranging from teaching to Wall Street before coming to Philadelphia. Although many students come from the Boston-to-Washington corridor, there are also many from California and the rest of the United States. A spirit of cooperation and enthusiasm and a continued interest in medicine and nonmedical topics tie the students together.

Admissions/Financial Aid

Applications to Penn are made through the universal AMCAS application and are reviewed by a committee of faculty members and students. Applicants visit in large group sessions (many on Saturday mornings). Each applicant has a student-led tour, a presentation on the curriculum, and two interviews. Interviews last 30 minutes, and interviewers (one student and one faculty member) are given only the front page and the essay of the AMCAS application. Most students find the interviews relaxed and pleasant, and the committee's final decision is based on interviewer opinions as well as transcripts, MCAT scores, and letters of recommendation. Most students find the Financial Aid Office staff quite helpful. In addition, Penn offers the

21st Century Scholars Program, which provides merit-based four-year full scholarships for a certain number of students (selected after admission).

Preclinical Years

Penn has recently revamped the preclinical and clinical curriculum in an effort to respond to student feedback. Previously, the preclinical first year was basic science classes (physiology, biochemistry, and anatomy, among others) taught in lectures and small sections. September through February of the second year consisted of a six-month "Bridge," which was a system-based curriculum in which students spent approximately one month learning the pathology, pharmacology, pathophysiology, and clinical cases of each organ system (e.g., cardiac). In response to students' lukewarm feelings about the first year and enthusiasm for the Bridge, a new structure, called Curriculum 2, has been developed. Preclinical studies now encompass September of the first year through December of the second year, and the entire time is organized in the integrated, system-based model.

Although the Bridge and the new curriculum mean packing a tremendous amount of information into a short time, students in the past have loved the Bridge, since subjects were well taught and (because things like cardiac physiology were taught by cardiologists, not laboratory physiologists) clinically relevant. Many classes are pass/fail, and students quickly learn to work together and teach each other. Thanks to technological advances, all lectures are now available on the World Wide Web. Even as the structure of classes changes, one constant is Penn's commitment to extraordinary teaching. Problem sessions in areas of study such as biochemistry are led by faculty members who take time to learn students' names, to work individually with students, and to focus on understanding concepts and being able to solve clinical problems, rather than merely memorizing facts. In spite of Penn's tradition of compacting the preclinical two years into fifteen months (now thirteen months), students have traditionally done well on boards and have always felt well prepared for the clinics.

Clinical Years

Under Curriculum 2, the clinical structure has changed. Students now enter clinics in January of the second year (instead of March) and, because of additions (such as more outpatient time and neurology, among others), have more required clerkships. The heart of the clinical sites are the Hospital of the University of Pennsylvania (HUP) and the Children's Hospital of the University of Pennsylvania (CHUP), which are located on the medical school campus. Internationally prestigious, tertiary teaching hospitals, both places also serve as primary-care centers for the inner-city area of West Philadelphia, which gives students the rare chance to see both complex, referral-center cases and less complex cases. Most people find the faculty and house staff members to be extremely interested in teaching and mentoring, and many faculty members actively reach out to students as mentors and encourage students to enter their field or work with them on research. In addition, students also do rotations at other affiliates, which include Pennsylvania Hospital and suburban Phoenixville Hospital, which is located in Reading and York, Pennsylvania.

Students take advantage of these community-based rotations, where there are often fewer students (in some cases no residents) and the chance to take a more active role. Clerkships stress basic understanding of and taking responsibility for patient care and, in comparison to other schools, only rarely require overnight call. Expanding what some of the more popular clerkships did in the past, Curriculum 2 now gathers students from all sites in a given clerkship for didactic sessions at Penn on Friday afternoons. This helps standardize the teaching among all sites, as do more technological tools like fake arms for practicing surgery and the use of standardized patients. Subinternships are also popular, and everyone does one to two. Most subinternships function as internship replacements and so take admissions and have cross-cover responsibilities. Students generally enjoy this busy month and feel that it solidifies their

knowledge and competency and allows them to go into residency feeling confident and prepared.

Because of the early start in clinics, students finish their required clerkships in the middle of the third year. This gives a full eight or nine months prior to applying for residency to do electives. This is particularly helpful for those torn between two fields, and it makes it easy to secure an adequate number of letters of recommendation. Because of this extra time, many students spend six to nine months on another project, such as traveling or doing research. In addition, taking a "year out" is encouraged, and approximately 25 percent of the class takes time from M.D./Ph.D. work to work on a project, do medicine abroad, get an M.B.A., or be at home with a child. The administration is supportive of all of these plans. Applicants traditionally do well in the match, with more than 90 percent getting one of their first three choices. Many students in fields such as medicine, dermatology, and pediatrics choose to stay at Penn; students find they are competitive applicants all over the country, and the range of programs they choose is enormous.

Social Life

The array of student activities is broad and always changing. There is a weekly free clinic for the homeless that was developed by students and staffed by first- and second-year students. CHUP offers theater activities with children. Every winter, large numbers of students from fourth to first year drop everything and rearrange call schedules to spend six weeks preparing *Spoof,* a musical comedy making fun of the medical school. Because Penn has other large graduate schools, there are plenty of chances to meet people either socially or through interdisciplinary summer projects like Bridging the Gaps. Music, museums, shows, restaurants, and cultural activities abound. Approximately one third to half of the students choose to live in West Philadelphia, near Penn, where rents are cheaper; most of the rest live a 20-minute walk away in Center City. Others choose the suburbs.

For good reasons (price, location, space), few people live in the dorms. Center City rents are higher (about $1,100 for a spacious two-bedroom in a high rise, less in a brownstone), and indoor parking runs $75–$100 a month, but many enjoy the proximity to such attractions as restaurants and stores. From a safety standpoint, walking alone at night in either

Center City or West Philly is not advisable, although Center City is generally felt to be safer than West Philadelphia. Penn runs a quick and convenient van service in both places at night. Frequent city buses and classmates' willingness to walk people home make getting around easier. The proximity to the Jersey shore, the Poconos, New York City, and Washington, D.C., make Philadelphia a palatable option for those who miss the wilderness or the activity of a big city. Many students take advantage of the Amtrak station 15 minutes from campus.

The Bottom Line

Overall, the majority of students enjoy their more than four years at Penn. They learn top-notch medicine from excellent teachers in fantastic hospitals, and the flexible curriculum gives them the time to explore medicine, choose a career, travel, and pursue other interests. Perhaps more lasting, students find that they have made friends for life, found mentors, and experienced true collegiality. The grounding in medicine, the superb clinical experiences, the faculty and administration's support, and the emphasis on balancing personal lives with medical careers are some of the School's most outstanding features. Few, if any, students regret the choice to come to Penn Med.

UNIVERSITY OF PITTSBURGH SCHOOL OF MEDICINE

Pittsburgh, Pennsylvania

Students Receiving Financial Aid: 19%
Applications: 452
Total Number of Women Students: 326 (47%)
Total Number of Men Students: 367 (53%)
World Wide Web: www.dean-med.pitt.edu/

Contact: Graduate Studies Administrator
4200 Fifth Avenue
Pittsburgh, PA 15260
412-648-8957

The University of Pittsburgh School of Medicine (Pitt Med) has built a reputation as an internationally known center of research and advanced clinical methods. Despite this tradition, the School has also made a significant number of changes to its curriculum to keep pace with modern times.

Preclinical Years

In the wake of Harvard Medical School's progressive New Pathway program that was inaugurated in the mid-1980s, several medical schools attempted to restructure their curricula to decrease the amount of time spent in lecture halls and increase the amount of group-based learning situations. With these philosophical underpinnings, the University of Pittsburgh School of Medicine launched its innovative New Curriculum in the fall of 1994.

The curriculum at Pitt Med is centered on "Problem-Based Learning" (PBL). Course work during the first two years is varyingly but inevitably based on the PBL concept; some courses may only have one PBL session per week, whereas others are conducted completely in PBL, with very minimal lecture time. Each PBL session is divided into two 2-hour meeting times. Each PBL group consists ideally of nine students who remain together as a PBL group for approximately three months at a time. Supervision is carried out by a facilitator, whose role is to provide information when asked but otherwise to refrain as much as possible from lecturing. During the initial meeting, students review a preprovided, standardized history and physical, along with a minimal diagnostic work-up. One student is designated as "scribe" and documents pertinent information as the remaining students read through the case. The goal of the session is for the students to generate hypotheses and learning objectives for the second "resolution" session. Ideally,

each student is given a general learning issue to explore in detail and is expected to return to the resolution session (usually two to four days later) able to present 5–10 minutes worth of information, with published articles, slides, and other tools as appropriate. During the resolution session, the case is read through again, with students providing the necessary supplemental information via presentation and/or discussion as learning issues present themselves.

The benefit of the PBL system during the first two years of traditionally lecture-based instruction is that it greatly reduces the amount of time spent passively learning information in the classroom. The resultant time spent out of the classroom is referred to as "Self-Directed Learning" (SDL) time and is spent studying, participating in extracurricular activities, or sleeping. An additional bonus is ten weeks of study time (seven weeks of a morning PBL offering entitled Integrated Case Studies followed by three full weeks of free time) to prepare for USMLE Step I.

The PBL system is not the only innovation present in the Pitt Med curriculum. The first two years are divided by course content and structure into two general blocks, the Basic Sciences block (the first eight months of the first year) and the Organ Systems block (the remainder of the first year and the entire second year). Students take one major class at a time; all course work, five days a week, is dedicated to this subject alone. For example, gross anatomy, a subject usually taught for two thirds of the first year at most schools, is allotted just five weeks in the New Curriculum. During the Organ Systems offerings, the histology/pathology, physiology, and clinical pathophysiology of each organ system is presented simultaneously in an integrated fashion. As might be expected, people have varying opinions on whether course work is taught and retained better in an intensified fashion over a shorter period of time or in the traditional manner. To make sure students retain the information learned, cumulative examinations are held at the end of each subdivision such that course material is studied twice for examination purposes.

In reality, some courses at Pitt Med would be better served if they were taught spread out over the traditional time frame. Anatomy clearly cannot be learned in any meaningful fashion when presented over five weeks; similarly, pharmacology, although well taught, is inadequate as only a biweekly course taught over five weeks. Nevertheless, certain courses, such as biochemistry and microbiology, deserve recognition for distilling their subject matter to the medically relevant without sacrificing either thoroughness or scientific accuracy. Similarly, the Cardiac/Renal/Pulmonary Organ Systems block does an outstanding job of fitting what many would consider the core of internal medicine and pediatrics into twelve weeks of clinical pathophysiology steeped in the basic sciences of anatomy, physiology, and histology.

Clinical Years

The third- and fourth-year clerkships are varyingly flavored with the PBL philosophy but are similar to those at other institutions with similar hospital facilities. The pediatrics rotation is based at the highly regarded Children's Hospital of Pittsburgh. Teaching in this rotation is exceptional and is no doubt the result of its dedicated residents and equally accessible, first-rate faculty. The obstetrics/gynecology rotation is taught at the Magee-Womens' Hospital, a nationally known center for both research and clinical care. The didactic portion of the rotation is conducted in PBL fashion, with four sessions per week and an essay examination at the end; clinically, students spend two weeks each on outpatient gynecology, gynecological surgery, and labor and delivery services. Another well-taught rotation is psychiatry, which is conducted at a prestigious research facility, the Western Psychiatric Institute and Clinic, in two 3-week inpatient blocks with superimposed outpatient and ER experiences. This rotation is popular because inpatient teams consist only of an attending physician, a single resident, and one or two medical students. This allows for significant attending contact and excellent teaching.

Internal medicine is subdivided into four weeks of inpatient and outpatient medicine; inpatient experi-

ences vary greatly, depending on whether the student is assigned to Montefiore Hospital (a private hospital with a more traditional approach) or the Oakland VA hospital, which, as might be expected, offers a more hands-on, unorthodox experience. The family practice rotation runs four weeks; certain hospitals, such as St. Margaret's Hospital and Washington Hospital, deserve special mention as exceptional combination inpatient/outpatient experiences. Surgery consists of six weeks with two- to three-week blocks in general, trauma, vascular, GI, and gynecological surgery. This rotation is hospital, resident, and attending dependent. Specialty surgery at Pitt Med is taught over six weeks as a required offering entitled Ambulatory Subspecialties and is a low-key, comprehensive experience.

Apart from required courses in neurology, radiology, anesthesiology, basic science, and an additional four weeks of medicine (usually spent in critical care), the fourth year is primarily for exploring career choices via electives and residency application and interviewing. The Department of Pediatrics is supportive of Pitt Med pediatrics applicants, whereas the quality of advice offered by other departments is often a function of the specific faculty member chosen as one's adviser. In recent years, the most popular residency programs chosen by students have been in emergency medicine, pediatrics, family practice, internal medicine, and obstetrics/gynecology. Generally, the top 5–10 percent of students in each class match at nationally ranked residency programs, whereas the remainder usually get their first or second choices. Failure to match is a rare occurrence and is usually limited to highly competitive disciplines such as the surgical subspecialties.

Social Life

For a small city on the fringe of the Midwest, Pittsburgh offers a surprising, often eclectic, array of options for those interested in gourmet food, microbrewery beer, the latest alternative band, or simply an affordable night out. Restaurants abound in Pittsburgh and include a number of authentic Asian, Middle Eastern, French, German, and Spanish kitchens, as well as standard meat-and-potatoes fare. Pittsburgh also houses a variety of bars and clubs with venues for seeing live bands, dance clubs catering to a number of different music styles, and pubs that manufacture a wide selection of beers and ales. Sporting events are also accessible in Pittsburgh, since the city is home to a number of top professional and college teams.

Campus social life generally centers on clubs and intramural activities, where people of similar interests can meet and go elsewhere to cultivate those interests. Outdoor activities such as hiking, rock climbing, canoeing, and skiing are also popular, given the city's proximity to the mountains, hiking trails, lakes, and ski slopes of southwestern Pennsylvania and nearby West Virginia. Students also take frequent road trips to nearby cities, including Washington, D.C., which is 3 hours away.

The Bottom Line

Pitt offers students an opportunity to experience a "New Curriculum" and an old tradition of clinical excellence. Despite some inadequacies in the revised approach to basic sciences, the School offers top-notch clinical training.

UNIVERSITY OF ROCHESTER SCHOOL OF MEDICINE AND DENTISTRY

Rochester, New York

Applications: 4,560
Size of Entering Class: 100
Total Number of Women Students: 381 (47%)
Total Number of Men Students: 437 (53%)

World Wide Web: www.urmc.rochester.edu/smd/
Contact: Dr. Lowell Goldsmith, Dean
Wilson Boulevard
Rochester, NY 14627-0250

The University of Rochester School of Medicine and Dentistry was founded in 1920 as the first institution in the country to house both the medical school and teaching hospital in the same building. This innovative approach to medical education has continued throughout the past eighty years, culminating in the recent construction of advanced medical education facilities and the implementation of a cutting-edge, holistic (biopsychosocial) medical curriculum.

Rochester's student body can best be described as diverse. With no preference for New York State residents, the students at Rochester represent approximately half of the United States. Admission is fairly competitive, with 4,000 applications received and 700 interviews conducted to generate a class of 100. Tuition is high at $26,750, but this is offset by the relatively low cost of living in Rochester and the fact that 80 percent of students receive financial aid.

The atmosphere at Rochester has been described by students as down to earth and noncompetitive, while the School itself has a collegial, noncompetitive, supportive learning environment. This is fostered by a grading system of honors/satisfactory/fail, which encourages students to work together as a team, reinforcing the interdisciplinary team approach necessary for patient care.

Preclinical Years

Rochester has recently implemented a new, innovative Double Helix curriculum. The Double Helix motto is "integrating basic science and clinical medicine through a four-year biopsychosocial curriculum," which is achieved through a process of active, student-centered learning.

The most tantalizing aspect of this curriculum is the early clinical exposure, starting in the first few weeks of school. Introduction to Clinical Medicine, a course taught in most schools directly prior to clerkships, is taught in the first semester at Rochester. Students are exposed early to the history and physical exam and then build upon these skills in a primary care ambulatory clerkship, which lasts through the second half of the first year and the entire second year. Here, students get primary-care and subspecialty exposure that coincides with the basic science being taught at that time.

Basic science lectures during the first two years are limited to 2 hours per day, with the remainder of the time spent in labs, small groups, and problem-based learning (PBL) exercises. As with most schools, the quality of the lectures varies; however, for the most part, the lectures are interesting and even entertaining. One physiology lecture uses a video of Syracuse University basketball coach Jim Boeheim doing the macarena as an example of gated-ion channels in the heart.

Rochester's new Research and Education Building provides unique opportunities for the small-group and PBL experiences. Housed in this 240,000-square-foot building are state-of-the-art rooms designed specifically for medical students. Each room is equipped with a conference table, marker boards, and a networked computer and printer, along with network hookups for individual laptops. Also included in each room is a full exam room, including wall-mounted equipment, medical supplies, and an X-ray view box. This allows students to discuss a particular disease and then exam a patient with the disease to reinforce vital concepts and details.

The typical day during the first two years at Rochester includes lecture and small groups in the morning and two afternoons of clinical exposure; two afternoons for electives, free time, and humanities seminars; and one afternoon for a biopsychosocial integration conference to complete the week's activities. Elective time can be spent in a variety of ways, from catching up on sleep to formal classroom electives to volunteering at a local homeless shelter or city school.

Clinical Years

Under the new curriculum, students are given until December of the fourth year to complete their inpatient clerkships in adult medicine (internal medicine, family medicine, and surgery), women's and children's health (pediatrics and obstetrics/gynecology), mind/brain/behavior (which integrates psychiatry and neurology) and urgent/emergency care. With the deadline for required clerkships set at the middle of the fourth year, students are given a great deal time before the match to explore various rotations in a wide variety of primary-care and subspecialty electives. After the match, students participate in a sophisticated, intellectual series of PBL cases as well as a number of electives in successful interning to prepare for residency.

Clinical time is spent at one of several Rochester area hospitals, which include Strong Memorial Hospital (SMH), Rochester General Hospital (RGH), the Genessee Hospital, Highland Hospital, St. Mary's Hospital, and Park Ridge Hospital. Activities and duties are different at each hospital and depend primarily on the residents and/or attending physicians with whom a student works. SMH is connected to the medical school and is the main tertiary/trauma care center for a large portion of central New York State, thus offering exposure to the widest variety of the diseases. Highland and Genessee are smaller hospitals that emphasize a more primary-care experience.

Choosing a site at which to do a clerkship depends on individual goals, preferences, and prior experiences. For example, SMH and RGH give students an idea about the life of a surgical intern, including overnight call shifts and repairing lacerations in the emergency department. Genessee and Highland offer more hands-on experience. In most clerkships, students are given a great deal of responsibility as important members of the functioning health-care team.

Throughout the clinical years, primary-care education is emphasized through the biopsychosocial curriculum, and more than half of each year's graduates match in a primary-care field. Students not only learn the practice of evidence-based medicine but also develop the humanistic, relationship-centered art of medicine. At other health-care institutions, Rochester graduates are well-known for their ability to listen and create a bond with patients.

Social Life

Rochester is known as the "Imaging Center of the World," with corporate headquarters for Eastman Kodak, Xerox, and Bausch and Lomb located downtown. Although the city itself has only 250,000 people, the metropolitan population of more than 1 million people, along with the economic surge spearheaded by these three companies, provides all the amenities of a big city coupled with a low cost of living, little traffic, and clean air.

Contrary to popular belief, Rochester's climate does not resemble Antarctica. It does snows, but temperature and snowfall are moderated by nearby Lake Ontario. In fact, Rochester's location is perhaps its biggest draw. Located on the southern shore of Lake Ontario, almost all types of outdoor sports are available within a 1 hour's drive, whether it's kayaking on the Genessee River, taking a leisurely hike along the historic Erie Canal, or skiing at one of the area resorts.

Culture- and arts-minded students never run out of things to do in Rochester, with the Memorial Art Gallery, George Eastman House, the Rochester Museum and Science Center, and the Strasenburg Planetarium. The world-renowned Eastman School of Music has several performances each week that are free to students.

Although Rochester lacks a professional sports team, there are several minor league teams that are avidly supported by the community. They include the Red Wings (baseball), Amerks (hockey) and Raging Rhinos (soccer). There are also several bars, pubs, and dance clubs that students frequent for stress relief.

Athletic facilities at the School were recently renovated. The Medical Center Athletic Club houses squash/handball courts, basketball/volleyball courts, a weight room, and rooms for aerobics and kickboxing classes. Additional facilities, located on the undergraduate campus just across the road, include an indoor/outdoor track, tennis courts, and a pool.

Medical school–sponsored events are also popular with the students. Annual events include first-year and fourth-year class plays, which allow the students to poke fun at the faculty and medical student life, and the spring semiformal, where students can dance the night away with deans and professors.

A great deal of housing is available for medical students. Some prefer on-campus housing, which ranges from an apartment tower adjacent to the School to town-house–like units located a short walk away. Off-campus housing is also readily available in the residential neighborhood coined the "White-Coat Ward," which is near the School. One-bedroom apartments range from $350 to $500 per month, and two- and three-bedroom apartments/houses cost anywhere from $450 to $800 per month.

The Bottom Line

The University of Rochester is the place for students who don't mind some snow and who value a medical education that emphasizes the human aspect of being a physician in a student-centered atmosphere.

UNIVERSITY OF SOUTH ALABAMA COLLEGE OF MEDICINE

Mobile, Alabama

Tuition 1996–97: $14,000 per year
Total Number of Women Students: 119 (39%)
Total Number of Men Students: 187 (61%)
World Wide Web: southmed.usouthal.edu/index.
   html

Contact: Dr. William A. Gardner, Jr., Interim Dean
307 University Boulevard
Mobile, AL 36688

The last word that comes to mind in describing the students at the University of South Alabama College of Medicine is cutthroat. The student body is best described as diverse, friendly, helpful, and dedicated to learning medicine. On the first day of orientation, students are taught the importance of working together as a team, which serves as the foundation for the intimate relationships forged among classmates during four years at South. Upon entrance, students are assigned a second-year medical student to serve as a mentor until fourth year, when a clinical faculty member takes over guidance. A mentor is chosen based upon shared interests and goals. They are always available with copies of their notes, helpful texts, favorite high-yield review books, old tests, and the best advice on how to survive each year. Class size is small, so students have easy access to faculty members, who are readily available for personalized help or discussing favorite topics. Students and faculty members get to know each other.

Admissions/Financial Aid

As South Alabama is a public, state-supported medical school, the majority of the student body is composed of state residents. Each year, approximately 1,000 students (both in and out of state) apply, and seventy gain admission. Attaining admission to South is similar to any state school; grades and MCAT scores are certainly important, but extracurricular activities are equally valued. Applicants are advised to be themselves on interviews; the best strategy is to be confident and honest.

Of interest to underrepresented minorities is South's BEAR program. This is a biomedical enrichment program for premed students who are members of minority groups whereupon admission is granted to qualified students who complete it.

Yearly tuition is approximately $8,000 per year for state residents and $14,000 for out-of-state residents. Financial aid is need-based and available to all who qualify, and most students receive federal financial aid. The financial aid officer works closely with students who may choose to apply for the approximately fifty available scholarships.

Preclinical Years

The first two years of medical school are rigorous. The first-year curriculum at South focuses on topics in anatomy, biochemistry, and physiology. The bulk of the course work is didactic, but problem-based learning is included in several seminar-type sessions throughout the first year. There is significant lab work associated with gross anatomy and histology, but lab groups are small, with abundant interaction with faculty members. Labs correlate tightly with lecture material, providing the advantage of reinforcing the material taught in the classroom. With such small lab groups in anatomy, every student participates in the dissection. There is also daily interaction with faculty members, many of whom come in during off hours to provide extra assistance. Best and favorite classes vary from student to student depending on their interests.

The second year changes the focus from learning normal anatomy and physiology to investigating disease processes and how they affect the body. Pathology is the largest course in the second year; it lasts seven months. Weekly labs entail evaluation of both gross and histological specimens. The volume of material to be covered and learned seems impossible at first, but the high clinical correlation of the course work piques student interest and serves as an excellent motivator. At South, most students say they find the second year more interesting, and they tend to perform better scholastically despite the increase in workload. As always, faculty members are readily available to provide students with any assistance they may need.

Exams at South are conducted in blocks. Every three to four weeks there is a span of two to three days when exams are administered. Many students appreciate this format, as it forces them to keep current with material being taught in each class.

During the summer before or between the first and second years, students have the opportunity to engage in a research project with either a basic science or clinical faculty member. Awards are given for the best presentation and poster, and a few students have presented at national conferences or have had their work published.

Clinical Years

During the third year, students rotate through the medical center, Knollowood Park Hospital (a former private hospital), and Children's and Women's. The clinical experience at South Alabama is often cited as the most rewarding. Many graduates state they have found themselves well prepared for their internship year once they move on to their residency. Clinical education begins in the first year with the physical diagnosis course. This class focuses on teaching students how to conduct physical exams as well as practicing on each other under supervision of a fourth-year student. During the second year, students expand upon what they have learned through progression into Introduction to Clinical Medicine. Here, students are responsible for interviewing patients at the medical center, conducting an exam, and presenting history and physical to a clinical faculty preceptor. Students also learn how to formulate a differential diagnosis and how to decide what appropriate next steps should be taken when conducting a patient work up.

Third-year students are considered members of the team. They are assigned patients to follow and learn to admit them to the hospital, write orders and progress notes, and even do procedures. Third-year students are asked for assessments and plans of care. Students gain extensive exposure to procedures such as spinal taps, inserting lines, drawing bodily fluids, putting in chest tubes, suturing, and delivering babies. The philosophy at South emphasizes learning through experience.

Favorite classes vary and depend upon student opinions and interest areas. Psychiatry is the smallest program at South. Medicine, family practice, and pediatrics are well liked. Students either love or hate surgery and ob/gyn. The hours are long, some of the faculty members can be difficult, and expectations of students are the highest. However, students always scrub in for surgeries in these rotations, and there is the greatest opportunity to do procedures. The performance evaluation for this year is based on a subjective component and the miniboard exam taken at its conclusion. The fourth year requires that students take five courses, including an acting internship. The remainder of the year serves as an opportunity to visit other medical centers, in particular for specialties not offered at South.

More than 90 percent of graduating seniors match in their first-choice residency program each year. Sixty-five percent of South Alabama graduates choose primary-care residencies. Student-oriented faculty members are always available for advice on career choices, to reassure students through the residency match process, and to organize class meetings to enable students to complete needed paperwork. There is also generous time to take off to interview for residencies. Rarely, if ever, has a conflict arisen in which a student has been unable to schedule an interview at their convenience.

Social Life

Mobile is a small city 2 hours away from New Orleans. There are many restaurants with live jazz-band music during dinner as well as bars and nightclubs for entertainment. The Florida panhandle is also close and offers white sand beaches within a 2-hour drive. Classes often plan activities together, and trips to New Orleans to catch the Jazz Fest or Mardi Gras are not uncommon. Some classes plan annual Halloween parties, Crawfish Fests, disco revivals, canoeing trips, and even travel to other countries. Housing is inexpensive; students can buy property for approximately $60,000–$80,000 and can rent one-bedroom apartments for less than $400 monthly.

The Bottom Line

The University of South Alabama is a small school known for its congenial faculty and close-knit students. Students interested in studying in a more intimate environment with ample hands-on experience should consider South. Although there is more emphasis on the clinical experience than on research, South graduates are well prepared to pursue any chosen career.

UNIVERSITY OF SOUTH CAROLINA SCHOOL OF MEDICINE

Columbia, South Carolina

Tuition 1996–97: $22,550 per year
Size of Entering Class: 72
Total Number of Women Students: 194 (46%)
Total Number of Men Students: 230 (54%)

World Wide Web: www.med.sc.edu/
Contact: Dr. Larry R. Faulkner, Dean
Columbia, SC 29208

The University of South Carolina (USC) School of Medicine is a medical school with a lot of appeal. Aside from the obvious benefits of attending a university whose mascot is the "Gamecock," one has the opportunity to learn medicine in a competitive yet friendly atmosphere prized by students. The majority of students come from within the state, and many know each other before matriculation. Everyone, faculty and staff included, becomes "family" soon. Among other things, it is this camaraderie that instills a love for the School that lasts long after graduation.

The USC School of Medicine began in 1977 as an effort to improve the health of people who live in South Carolina. Most students elect to do this by becoming practicing physicians as opposed to going into research, but ample opportunity is available should one choose that avenue.

Preclinical Years

The course work at USC is divided into two relatively traditional years of preclinical work and two years of clinical work, although students have exposure to patients early on. The preclinical years at the University of South Carolina are spent in the attractive and well-equipped campus located on the site of the Dorn VA Hospital. State-of-the-art classrooms are newly renovated and comfortable. In the first and second years, students are graded on an A to F scale in all classes. USC students are competitive in an affable manner.

USC approaches the learning process through an innovative combination of lectures, labs, and small groups. While a great deal time is spent sitting listening to lectures, an equal amount of time is devoted to hands-on learning. The preclinical faculty, for the most part, like to teach. They are readily accessible and student friendly. Due to the small size of the classes (the average is in the mid to low seventies), the

students and professors get to know each other. There are no courses that students uniformly hate in the first couple of years, but some courses are obviously more popular than others. The pharmacology and neuroanatomy courses are consistently student favorites.

One of the most unique aspects of the first two years at USC is a course entitled Introduction to Clinical Practice (ICP). This course combines biopsychosocial issues, sexual education, preventive medicine, physical diagnosis, geriatrics, biostatistics, common clinical problems, alternative medicine, ethics, and epidemiology in an integrated course that lasts the first two years of school. Through this course, students have the early opportunity to meet patients in a nerve-calming, small-group setting; receive instruction in taking blood pressure; or discuss whether an experiment in a journal article was well-planned. ICP has recently been revamped to include problem-based learning. Through this case-based aspect of the course, students are able to interact with each other and with faculty members to figure out what ails patients.

First- and second-year students are in class from 8 a.m. to 5 p.m. on Mondays, Tuesdays, and Thursdays, and from 8 a.m. to 12 p.m. on Wednesdays and Fridays. Nonetheless, there is ample opportunity for electives. Students can choose from more traditional experiences, such as emergency medicine and surgery or humanities courses, such as literature in medicine. For those students who haven't had enough medicine during their first year, USC provides paid summer clerkships. While all students are not guaranteed to receive one of these, there are usually enough to go around. Opportunities have ranged from conducting physiology research on hyperbaric oxygen treatment to shadowing bone marrow transplant physicians. Students feel well prepared after their first two years.

Clinical Years

During the clinical years at USC, approximately one dozen volunteer members of the class travel 90 miles to the Greenville (South Carolina) Hospital System. This program has been popular with upstate South Carolina natives who enjoy returning to their homeland. The students who travel to the Greenville hospital program experience satisfaction that is similar to that achieved by those who remain in Columbia. These expatriate students spend their third and fourth years "abroad" and then return to Columbia the month before graduation.

The majority of the students at USC stay at home in Columbia for their third and fourth years. The students have experience at a number of hospitals in the Columbia area. The majority of the early mornings and late nights experienced by third- and fourth-year students are spent at Palmetto Richland Memorial Hospital, a large public regional community hospital. Students also get to spend time at the Dorn Veteran Affairs Medical Center, the William S. Hall Psychiatric Institute, and the Moncrief Army Community Hospital.

Students in both the Columbia program and the Greenville program experience the same third-year curriculum, which consists of eight weeks each of surgery, pediatrics, internal medicine, family medicine, obstetrics/gynecology, and psychiatry. Students are often well acquainted with faculty members (particularly in internal medicine and family medicine) before reaching the clinical years. Also, through ICP, students have had an opportunity to become comfortable performing histories and physical exams long before they are ever on call. Again, there is no across-the-board consensus of what is the best or worst, although the pediatric attending physicians are constantly cited as outstanding teachers. Most students find surgery and internal medicine to be the most challenging yet most enriching.

Because of Columbia's location, students get exposed to a wide variety of patient types. Columbia is large enough to have its share of urban medical problems and is also minutes from rural South Carolina. As a result, one patient may be a college professor, the next may be a farmer, and a third may be an inner-city resident. With the added exposure of Moncrief Army Hospital and Dorn VA, the variety of patients increases even more. Primary care is considered important at USC, and a large number of USC graduates go into primary-care fields. As a result, opportunities have been established to provide students with more exposure to varied types of practices. For example, many students with an interest in rural medicine spend a portion of their family medicine rotation in the more bucolic setting of Winnsboro, South Carolina.

While the third-year curriculum is basically set in stone, the fourth year allows for many electives both at and away from USC. Students are often stressed out by their search for a residency but still manage to enjoy this year. They generally match in one of their top few choices, and few are dissatisfied. Another unique aspect to USC is the final portion of the fourth year, dubbed Capstone Month. This event is a time when the entire class gets back together officially for seminars that may help them later on in their medical careers and unofficially to play golf.

Social Life

Students enjoy a number of medical school–sponsored events, including oyster roasts, minor league baseball game socials, holiday parties, and intramural athletics. The climate is hot in the summer and mild in the winter. Columbia is large enough to support a ballet company and an excellent zoo but small enough to still be neighborly. In addition to the medical school, Columbia is also home to the University of South Carolina main campus and the bars and nightclubs that cater to its students. Medical students have access to all the facilities and extras of the main campus, including tickets to SEC football and basketball games. For those who enjoy the outdoors, Columbia is a short drive from Lake Murray and a number of state parks and approximately 2 hours from both the beach and the mountains. It is a safe and affordable place to live and has nationally recognized public schools.

The Bottom Line

USC students are happy with almost every aspect of their education. The academics are good, and the lifestyle is enjoyable. Everyone strives to make USC a comfortable but challenging place. Best of all, students really like each other. The only downside to USCSOM is its age; because it has only been around for about twenty years, it is not yet as well-known as some other institutions.

UNIVERSITY OF SOUTH DAKOTA SCHOOL OF MEDICINE

Vermillion, South Dakota

Size of Entering Class: 50
Total Number of Women Students: 209 (58%)
Total Number of Men Students: 154 (42%)
World Wide Web: www.usd.edu/med/
Contact: Dr. Harry E. Settles, Interim Dean,
Student Affairs

414 East Clark Street
Vermillion, SD 57069-2390
605-677-5233

Established in 1907, the University of South Dakota School of Medicine (USDSM) is South Dakota's only medical school. Its primary objective is training family practice physicians to serve the rural areas of the state. USDSM has topped all medical schools for the past four years in placing the most graduates in family practice residencies. This is partially attributed to the significant exposure to family medicine during a student's four years at USDSM. Most graduates match at residencies in the Midwest, and many return to South Dakota to practice.

USDSM has one of the smallest class sizes in the nation at fifty. The average age of the students varies from year to year. One year the average age was close to 30, while the next year it was 23. Most students are from South Dakota, although out-of-state students do enroll. Approximately 50 percent of each class consists of women; this has been the norm for several years.

Preclinical Years

The first two years of basic science education are located on the University of South Dakota campus in Vermillion. The best part of the preclinical years is the professors. They know students and their spouses or significant others by name; consequently, they also know when students skip class. Class attendance is required in many classes during the first and second years. USDSM still uses the A–F grading system. This tends to make the atmosphere more competitive.

Students are initiated in the first year with biochemistry and gross anatomy. Because of the small class size, medical students take anatomy with physical therapy, occupational therapy, and physician assistant students. The first group of finals comes just before

Thanksgiving; then physiology and histology begin. Physiology continues until the end of the year (which is the first week in May). Neuroanatomy starts when histology ends, which is in February. Students claim that neuroanatomy is the most organized course they have ever taken. Throughout the first year, students are required to take introduction to clinical medicine, which is really a sociology class in medicine. The class is held on Wednesday afternoon and is found to be a nice reprieve from "real" classes.

During the three months between first and second year, many students take part in a family medicine preceptorship and gain valuable clinical experience. Part of the program requires students to undertake a project relating to family medicine (e.g., writing a paper on nutrition for the *South Dakota Journal of Medicine* or assisting in the organizing of National Primary Care Day). However, a significant number of students use this time to recuperate and prepare for the second year. Several students in one class spent the summer traveling through Europe.

Second year begins and ends with pathology, which many students actually enjoy but find to be the most difficult preclinical course. Pathology is wrought with specimens and slides but is moving toward more problem-based learning. Microbiology is over by October, and pharmacology lasts until April. All tests in pharmacology are comprehensive, which is good training for the USMLE in June but becomes absolutely painful while trying to memorize 500 pages for a single test. The second year ends academically in April, after which second-year students are required to spend four weeks in a rural setting learning family medicine. This is great exposure to clinical medicine and gives students a chance to truly understand what it means to "take call."

Clinical Years

The class divides into three groups during the clinical years. Twelve students go to Rapid City (population 50,000), twelve to Yankton (population 12,000), and twenty-six to Sioux Falls (population 120,000). Social activities and nightlife get much better after one leaves Vermillion, although it doesn't compare to big cities. Rapid City and Sioux Falls have very similar clinical programs, including six separate clerkships and an ongoing radiology course. Yankton, on the other hand, has incorporated a longitudinal clinic into the third year. Rather than completing individual clerkships, students in Yankton have a variety of patients they see each day in the clinic. Students then follow these patients to such areas as the wards, surgery, and labor and delivery, a structure they find enjoyable.

USDSM students have a much greater opportunity for hands-on learning during the third and fourth years compared to other schools, since there are few residents to get in the way. Rather than having to stand against the wall watching the residents perform surgery, students take part in the procedure and learn firsthand.

Since students are spread throughout the state during the third year, PicTel has proven extremely beneficial. PicTel is a system in which students at various sites are broadcast over a television screen at the same time. Students in Rapid City see the Sioux Falls students on their screen and vice versa. Students thereby interact audiovisually. In this way, physicians around the state can provide lectures for students in different locations.

Social Life

The main university campus is located in Vermillion, a town of 10,500, including the approximately 7,000 students. Although the town is small, there are many advantages to attending medical school in Vermillion.

First, Vermillion is centrally located. Sioux Falls, South Dakota's largest city, is 1 hour away, while Omaha is only 2 hours away. Next, because Vermillion is so small, the whole town revolves around the students, with restaurants offering good prices and stores having sales especially for the students. Finally, Vermillion is home to the state's only medical school, only law school, and the DakotaDome, which accommodates many sporting events throughout the year.

South Dakota lacks a spine-tingling social scene, but because class size is small, numerous parties are organized and well attended throughout the year. For example, after the first anatomy practical exam, all the first-year students organize a huge celebration (although they've only just begun). There are Christmas formals, cookouts, and a "Boards Are Finally Over" party. In the winter, students make a yearly road trip to the Black Hills of western South Dakota for downhill snow skiing.

In South Dakota, high-quality housing is inexpensive. A two-bedroom apartment in a nice location runs $450–$500 a month. New town houses with two bedrooms and a garage rent for $700 per month. A car is a definite necessity, as everything is so spread out. Weekend getaways to the Twin Cities or Lake Okoboji are often enjoyed by students looking for relaxation.

Financial aid is available to all students and varies from student to student, depending on yearly income, outside assistance, and other factors. Many scholarships are available throughout the four years, based on grade point average and extracurricular involvement. Average indebtedness varies, with many students owing approximately $60,000.

The Bottom Line

USDSM offers excellent hands-on experience and exposure to family medicine, although some graduates do pursue specialty fields. The small class size allows classmates, professors, and attendings to get to know each other well, and the environment is not particularly competitive.

UNIVERSITY OF SOUTHERN CALIFORNIA SCHOOL OF MEDICINE

Los Angeles, California

Tuition 1996–97: $30,468 per year
Size of Entering Class: 152
Total Number of Women Students: 422 (46%)
Total Number of Men Students: 505 (54%)

Contact: Dr. Stephen J. Ryan, Jr., Dean
University Park Campus
Los Angeles, CA 90089

The image of the University of Southern California (USC) School of Medicine is inseparable from that of the Los Angeles County Hospital, known also as television's "General Hospital." Established in a crude adobe house in 1858, the hospital has since grown into one of the largest county medical centers in the United States, along the way becoming affiliated, in 1885, with USC. In 1932, the small house was converted into the building fondly referred to as the Big House. USC students most cherish their experiences within the 13-foot–thick walls of the Big House. They also appreciate the spectrum of activity offered by Los Angeles.

Preclinical Years

The typical week for a first-year student includes half days of gross anatomy and microanatomy labs and Wednesday afternoons off. Through Introduction to Clinical Medicine (ICM), students begin seeing patients on the first day of school and learn how to take a full medical history. The remainder of the school week is spent in lectures or in small-group, problem-solving sessions. Lecture hours are long but interspersed with the various teaching styles of each instructor, small-group discussions, and labs. Professors distribute handouts a few days before each lecture, and this, combined with a student-run transcript service, convinces some not to attend certain lectures.

Students' academic lives are centered in the multidisciplinary lab groups (MDLs) of twenty-five students, where each student has his or her own desk with Internet access for a laptop and cabinet space large enough to store books and food. Each MDL also has two computers with Internet access, a slide projector for those endless microanatomy and pathology slides, a chalkboard, and student mailboxes. A student lounge on the same floor offers leather couches, a big-screen TV, a Foosball table, refrigerators, a telephone, and a printer for the MDL computers.

USC's curriculum is organ based. Exams come after the completion of each organ system, approximately every six weeks, in groups of five exams spread out over a week. The grading scale is honors/pass/fail. Although this grading system does not promote competition, students complain about it because it provokes pressure by emphasizing grades. While there has been some discussion about changing to a pass/fail system, there are no signs the School will do so any time soon.

Summer vacation between the first and second years lasts eight weeks, during which time many students do research sponsored by grants and stipends available through the student curriculum office and other organizations. Some students complete preceptorships with a specific doctor, especially if they are already considering certain specialties. Other students choose to travel, work, or relax.

The second year is much like the first, except it is one floor below. ICM meets once a week for 4 hours; during this year, students perform full physical examinations. The second year usually ends around the third week of May, and third year begins in the first week of July. In this interval, students use the time to study for Step I of the USMLE, vacation, or worry about the upcoming clerkships.

Faculty members at USC are excellent, with several wonderful lecturers. Most of these professors are easily accessible, especially because their offices are in the same building as the lecture halls. Another source of help is the popular Medical Scholars Program, in which first-year students work together and with a second-year student instructor to review and learn material. Nearly all first-year students participate.

There is no shortage of study space. The library, only 100 feet away from the lecture halls, offers three levels of material and quiet study areas. Students can also study at their desks in the MDL or outside in the quad.

Clinical Years

The majority of specialty rotations during the clinical years are spent at the Big House. At USC, meeting and treating patients with rare diseases is common, and the clinical experience is essential. Students are responsible for a significant amount of patient care and receive a valuable hands-on medical education. Unfortunately, the tremendous volume of patients can also overwhelm ancillary services staff members, leaving students and residents to do part of the work. The benefits outweigh this extra effort.

Although primarily linked to the Los Angeles County Medical Center, which includes the General Hospital and the Women's & Children's Hospital, the medical school is affiliated with numerous other hospitals. USC University Hospital, USC/Norris Cancer Hospital, and the Doheny Eye Institute are all on the medical school campus. Huntington Memorial Hospital in Pasadena, Children's Hospital of Los Angeles in Hollywood, Rancho Los Amigos Rehabilitation Hospital in Downey, and Cottage Hospital in Santa Barbara are popular places to do some required rotations and several selective rotations (see below). Several county clinics at the medical center and throughout the nearby community offer outpatient primary-care experiences.

Seven clerkships are required in the third year: internal medicine, general surgery, pediatrics, obstetrics and gynecology, psychiatry, family medicine, and surgical subspecialties. Each rotation lasts six weeks. In the past, students have voiced complaints about the lack of structure and adequate teaching in certain rotations. There has been a tremendous improvement in this regard, however, and students are currently satisfied with their third-year experience. In the fourth year, there are two additional requirements: six weeks of internal medicine and four weeks of neurology. All these core clerkships are graded on an honor/near honor/pass/fail system. This scale is somewhat imprecise and frustrating for students, but there is hope that it will soon change with elimination of the "near honor" category.

The remainder of the clinical years is divided into selectives, electives, and vacation. Three selective clerkships are chosen from among a long list of options at USC's affiliated hospitals. Emergency medicine, medical intensive care, endocrinology, and dermatology are popular rotations. Students also schedule four elective clerkships, which may be done anywhere in the world. Research rotations are considered elective credit. These rotations are graded on a pass/fail basis. Finally, students may schedule their fourteen weeks of vacation throughout the third and fourth years.

USC students do well in the match. In 1998, 72 percent of seniors matched to one of their top three choices. Eighty-three percent of the class matched to positions in California, with 72 percent in southern California. Fifty-eight percent of the class went on to primary-care programs.

Social Life

Los Angeles offers an endless array of places to see, visit, and explore. The mountains, beaches, desert, nightlife, and diverse cultures give Los Angeles its character and fun-filled image. In the middle of February, the sun shines, the air is crisp, and the ambient temperature is in the mid-70s.

On-campus housing is extremely limited. Most students live 10 to 15 minutes from campus in locations such as Monterey Hills, South Pasadena, and Alhambra and commute to school by car, which is an absolute necessity. Students tend to share apartments or houses with classmates, with the average rent per person averaging approximately $700 per month.

The medical school shares the health sciences campus with the nursing, pharmacy, occupational therapy, and physical therapy schools. There are numerous opportunities to interact. At night, students usually drive to Pasadena, Santa Monica, or Hollywood for entertainment. Numerous student groups organize events, including community outreach programs, lectures, athletic/outdoor activities, and social events such as barbecues, talent shows, beach parties, and evening formals.

The Bottom Line

USC offers students an excellent education with great clinical exposure and a lifetime of wonderful memories of the city of Los Angeles and all it has to offer.

UNIVERSITY OF SOUTH FLORIDA COLLEGE OF MEDICINE

Tampa, Florida

Tuition 1996–97: $28,109 per year
Students Receiving Financial Aid: 18%
Applications: 1,913
Size of Entering Class: 96
Total Number of Women Students: 175 (37%)
Total Number of Men Students: 293 (63%)

World Wide Web: www.med.usf.edu/
Contact: Joseph J. Krzanowski, Associate Dean
for Research and Graduate Affairs
4202 East Fowler Avenue
Tampa, FL 33620-9951
813-974-4181

The College of Medicine, founded in 1971, is one of four colleges that comprise part of the University of South Florida (USF) Health Sciences Center. The College maintains academic teaching links with several other institutions in the area, including H. Lee Moffitt Cancer and Research Institute. Medical students have the opportunity to earn a dual degree in the M.D./M.B.A. or the M.D./Ph.D. programs. Tuition ($10,500 per year for Florida residents) is cheap, as is the cost of living. Students have a unique opportunity to actually enjoy their medical education through the myriad of social activities that the Tampa Bay area and the College of Medicine have to offer.

Out of 4,000 applicants, USF matriculates ninety-six students each year; 36 percent are women, and 6 percent are members of minority groups. The College of Medicine considers all aspects of a student's application; however, MCAT scores and mean GPA are particularly important to the admissions committee. It is also important to know that only Florida residents are eligible for acceptance. The admissions office has recently become particularly interested in recruiting more women and members of minority groups. USF also offers an early acceptance program (by completing three years of undergraduate work) and an early decision program (students must have a minimum GPA of 3.4; the average MCAT score for successful early decision applicants is higher than 9).

USF tuition is $10,500 per year. Many students receive considerable financial assistance with scholarships, grants, and deferrable loans (such as MedLoans and Perkins Loans). There are also several summer opportunities for medical students to earn grants and stipends while participating in groundbreaking research. Nearly all of the medical students live in nearby private apartments, which average approximately $500 per month. The financial aid office staff members are personable and supportive.

Although there is no "typical" student profile at USF, it is fairly apparent that the admissions committee tends to prefer applicants with interesting life experiences and diverse backgrounds. For example, an applicant with qualifying scores and grades who participated in collegiate sports would get noticed, as would someone with peace corps experience. In addition, the mean age of entering students varies from year to year but usually falls anywhere between 24 and 30 (the average age is 26).

Preclinical Years

The curriculum at USF is fairly standard, with a great deal of time spent behind thick textbooks. Exams are given in "blocks," which means students study for three weeks nonstop, then take tests on everything covered during that time. Such a format provides more free time after and between the intense studying periods. Recently, USF adopted a paperless system for educating students. Everyone is required to utilize laptops during lectures and for class assignments. The first computer administration of the USMLE licensure exam begins in 1999. There are even senior electives in making Web pages, surfing the Internet, and creating unforgettable high-tech presentations. The College has spent an impressive amount of money updating their media equipment, making lectures seem more like an infomercial than mere regurgitation.

A serious advantage USF offers is early clinical exposure. Students start examining real patients in the first semester of their first year. Students can make money over their first summer by performing health exams on patients in the community and at the medical clinics on campus. Experience with clinical procedures is abundant.

At the end of the second year, students take the USMLE Step I, and mean scores are usually around 215 (above national average), with impressive pass rates (90–100 percent in recent years). An excellent review course is offered to all students, although it does cost about $700.

Clinical Years

Students rotate through six junior clerkships lasting eight weeks each during the third year. These include medicine, obstetrics/gynecology, pediatrics, psychiatry, family practice, and surgery. Most clinical clerkships are done at the local VA hospital (which has 500 beds and is reported to be one of the busiest VA hospitals in the country) or at Tampa General Hospital (900 beds), which is located 12 miles away on an island. The training is superb, since Tampa is a big city and the hospitals are always packed. Despite obstetrics/gynecology and surgery being touted as the most grueling areas, a large percentage of USF graduates go into these two specialties. On the other hand, graduating classes nearly always maintain more than a 50 percent rate of participants entering into primary-care fields. Senior students take ten rotations of four weeks duration each, and of these, only three are specified (medicine, surgery, and neurology). The rest are electives, and USF has a vast array of choices, from medical Spanish or ethics to externships in Australia or Germany. Compared to many other medical schools' curricula, the fourth year offers less time off. In addition, students are required to take the USMLE Step II in the fall of their senior year, instead of having the option to take it later.

Residency matching is a stressful time for every student, and developing a good relationship with a professor in a chosen field of interest is therefore a priority at USF. By establishing formal advisers, the Dean recently made it easier for students to identify faculty members who are particularly interested in helping students with letters of recommendation and the application process. Students have matched successfully in competitive specialties such as neurosurgery, plastic surgery, ophthalmology, dermatology, otolaryngology, and orthopedic surgery. It should be noted, though, that USF currently does not have orthopedic surgery or emergency medicine residencies, and matching in either of these fields may be more difficult for some applicants. Overall, 86 percent match at one of their top three residency choices.

Social Life

Student quality of living is outstanding at USF. The College is located close to many beaches, parks, and city life. Ybor city is becoming quite famous in the area for its active night life and artistic flare, as well as for ethnic and culinary diversity. The weather in Tampa is warm nearly all year round. In fact, students usually attend class in shorts and sandals, except for the occasional brief cold spell, when the temperature plummets into the 60s.

Sports and recreation are a common denominator of USF medical students, and the school sponsors several events annually for everyone to enjoy. Outside of those events, students take part in class-organized "block" parties to encourage camaraderie and take advantage of the weather. Professional sports teams include football (the Tampa Bay Buccaneers, in their new football stadium), hockey, soccer, and baseball. The New York Yankees' spring training grounds are also in the area. Tampa also offers a performing arts center, a variety of big-name music concerts, several shopping malls, water sports, hiking, camping, and unlimited bicycling locales across the flat Florida geography. Miami is approximately 4 hours by car to the south, and the Florida Keys are about 3 hours farther.

The Bottom Line

USF College of Medicine offers the young-at-heart student a chance to obtain an excellent medical education with outstanding clinical exposure while enjoying an unsurpassed quality of living. The students are not adversarially competitive with each other, and faculty members are approachable and friendly.

UNIVERSITY OF TENNESSEE, MEMPHIS, COLLEGE OF MEDICINE

Memphis, Tennessee

Tuition 1996–97: $19,248 per year
Students Receiving Financial Aid: 81%
Applications: 900
Size of Entering Class: 165
Total Number of Women Students: 227 (35%)
Total Number of Men Students: 420 (65%)
World Wide Web: utmgopher.utmem.edu/
medicine/

Contact: Nelson Strother, Assistant Dean,
Admissions and Student Affairs
800 Madison Avenue
Memphis, TN 38163-2
901-448-5560

Nestled in downtown Memphis, Tennessee, land of Elvis the King and pork barbecue of every persuasion, The University of Tennessee (UT) College of Medicine is committed to training physicians who are dedicated to public service. From that first day in August to graduation day, students are taught by loyal UT alums of several generations who play an active role in continuing that legacy through medical education and community practice. However, tradition has not stifled UT's conviction to tailor medical education to the needs of the future physician.

Preclinical Years

As recently as three years ago, the curriculum consisted of a typical classical curriculum (i.e., anatomy, pathophysiology, etc.) taught in lecture format with laboratory supplementation. Each course had an independent syllabus, and performance was measured using multiple-choice questions that were evaluated with a letter-grading system. Today, the curriculum is radically different. Instead, the emphasis has shifted away from memorization of facts toward a more integrated approach to learning. Clinical skills are introduced as early as the first year in conjunction with anatomy; disease processes are taught from the perspective of pharmacology, pathophysiology, and pathology at the same time. Community work is required on a monthly basis.

All of these changes are geared toward addressing the common complaint that preclinical work has no relevance to the role of future physician.

In addition, exams, previously given monthly, are now administered less frequently (at midterm and

at the end of the semester) to encourage students to organize and consolidate large amounts of information as they will be expected to do in residency and in their clinical years. Some exams are now given on computer in the same way USMLE will be administered, and the goal is to eventually administer all testing on computers. Exams are still letter graded. M4s are expected to work with M1s on simple physical examination skills in preparation for their roles as teachers when they begin residency.

There are active plans to convert to eighteen months of preclinical work, versus the twenty-four months that exist now, by August 2000. Of note, UT's curriculum has separate courses in preventive medicine, behavioral medicine, and nutrition. These too will be merged into one course concentrating on these health promotion topics.

In 1992, the Underserved Areas Clinical Scholars Program was initiated in response to the growing need to train more primary-care physicians and to encourage them to practice in underserved communities of Tennessee. In exchange for a community's sponsorship, which consists of a $20,000-per-year grant to cover tuition, fees, educational expenses and other costs, a student chooses a primary-care specialty and contracts to practice in that community for at least four years, one year for each year of grant support. This arrangement was originally popular among students, with up to 25 percent of the student body matched with an outlying community in need. More recently, with the changes in managed care and TennCare, the state-funded managed-care system, this arrangement has become less feasible for outlying community health organizations, and the program is being appropriately reduced.

Though not officially espoused by the administration, there is an elaborate student-officiated note system that provides outlines of all lectures for a semiannual fee. Each participant is responsible for taking notes for an assigned lecture approximately two to four times per semester. Or students can hire someone who takes their turn for a small price (during exam time, the going rate can be as high as $150 for a lecture). Thus, there are moonlighting opportunities for good note takers. However, the notes must be in top shape and according to highly specific standards outlined in the *Notetaking Handbook* and policed by the Quality Control Board, which doles out fines for suboptimal notes.

In the summers and during the year, most students take advantage of the mentoring programs set up by the various medical specialty student organizations (such as the Family Practice Student Association and the Internal Medicine Student Association). They pair a student with a community physician, and the student observes how a physician runs a practice. Often there is a small stipend. Of some prestige is the job of "suture tech," which involves working at the old "Green Desk" or the trauma assessment area through the night. At this position, students gain massive exposure to suturing.

There are any number of student organizations, including a local chapter of AMSA, for the purpose of sharing community service opportunities, public policy campaigns, common extracurricular interests, or social support. If students have the time, there are many extracurricular activities, but most people find themselves studying extensively at the library or at the Graduate Education Building (GEB). The student support staff is excellent. Professors are dedicated to helping students through these challenging years, and both professional and peer tutors offer additional instruction.

There is a five-year program that expands the preclinical years into a three-year curriculum for those with extenuating circumstances. Approximately 5–10 percent of students take advantage of this. When this is complete, students celebrate with "Countdown," four weeks set aside to poke fun at professors and each other, to see the infamous Dr. Jones video, to have one last hurrah and several beverages before undertaking Step I of USMLE, and to say farewell to the lecture halls and laboratories of the GEB.

Clinical Years

The clinical years are the strongest part of UT's curriculum. The six core clerkships, usually completed in the third year, form the foundation of the clinical years. This consists of two months each of family medicine, medicine, pediatrics, surgery, ob/gyn, and psychiatry; twelve intense months of overnight calls, clinics, and ward services; and much more. Many rotations are also available in Chattanooga and Knoxville. The fourth year has its own set of requirements, as well as plenty of elective and vacation time to interview or to engage in much-needed rest and relaxation.

Most training takes place at the MED, a public hospital located in the middle of the medical center, which also includes the prerequisite VA and children's hospital (LeBonheur) as well as the Birthplace, the Bowld, the UT teaching hospital, and various private institutions. The high-risk patient population derives from Memphis and various surrounding counties, thereby exposing students to common and uncommon conditions.

Students are an integral part of every team. "See one, do one, teach one" even applies at the student level. Reading when there is work to be done is frowned upon. Clinical experiences are varied and unforgettable. Students take call with the surgery residents (24 hours on/24 hours off) at the trauma center, and it is here that students gain shock-trauma-team seasoning while caring for gunshot wounds, shotgun wounds, and motor vehicle accidents. Students also participate in emergency procedures such as going to the roof to meet the Heliport. They also manage the triage area with the OB intern at the Birthplace, a high-risk pregnancy care center where it is not uncommon to deliver a baby in the parking lot, take care of a patient with twins in preterm labor with gestational diabetes, do a side of a tubal ligation with a resident, and learn to do ultrasound measurements in the same night.

There is no lack of role models as students move from clerkship to clerkship. UT faculty members are dedicated to teaching and to making their students and residents adroit clinicians. During medicine clerkship, students meet twice weekly with the chair of the internal medicine department, Dr. Schaberg, for morning report and then student case presentations. During these conferences students challenge each other with unusual cases. Also during medicine clerkship, Dr. Lewis inspires students during rounds with his off-the-cuff "chalk talks" and his stories of how he "coded" Elvis as an intern.

Students attend pediatrics morbidity and mortality (M&M) conferences, where bad outcomes are reviewed and discussed. Students have the opportunity to train with internationally prominent oncologists at St. Jude Children's Research Hospital, which houses the immunology lab of Dr. Peter C. Doherty, 1996 co–Nobel laureate in medicine. Most students complete their clinical training in family medicine in an outlying rural community.

Though there are training sites in Memphis, students opt for the autonomy, variety, and challenges offered by training in these less privileged, nonacademic centers. The residents who train at UT are both teachers and advocates. Students spend long hours with teachers, who give career advice outside the classroom.

The M4 year is markedly more leisurely, and there is time to further explore future career possibilities as well as to try the new and unusual. The requirements include two JI's (junior internships), during which students practice the responsibilities of a full-fledged intern, and rotations in ambulatory medicine, surgical subspecialties, and neurology. Popular electives include radiology and skin oncology (where students can see Mohs surgery performed in the office). Less popular, but immensely fascinating, is the hypnosis elective, during which Dr. Battle allows students to attempt a simple hypnosis.

When applying for residencies, the Dean's Office is accessible 24 hours a day for advice, troubleshooting, and support. The Dean's Office also offers, with few exceptions, completion of applications, writing of the Dean's letter, planning travel to interviews, and matching students to a residency program.

Social Life

Memphis is a growing community, with remarkably diverse options available in cuisine, entertainment, theater, and athletics. In spring 2000, students will be able to see the Redbirds compete with other AAA baseball teams in the new downtown stadium. The Orpheum Theater hosts major Broadway shows and sponsors a classic film festival every summer. The Germantown Performing Arts Center recruits smaller,

more eclectic performances. Students who are willing to explore find all the opportunities and attractions of many major cities without the traffic and hassle. Students can get to any spot in Memphis on the I-240 loop in less than a half hour.

Most students live off campus at any of the various apartment complexes in the midtown/downtown area; some even venture out to the suburbs for more space and quiet and less crime. Life is affordable in Memphis, with apartments, groceries, restaurants, and shopping in every price range imaginable. Downtown offers upscale living at any of the high-rises dotted along the Mississippi River or on Mud Island, where one can find rowhouses and resort-like apartments complete with pizzerias, grocery stores, coffeehouses, and elementary schools. Midtown guesthouses in Central Gardens offer residential surroundings a few blocks away from the Cooper/Young District, where street festivals, poetry readings, open-air bars, and tattoo parlors abound.

Students share the campus with the other colleges, including biomedical engineering, dentistry, allied health, graduate health, pharmacy, and nursing.

There are many opportunities to mingle with students of other colleges, though most find their closest friends among immediate classmates secondary to time constraints and intrinsic similarities. The Fitness Center offers a full workout facility as well as yoga classes; an outdoor adventures program for backpacking, kayaking, and rock-climbing enthusiasts; and opportunities for SCUBA certification. The Office of Student Life is constantly advertising discounts for students and UT staff at local businesses as well as organizing schoolwide social events. There are bars in the Pinch District, and attractions such as the FlyingSaucer, Overton Square, and Hollywood Raiford's abound.

The Bottom Line

Fifty percent of graduates stay in Tennessee for residency. In a recent survey of residency program directors across the country, 90 percent of whom responded, UT graduates were ranked in the upper half of their residencies for overall performance. The work ethic and clinical skills cultivated during medical school training at UT are both subjectively and objectively commendable and form an excellent foundation for whatever medical career path is chosen.

UNIVERSITY OF TEXAS HEALTH SCIENCE CENTER AT SAN ANTONIO

San Antonio, Texas

Tuition 1996–97: $19,650 per year
Applications: 3,159
Size of Entering Class: 200
Total Number of Women Students: 340 (42%)
Total Number of Men Students: 474 (58%)
World Wide Web: www.uthscsa.edu/

Contact: Dr. David J. Jones, Director of
Admissions
7703 Floyd Curl Drive
San Antonio, TX 78284-6200
210-567-4515

Nestled in the heart of south Texas, a land rich in Hispanic roots, the University of Texas Health Science Center at San Antonio (UTHSCSA) has humorously been referred to as "Juan Hopkins." The warm people, flavorful Mexican food, mixture of Spanish colonial and modern architecture, and regional activities all influence the educational experience. UTHSCSA is situated on 100 acres at the foot of the beautiful Texas Hill Country and is composed of five schools.

The University's mission is fourfold: education, research, patient care, and community service. Since its beginnings in 1959, UTHSCSA has maintained a strong commitment to community service, made possible through state funds and partnerships with groups such as the World Health Organization. UTHSCSA has a special role in providing health care and education to the south Texas/Border Region. Research activity is broad and includes participation in the global gene-mapping project, artfully expressed in the aluminum sculpture "Double Helix" adorning the front entrance.

UTHSCSA is one of four medical schools in the University of Texas System. One central application form, available from the central application center in Austin, can be used to apply to all four schools at the same time. This prevents hassles and is also economical—for all four schools, it is $60 for Texas residents and $110 for nonresidents.

The four medical schools have different emphases in their admission criteria. In addition to grades and accomplishments, UTHSCSA also takes into account factors such as bilingual ability, desire to serve in a medically underserved region of Texas after graduation, coming from an area of residence that has been designated medically underserved (especially in south Texas), and socioeconomic history (educationally or economically disadvantaged students are encouraged to apply). As with the other three schools, state law mandates that 90 percent of the students must be Texas residents.

Tuition at UTHSCSA is $6,550 for Texas residents and $19,550 for nonresidents. More than 90 percent of students who apply for financial aid receive it.

Social groups do form within each class, but because intergroup friendships are so common, the social setting is not "cliquish." The general feel is based on camaraderie and cooperation rather than competition. The student body is large and diverse: each class consists of approximately 200 students of various ethnic and educational backgrounds, which range from biochemistry to creative writing. A number of students attend after having pursued other careers, such as engineering, teaching, or law. The average age of entering classes is 24 or 25. UTHSCSA is strong in primary-care education: more than half of the 1998 graduating class (57 percent) chose primary-care fields.

Preclinical Years

Within the traditional two years of basic science, UTHSCSA has recently added the interdisciplinary Clinical Integration Course (CIC). This course integrates clinical thinking and physical examination skills with basic science education, creating a smooth transition from classroom to clinical setting.

Along with CIC, the first year consists of the usual courses in gross anatomy, biochemistry, microbiology, histology, physiology, and neuroscience. The first summer vacation is the longest, at two months. Students take advantage of this break to travel, relax, or participate in summer research while studying for the USMLE.

Second year is organized into organ system modules, such as the cardiovascular system, the reproductive system, and so on. Each module lasts about five weeks and is followed by one main exam. A clinical integration course and behavioral science/psychopathology course are taught alongside the organ systems throughout the year.

UTHSCSA uses a letter grading system, which is controversial among students. Although it does not foster competitiveness (tests are not curved), some dislike it because it shifts the primary focus from learning to making good grades. However, others like it because they contend it helps protect against laziness and complacency.

Clinical Years

The third year is a time in which the program becomes more rigorous. At UTHSCSA, this year is comprised of required clerkships in surgery, pediatrics, family practice, internal medicine, ob/gyn, and psychiatry. Students rotate throughout the year in groups of twelve and thirteen; these groups are formed at the end of second year. This system lets students choose their colleagues and allows the group to vote collectively on the order of their rotations.

Inpatient rotations are generally done at Bexar County Hospital (a University Hospital housing 547 beds) and the Audie Murphy Veterans Administration Hospital (633 beds), while outpatient rotations are done at the downtown clinic (Brady Green). The patients seen in the University system consist of a largely underprivileged, predominantly Hispanic population. Bilingual abilities are an asset, and those fluent in Spanish are often called on to translate. UTHSCSA provides ample opportunity to learn about medical problems commonly found in Hispanic people, such as diabetes and its complications, as well as cultural issues.

Students can also choose to work at Santa Rosa Children's Hospital or at one of the local military hospitals (Brooke Army Medical Center or Wilford Hall Medical Center). Many enjoy rotating through the military hospitals because of the excellent teaching, less stressed residents, and experience with a different patient population. In family practice, students can work at a community hospital in the neighboring towns of Corpus Christi, Harlingen, McAllen, or Laredo. This is another chance to experience health-care delivery in a different environment, and it is particularly beneficial for those interested in community or rural medicine. Some take advantage of this rotation to spend time at the beaches of Corpus Christi, while others pursue an interest in border-town life.

The amount of responsibility allotted to medical students at UTHSCSA depends on the rotation and an individual's interest and perceived level of competence. In psychiatry, third-year students essentially serve as interns, whereas in surgery, students typically only watch operations and make daily rounds on their patients.

The fourth year brings back memories of what life was like before medical school; students finally have some discretionary time. The home stretch includes only three more months on campus (in surgery, internal medicine, and primary care) and four months of electives, which can be anywhere in the world. The rest is vacation time. Many use a long winter break to interview for residency; others save up their vacation months for just that—vacation.

Social Life

A city of nearly 1 million inhabitants, San Antonio still possesses small-town charm while offering the advantages of a big city. Although a car is needed to comfortably get around, it is a convenient place to live: reasonable traffic, cheap rent, many grocery and department stores, a beautiful public library, several art and historical museums, botanical gardens, and authentic Tex-Mex food. The Alamodome, a 175-foot-tall structure with a 9-acre dome roof, houses sporting events and concerts, and the Majestic Theater lends a historical flavor to the shows. Every April, tourists and San Antonians alike celebrate Fiesta, a citywide, week-long south Texas Mardi Gras in downtown San Antonio. Tourism is a big industry, with the Alamo, San Antonio missions, Sea World, El Mercado (Market Square), and Tower of the Americas.

El Paseo del Rio (the Riverwalk) is a perennial favorite. People everywhere are attracted to the lyricism of this serpentine man-made river, which was initially a flood-control project. The Riverwalk is lined with trees, shops, restaurants, and bars. It rests one flight of stairs below the center of downtown San Antonio. There are also hiking trails in the surrounding Hill Country, and students can go tubing down the rapids of the Guadelupe River and take in the crisp air and delicate colors of a sunset from Enchanted Rock, the second-largest natural rock formation in the U.S. Many enjoy spending the weekend in Austin to experience live music, liberal people, and alternative lifestyles.

Intramural sports are popular, and there are also tennis courts and a half-mile track on campus. The weight room is modest but complete and open to all students.

The cost of living is very reasonable in San Antonio, and this may well be why students with families are drawn to UTHSCSA. As there is no campus housing, students can choose from a variety of apartments, condominiums, and rental homes near the medical center. One-bedroom apartments rent for $400 to $550, two-bedroom apartments for $600 to $900, and three-bedroom houses for $800 to $1,200. Students seeking roommates can easily arrange this through the Office of Student Services. The crime rate is low in northwest San Antonio, making the medical center area ideal for single and family living.

The Bottom Line

UTHSCSA offers a good medical education for a low price in a distinctive and affordable city flavored with Hispanic culture.

UNIVERSITY OF TEXAS HEALTH SCIENCES CENTER MEDICAL SCHOOL

Houston, Texas

Tuition 1996–97: $20,250 per year
Applications: 3,253
Size of Entering Class: 200
Total Number of Women Students: 375 (45%)
Total Number of Men Students: 461 (55%)
World Wide Web: www.uthouston.edu/

Contact: Dr. Albert E. Gunn, Associate Dean for Admissions
PO Box 20036
Houston, TX 77225-0036
713-500-5118

The Texas Medical Center, a conglomeration of medical institutions surrounded by Rice University, Hermann Park, the Houston Zoo, and the Museum District, is located in the heart of the sprawling but friendly city of Houston. Within the Texas Medical Center, which is the largest medical center in the U.S., lies the University of Texas at Houston Medical School (UT-Houston). In its thirty years of existence, UT-Houston has already begun emerging onto the national scene, having garnered a Nobel Prize laureate and featuring clinical programs geared for excellent training in primary care as well as specialties.

Preclinical Years

UT-Houston's first semester is by far the longest and hardest semester. Students toil in the gross anatomy lab three afternoons per week and the histology lab the other two afternoons per week. In the morning hours, they learn the fine details of medical biochemistry, gross anatomy, developmental anatomy, and histology. The School serves a fairly standard course of classes in the preclinical years, which is now integrated with problem-based learning and exposure to patient care starting in the first semester. Most students welcome the opportunity to participate in preceptorships during the first year.

Although the first semester is demanding academically, UT-Houston is imbibed with a collaborative, friendly spirit. Students are not ranked, study groups abound, and both teachers and the administration are friendly, receptive, and accessible. Upper-level students serve as tutors, free of charge. Classes are, for the most part, well attended, but for those who miss class, all lectures are videotaped and can be viewed at any time, a distinct advantage over the previously used transcript.

Exam questions stem mostly from lectures and comprehensive class syllabi. In the past, exams were administered once a month over a two- or three-day block, which resulted in frequent exams crowded into the span of several days. The schedule has now changed, at the urging of students, to exams once every five to eight weeks given over a one-week block. More study time has also been allocated for final exams and the USMLE Step I.

By January, gross anatomy lab is a fading memory, and microbiology, neuroanatomy, immunology, physiology, and genetics take center stage. Though physiology and neuroanatomy can pose problems for some students, most find the spring semester rejuvenating. More free time is available, and the search for summer opportunities begins. Most students pursue one-month preceptorships (in family practice, internal medicine, or pediatrics) or ten-week research stints either at UT-Houston or M.D. Anderson Cancer Center, all of which pay $500–800 per month. Numerous research opportunities exist, as the medical school and M.D. Anderson combined have the largest external funding for research of any institution in Texas. A unique program (the Pre-Entry program) to teach incoming first-year students during the summer is also available.

By the time second year rolls around, students feel comfortable with classes, which include pathology, pharmacology, behavioral science, physical diagnosis, and clinical medicine. Students delve into the problem-based curriculum. Many venture, if they haven't already, into extracurricular activities such as specialty interest groups, organized medicine, and ethnic and religious organizations. The second year comes to a close with final exams and four weeks to study for the Step I exam.

Clinical Years

One of the advantages of being in the heart of the Texas Medical Center is the breadth of clinical experiences. Most rotations are completed at Hermann Hospital and LBJ Hospital, a county hospital. However, students also have M.D. Anderson Cancer Center, Texas Heart Institute, St. Luke's Episcopal Hospital, and Harris County Psychiatric Center at their disposal. LBJ offers extensive hands-on experience with an extensive amount of pathology. Rampant tuberculosis, cysticercosis, AIDS, and unchecked uremia are some of the diagnoses made on the indigent population present. Hermann Hospital, on the other hand, is a major tertiary referral center, with a mix of 50 percent private and 50 percent public patients. Its recent merger with Memorial Healthcare puts nine outlying community hospitals into its referral network and ensures its continuing financial stability in the managed-care era.

Third-year students are required to take core clerkships in medicine, surgery, pediatrics, psychiatry, obstetrics and gynecology, and family practice. Students usually get their first or second choices for particular rotations at specific hospitals. Those that want more autonomy and clinical experience usually prefer to do their rotations at LBJ despite the larger time commitment. Teaching at the other hospitals tends to be better, and more extensive ancillary services allow students to study for the National Board shelf exams, which are given after every clerkship and contribute a significant amount to the final grade.

Particularly strong and popular rotations include internal medicine (especially cardiology, rheumatology, and endocrinology), transplant surgery, trauma surgery (with three LifeFlight helicopters), and psychiatry. For those interested in primary care, which is the major thrust of the medical school, the curriculum provides an ideal set of rotations and extracurricular opportunities. For example, a number of ambulatory care experiences are available throughout Houston for both adult and pediatric care.

The faculty members are committed to teaching, and the majority serve as mentors. Students also find numerous opportunities for learning about the various specialties, and approximately 40–50 percent enter specialty residencies. As the Texas Medical Center is a major tertiary-care center, the specialty services are busy and provide an ideal learning environment.

Fourth-year students are given more flexibility in the form of four months of electives and two months of vacations. International electives in China, Mexico, India, and South America complement the usual offerings of subinternships, specialty electives, and ICU care. Some use elective time to finish work on theses for Ph.D or M.P.H. degrees, which are offered in the Texas Medical Center.

Social Life

As a major metropolitan city, Houston has a vibrant social scene yet stays true to its Southern roots of hospitality and geniality. There's something to do on just about any occasion, whether it's restaurants, movies, operas, plays, or sporting events. Houston is ethnically diverse, a blend which is reflected in the student population at UT-Houston. The social scene at the medical school centers on the Rice Village, a vintage shopping arcade with shops and restaurants.

The average age of entering students is slightly older than 22, but a number of students are entering their second professions or are in their thirties. Nearly half of the entering class is married, and many have children. By Texas law, at least 90 percent of incoming students must be Texas residents, and most students plan to stay in Texas for residency. Students participate in numerous extracurricular activities and intramural sports. A retreat for the first-year class is planned and carried out by the second-year students one week prior to the start of the fall semester.

One of Houston's main attractions is the low cost of living. A one-bedroom apartment can run from $400 to $600 per month. Most live in Condoland, an area of apartments and condos located about 3 miles from the Texas Medical Center, which features good security and a low crime rate. Houston, too, has recently seen its crime rate sharply decline. An on-campus option exists, though it is more expensive ($700 per month for a one-bedroom apartment). While there is a reliable shuttle bus system in place between the Texas Medical Center and Condoland, public transportation in Houston and surrounding areas is inconvenient and not well-suited for a sprawling city. Having a car is a must for enjoying the city beyond the medical center.

The Bottom Line

UT-Houston is a young public medical school that offers excellent clinical training in the friendly and livable city of Houston and is poised to become nationally recognized within the next five years.

UNIVERSITY OF TEXAS MEDICAL SCHOOL AT GALVESTON

Galveston, Texas

Applications: 3,216
Size of Entering Class: 200
Total Number of Women Students: 341 (42%)
Total Number of Men Students: 479 (58%)
World Wide Web: www.utmb.edu

Contact: Dr. Billy R. Ballard, Director of
Admissions
301 University Boulevard
Galveston, TX 77555
409-772-1441

During its history, the University of Texas Medical Branch at Galveston (UTMB) grew from one building, twenty-three students, and thirteen faculty members into the nation's ninth-largest health-care complex, with more than seventy major buildings, 2,800 students, and 1,600 faculty members.

Graduating its first class in 1892, UTMB's 100-acre campus now houses four schools: the Schools of Medicine, Nursing, and Allied Health and the Graduate School of Biomedical Sciences. Included in this complex are the Institute for Medical Humanities, the Marine Biomedical Institute, and the Shriners Burns Hospital, a $40-million facility also affiliated with UTMB.

UTMB has undergone a major overhaul of curriculum, complete with new educational direction, new student programs, new services, renovated small-group tutorial rooms, and a $2.7-million field house, to name a few of the more prominent improvements.

With feedback coming from high administrative levels, faculty members, and students, the curriculum underwent close scrutiny and restructuring. The end result is a pilot project called the Interactive Learning Track (ILT) that was initiated in 1995 with twenty-four beginning medical student volunteers from a class of 200.

ILT students learn early on how to take initiative. This is accomplished by greater student-faculty interaction. Tutorial classes ensure that students grasp long-term knowledge. Early clinical experience allows students to develop practical skills.

Every year since 1995, a new batch of students has moved through the experimental curriculum for their first two years, and by doing so, have pointed the way toward radical changes in the way medicine is taught at UTMB.

The idea is that once concepts about a new curriculum are formulated, they eventually can be implemented for the entire incoming class. This has now happened to some extent. Twenty-four students still enter a more intense Interactive Learning Track, but all 200 of UTMB's incoming students reap a more active, student-centered curriculum that is constructed around problem-based learning, small groups, and greater faculty-student interaction. As the curriculum develops, more changes are anticipated.

Admissions/Financial Aid

Only 10 percent of each class is filled by nonresidents. Older applicants and members of minority groups are encouraged to apply. Approximately 15 percent of each class are represented by members of minority groups. UTMB is seeking to enroll students from disadvantaged socioeconomic and educational backgrounds.

Most students take out loans of varying interest rates and lengths, which the financial aid office gives on the basis of financial need. Scholarships are available for students willing to make a service commitment. A number of private donors offer scholarships, some of which are based on need and some on academic achievement. Scholarships are also available to disadvantaged students. The financial aid office helps students with fiscal planning and debt management.

Preclinical Years

The 176 students not on the Interactive Learning Track are in the Integrated Medical Curriculum

(IMC). Begun in August 1998, this track essentially takes what was learned from observing the achievements of the twenty-four volunteer students and changes it to fit a bigger student body. IMC students get a combination of passive and active and lecture-based and problem-based learning in a more structured environment.

As a state-owned medical center, the school's focus is on primary care. Ambulatory primary-care education is front and center throughout all four years. UTMB is one of fourteen medical schools nationally to receive a Generalist Physician Initiative Grant from the Robert Wood Johnson Foundation. The school used this grant to recruit as preceptors more than 600 physicians from Texas communities to share their firsthand experience with UTMB students.

With primary care at its core and a new approach to medical education shaping the curriculum, all 200 incoming medical students are involved in longitudinal primary-care activities. First-year students are introduced to clinical training situations in their first week and build on those experiences for the next two years. An Introduction to Patient Evaluation teaches them about patient examination. They then put those skills to use in a required Community Continuity Experience.

Clinical Years

Third- and fourth-year students are exposed to a general clinical education that combines both primary and tertiary health situations. Because all inpatient facilities and most of the outpatient facilities are owned by Texas and operated by UTMB, students benefit from this unique clinical learning environment. Instead of the possible differences that can occur between privately owned clinics and medical schools, in UTMB's arrangement both are more apt to be working in the same direction. Students gain clinical experience at eight state-owned hospitals operated by UTMB, the Shriner's Burn Institute, the Marine Biomedical Institute, and the Institute for Medical Humanities, plus a network of University-operated community practices and independent private practices statewide.

Patients come from multiethnic and diverse socioeconomic backgrounds. Students see an average of three to six inpatients during their clinical clerkships.

Third-year students take a multidisciplinary ambulatory clerkship of required clinical clerkships. A large part of the third year is taken up with rotations in community-based affiliated primary-care physician practices.

Fourth-year students take required four-week clinical clerkships in neurology, surgery, emergency medicine, and radiology/dermatology, plus a four-week acting internship that they can select from a number of disciplines.

UTMB allows students to choose electives to fit career goals and to take them on campus or at other institutions. Electives can be taken in other countries.

Medical students who want to delve into research from the beginning of their studies can do so in a summer research program between their first and second years. For students who are seeking a career in biomedical research, UTMB has a combined M.D./Ph.D. program in which students receive full funding.

A lot of interesting research is going on around UTMB; they include projects in space research, development of techniques for telemedicine, DNA repair at the Sealy Center for Molecular Sciences, and human research at the Whole Body Facility. Plans are in the works for a Level 4 Virology Center for the Department of Pathology's World Health Organization Center for Tropical Diseases and Tropical Medicine.

With the proximity of the Johnson Space Center, space flight is a natural direction for UTMB researchers to take. A $555,000 grant from NASA has boosted the study of different types of normal-cell and cancer-cell growth and the effect that a near-weightless environment has on it. In addition, under the auspices of UTMB, the University of Texas Health Science Center at Houston, and NASA Johnson Space Center, doctoral candidates interested in space life sciences can research long-duration space flight.

Social Life

An 1892 UTMB catalog quaintly described Galveston as "admirably suited" for students because of its "refined and hospitable people," its "mild and equable climate," and "favorable conditions for the performance of mental labor." The mental labor is still present, but much has changed since then. Galveston has become a busy seaside resort in addition to a renowned medical center. Students are also only a few hours' drive from Houston.

Students live close to miles of open beaches, myriad water sports, fishing, golfing, and tennis. A twelve-day Mardi Gras celebration swells the city with half a million partygoers.

The University also offers both dormitories and apartments.

The Bottom Line

Incoming UTMB students find themselves in the midst of a transformation in the way medicine is taught and practiced. Great effort has been made in the last few years to implement and facilitate radical changes. The beneficiaries are the medical students, and eventually their patients.

UNIVERSITY OF TEXAS–SOUTHWESTERN MEDICAL CENTER AT DALLAS, SOUTHWESTERN MEDICAL SCHOOL

Dallas, Texas

Applications: 3,174
Size of Entering Class: 200
Total Number of Women Students: 270 (33%)
Total Number of Men Students: 539 (67%)
World Wide Web: www.swmed.edu/

Contact: Scott Wright, Administrative Director of Admission Committee
5323 Harry Hines Boulevard
Dallas, TX 75235-9002
214-648-2670

Since its inauspicious beginnings as a small wartime medical college in 1943, the University of Texas (UT) Southwestern has emerged as one of the nation's top medical schools and leading biomedical research institutions. Southwestern has consistently placed in the top twenty of the *U.S. News & World Report* rankings for medical schools, and Parkland Memorial Hospital, the main hospital affiliated with the School, has been voted one of America's Best Hospitals for the past several years. Southwestern has four Nobel laureates, more than any other medical school in the world. Three of them (Michael Brown, Joseph Goldstein, and Alfred Gilman) actually give lectures to the students. In addition, the nationally respected clinical faculty members actively participate in the medical student's education and remain accessible. They have authored or coauthored some of the leading textbooks in their respective fields.

In keeping with the maverick spirit with which Texas was founded, Southwestern and the other medical schools in the University of Texas system (Galveston, San Antonio, and Houston) do not participate in the AMCAS application process. Instead, applicants must apply through the UT Medical and Dental Application Center in Austin. Southwestern admits about 200 students each year, and at least 90 percent of each class must be composed of Texas residents per state law. However, anywhere from one third to one half of each class includes students who attended college outside the state of Texas, from Stanford and UCLA to Duke and Princeton. This creates a fairly open-minded and cosmopolitan student body.

When compared to other medical schools, Southwestern has a lower percentage of women and members of minority groups in each medical school class. A recent and controversial court decision involving the UT law school, the Hopwood case, prohibits Texas state institutions from considering race or ethnicity as a factor when granting admission. The administration has recently made efforts in an attempt to legally circumvent this decision and attract more women and minority applicants.

Although tuition is relatively inexpensive, the other costs associated with living in Dallas (such as food, gas, and rent) and textbooks require some financial assistance. The financial aid department helps; approximately 84 percent of the students receive loans, and 49 percent receive some form of grant or scholarship assistance.

Preclinical Years

The teaching philosophy is "to produce graduates who are problem solvers, not merely receptacles of knowledge." The first two years consist primarily of lecture-based classes with exams. Some students have bemoaned the paucity of patient contact during the first two years, which consists primarily of scattered case-based learning sessions during the Introduction to Clinical Medicine (ICM) I course and simulated patient interviews during the second-year version, ICM-II. The most actual patient contact during the second year draws upon the strength of the residents of Southwestern's nationally respected internal medicine program, currently ranked eighth in the nation in the latest *U.S. News & World Report* rankings. In addition to giving students informal lectures, residents draw upon an extensive variety of patients in providing students with patients for demonstration of physical exam findings and write-ups for the ICM-II course.

The first year covers biochemistry, anatomy, cell biology, physiology, neuroanatomy, psychiatry, endocrinology, and the ICM-I course. Biochemistry and anatomy comprise the majority of the first semester. The grading system during the first two years consists of letter grades, with anything below a C considered failing. The letter-grading system serves to establish a formal academic pecking order and foster healthy, but not adversarial, competition. It forces students to study more than if the classes were pass/ fail, but it can be a source of tremendous stress. Generally, approximately 30–45 percent receive A grades, 50–65 percent achieve B$^+$ through B, and 5–10 percent attain C averages. A student-run scribe service, which costs approximately $100 to join, allows students who skip lectures to study on their own time. The Integrative Human Biology course and anatomy are generally regarded as the best classes of the first year, while the remainder of the year's courses are pretty much forgettable and seen more as an obstacle toward getting to the second year.

During the twelve-week summer break between the first and second years, students may do research, which includes a paid stipend and the opportunity to present their results at a student research forum later in the year. For budding surgeons and anyone else who made an A in anatomy, students can make some extra cash by serving as teaching assistants for the physician assistant's anatomy course.

Although the second year presents more of a challenge academically, the material is more interesting and clinically relevant compared to the banality of first year. Highlights of the second year include the microbiology, pathology, and pharmacology courses. Psychopathology is viewed as somewhat of an annoyance, with pop quizzes and required attendance. Pathology is given high marks for the manner in which the material is presented, a combination of lectures three days per week and small-group case discussions two afternoons per week. The course is run by Dr. Vinay Kumar, one of the coauthors of *Robbins Pathological Basis of Disease* (the path textbook used by the majority of medical schools). Dr.

Kumar leads one of the small groups and promptly responds to students' questions with long, quirky, and occasionally funny e-mail messages. Another course that earns the students' praise each year is pharmacology, which includes several lectures by Alfred Gilman, whose work on G proteins earned him the 1994 Nobel prize in physiology or medicine.

Students get a little more than one month to study for the USMLE Step I, which helps explain the above-average Step I scores. The School holds several meetings throughout the year on preparing a study schedule, how to study, and what books are recommended. Several professors hold review lectures.

Clinical Years

During the clinical years, students gain exposure to real patients and medical problems. The strength of the clinical experience is what makes Southwestern graduates highly competitive when it comes time to apply for residency programs. This strength stems largely from its residency programs and affiliated hospitals. Both the obstetrics/gynecology and internal medicine residency programs at Southwestern are ranked eighth in the nation by *U.S. News & World Report,* and Parkland has more baby deliveries than any other hospital in the nation. The residents essentially run the services at the public hospitals, and this translates into a hands-on learning environment where students can garner tremendous experience with procedures such as drawing blood, placing IVs, suturing lacerations, helping deliver babies, and performing chest compressions during codes.

The third year consists of internal medicine (twelve weeks), obstetrics/gynecology (six weeks), psychiatry (six weeks), surgery (eight weeks), family practice (four weeks), pediatrics (eight weeks), and four weeks of electives or off time. The majority of the internal medicine, surgery, obstetrics/gynecology, and psychiatry rotations are done at Parkland Memorial Hospital (961-bed county hospital) and the Dallas VA (557 beds). Children's Medical Center, located adjacent to Parkland, serves as the site of the pediatrics rotation. Students peek into the world of private hospitals during a portion of their internal medicine, psychiatry, and/or surgery rotations at St. Paul Medical Center (300 beds), Zale Lipshy University Hospital (146 beds), and Baylor Medical Center (865 beds).

Internal medicine is widely regarded as the strongest rotation, as students are exposed to a plethora of diseases ranging from the common (myocardial infarction, congestive heart failure, and diabetes) to the rare "zebras" (pheochromocytoma, Conn's disease, and Pott's disease). The opportunity to help deliver an average of eight to fifteen babies is viewed as one of the highlights of the obstetrics rotation, while the gynecology clinics can be overwhelming. Surgery is the most physically demanding rotation, with students taking call every third night, compared to every fourth night during obstetrics and internal medicine. Being on call means being on duty throughout an entire night, which is a source of both fatigue and pride for students.

The pediatrics rotation also receives high marks, both in terms of the patient variety and the amount of responsibility given to students. Although family practice is often viewed as a light rotation and given the nickname of "family vacation," most students generally enjoy it. Married students are given priority for slots around the Dallas area, while other students are sent off about 100 miles away to either Waco or Tyler for their family practice clerkships.

Letter grades during the third year are a combination of subjective evaluations and USMLE shelf exams given at the end of each rotation.

By the time fourth year rolls around, students tend to breathe a little easier, as all rotations during the fourth year are four weeks long and graded on a pass/fail basis. The fourth year consists of four required rotations and four selectives/electives. About the only stressful experience during the fourth year is the match. Students are paired with a faculty adviser, and Student Deans Waller and Wagner encourage students with passion to set lofty goals when applying for residency programs. Generally, more than 95 percent of the class matches at one of their top three choices.

Social Life

In Texas, the distance between places is big, and a large amount of driving is required. A car is an absolute must to get anywhere either for social or academic purposes. Most students live in one of the myriad of apartment complexes in Dallas, while a minority, usually the married students, make the 15–25 minute commute from nearby cities and suburbs such as Irving, Los Colinas, Plano, and Irving.

The public transportation system is inadequate for medical students' needs, although the recent installation of a light rail system that serves mostly commuters from outlying suburbs does offer some hope for the future.

Dallas has five professional sports teams (Dallas Cowboys football, Texas Rangers baseball, Dallas Stars hockey, Dallas Mavericks basketball, and Dallas Burn soccer). The Student Union offers discount tickets to sporting events and other events for the more culturally inclined, such as the Dallas Symphony, the Dallas Opera, and touring musicals. Zoos and museums abound in Dallas and nearby Fort Worth, with the nod generally going toward the Fort Worth's Kimball Art Museum and Zoo in terms of overall quality. Popular attractions include the 6th Floor Museum on the assassination of JFK (students can also visit the less publicized Conspiracy Museum nearby), Dallas Alley (Planet Hollywood, music, restaurants, and bars geared towards tourists), Six Flags Over Texas (amusement park in nearby Arlington), Deep Ellum (an eclectic mix of live music, bars, and tattoo parlors), and the Galleria (a giant mall). Dallas also possesses a spectrum of bars, particularly along the Lower Greenville strip. These serve as popular post-exam hangouts. Each class receives funding from the Student Affairs Office to hold class parties and other assorted class functions, such as trips to Texas Rangers games.

One of the most anticipated events at the end of the year is the annual senior film, which showcases the comedic talents of the departing seniors and soon-to-be-interns as they offer a satirical and hilarious look at last four years of medical school. Faculty members participate, and the administration contribute finances to ensure a better-than-cable production and a post-film fiesta. Budding directors and writers have a chance to hone their skills during the first- and second-year faculty roasts, which offer students a chance to vent their frustrations in a delightfully humorous fashion.

The Bottom Line

UT Southwestern offers nationally and internationally respected faculty members, cutting-edge research, tremendous hands-on clinical experience, warm and friendly administration, and a financial bargain in one of America's most exciting cities.

UNIVERSITY OF UTAH SCHOOL OF MEDICINE

Salt Lake City, Utah

Size of Entering Class: 100
Total Number of Women Students: 229 (33%)
Total Number of Men Students: 455 (67%)
World Wide Web: www.utah.edu/som
Contact: Dr. John M. Matsen, Senior Vice President for Health Sciences and Dean

201 South University Street
Salt Lake City, UT 84112-1107

Set against the backdrop of the spectacular Wasatch Mountains, the University of Utah School of Medicine offers an inexpensive, high-quality education. The majority of students are from the Intermountain West and are encouraged by the medical school to pursue careers in primary care and to practice in one of the region's medically underserved communities.

Preclinical Years

The preclinical years are tightly structured, with anatomy, physiology, pharmacology, and biochemistry dominating the first year and pathology, neuroscience, and microbiology consuming the bulk of the second year. The first year is a more rigorous version of undergraduate training except for one or two afternoons per week of clinical medicine. All of the courses are heavy in basic science and are designed to lay a foundation for the second year. One notable exception is the neuroanatomy course, which teaches the basic anatomy with frequent correlation to neurology and neurosurgical cases. The first year gives way to an obligation-free summer. This three-month block can be spent vacationing, but many students elect to stay in Salt Lake and work on a research project. Virtually any project with a basic science correlation is funded through the School of Medicine and results in a small stipend.

In the early fall, the second year begins with a trimester of pathology, pharmacology, and microbiology. The courses are clinically relevant, and although the workload is increased, the subject matter is more interesting. The remainder of the sophomore year is spent with well-organized, organ-based course work. The organ system courses stress pathology, medical diagnosis, and medical treatment but often overlook surgical topics such as ophthalmology and orthopedics.

The instructor's abilities are variable. Like most research-oriented institutions, Utah hires professors primarily because of their research skills and their ability to obtain large grants. Good teaching is merely a bonus. Fortunately, the better teachers assume the bulk of the teaching burden, and the instructors are required to write extensive course outlines. Nevertheless, the freshman-year outlines are often incomplete, and students must rely on a friend or the class note taker if they miss class. The sophomore year outlines are much better, and some are written like expert texts. Many of these outlines are several hundred pages in length and contain all the information from the lectures. Students can potentially obtain honors in a course without attending a single lecture. The vast majority of tests are multiple-choice and are graded on an honors/pass/fail system.

Clinical medicine during the first two years is limited to a course called The Art of Medicine one afternoon per week and a course called Patient in the Community one afternoon every other week. Interactions with patients are awkward at first, but the courses are good preparation for the clinical years. Optional clinical experience is offered on Saturday mornings at a student-run clinic for the homeless. This experience can be highly rewarding for students, since many indigent people get their primary medical care through the clinic.

Clinical Years

The junior year clerkships include all the traditional rotations: medicine, pediatrics, surgery, ob-gyn, family practice, and psychiatry. Only one month of the year is available for electives. Roughly two thirds of the year are spent caring for inpatients at the affiliated hospitals, and one third of the year is spent in an office or clinic setting. On all major inpatient rotations except psychiatry, students are expected to take overnight in hospital call every third or fourth night. Psychiatry call can be taken from home. Students are active members of the clinical team and get involved in early morning deliveries, Saturday night traumas, and late-night admissions. The year is bad for one's social life and sleep-wake cycle but is enjoyable and a solid preparation for internship. One notable drawback is the lack of organized didactic teaching sessions on all rotations except ob-gyn and pediatrics.

The senior year is tremendously flexible. The year has only a few requirements: four weeks of neurology, six weeks of primary care, twelve weeks of clinical rotations (neurology and primary care fulfill ten weeks), and two weeks of ethics. Scheduling is individualized and can include long research blocks (months), rotations at other institutions, and time off for interviews or vacation (several months are available). Because of this tremendous freedom, students can theoretically schedule the year so that they have every weekend and weeknight off. One famous course is clinical pathology (a.k.a. ski path). This course is taught on weekday mornings in February and allows one month of afternoon skiing in Utah's famous champagne powder. The only thing breaking up the fun of the fourth year is a required two-week ethics course centered on finding solutions to unanswerable questions and unsolvable cases.

Most clinical rotations are held at the University Hospital, VA Medical Center, and LDS Hospital. The University Hospital serves numerous indigent patients, LDS Hospital caters to privately insured patients, and the VA Hospital has older veterans. There are advantages and disadvantages to each hospital. The University offers a regional trauma center, hands-on obstetrics, a large ophthalmology center, and a state-of-the-art cancer center. LDS Hospital has a large number of surgical cases, a trauma center, excellent ancillary services, and appetizing free food, but there are few opportunities for student-assisted obstetrics and student-performed procedures. The VA is a new, modern hospital, but it is still short on ancillary services. Often students are responsible for blood drawing and other more routine support-staff tasks, though there are frequent opportunities for more involved procedures, including placement of central venous catheters and lumbar punctures. The atmosphere at all three hospitals tends to be relaxed

and laid back when compared to medical centers around the country.

Social Life

There are many recreational activities both on campus and in the surrounding area to supply diversions from the course work and clinical rotations. The medical school campus is located on the east side of the Salt Lake Valley, immediately adjacent to the foothills of the Wasatch Mountains. On-campus recreation sites include a golf course (the seventh hole is one block from the main lecture hall); miles of hiking and mountain biking trails, beginning at the Medical Center parking lot; and multiple campus recreational facilities. Seven world-class ski resorts are located within 45 minutes of campus, and several captivating mountain communities (such as Park City and Sundance) are found within 1 hour of campus. On long weekends or over trimester breaks, six spectacular National Parks (such as Arches, Zion, and Yellowstone) can be reached via a 5- or 6-hour drive. The School encourages students to spend their family practice rotation in a rural community in the Intermountain West (housing is provided by the School), which provides an additional opportunity to experience more of the region's varied and magnificent scenery.

The Intermountain region's population and customs define the student body. The School of Medicine primarily accepts students from Utah, Idaho, and Wyoming and subsequently leaves few positions for applicants from other areas. The student body contains a high percentage of married students with families (probably higher than any medical school in the country), several older students, and many members of the region's dominant religion, the Latter Day Saints (Mormon). Classes typically consist of only 25–35 percent women, and 10 percent of the students are members of minority groups.

Students are still able to find relatively inexpensive housing for individuals or families on or near campus. Housing prices have been steadily rising as the area's population expands and as the 2002 Olympic Games draw nearer.

The Bottom Line

The University of Utah School of Medicine is a wonderful place for family-oriented outdoor enthusiasts who are considering a career in family practice.

UNIVERSITY OF VERMONT COLLEGE OF MEDICINE

Burlington, Vermont

Applications: 7,257
Size of Entering Class: 94
World Wide Web: salus.med.uvm.edu/
Contact: Dr. Cathleen Gleeson, Director of
Admissions

Burlington, VT 05405-0160
802-656-2154

The University of Vermont (UVM) College of
Medicine is situated in the rolling hills, scenic
countryside, and autumn colors of one of the
country's most picturesque states. Taking advantage of
these optimal surroundings, the school has provided a
nurturing environment in which to learn medicine.
One of the things that sets UVM apart is its emphasis
on clinical experience: basic science is compressed into
a fairly intense 1½ years, followed by 2½ years of
clinical rotations.

Preclinical Years

The first 1½ years include ten major subject areas,
starting with gross anatomy, microscopic anatomy
(histology), and biochemistry. The course in anatomy
is a perennial favorite, with excellent teaching
augmented by anatomical models created in-house by
the faculty. This is followed by physiology,
microbiology, neuroscience, general and then systemic
pathology, psychopathology, and pharmacology. The
pathology department does a particularly outstanding
job, although histology, biochemistry, and
psychopathology often get below-average ratings.

The professors and other faculty members care
about teaching and are available to help students.
Their friendliness and dedication, however, do not
prevent them from writing difficult exams. Similarly,
the staff and administration seem to go out of their
way to make the time spent at the school as bearable
as possible. They get to know each student personally,
can be reached at any time, and can be counted on
for useful advice.

Starting almost from day one, UVM students
have a good deal of exposure to clinical medicine. The
first semester includes Doctoring Skills, a class on the
use of exam tools, interviewing skills, history taking,
and the fundamentals of the physical exam, practiced

on "patient instructors" hired to provide feedback to
students. After winter break, every student is assigned
to an area primary-care doctor for an afternoon every
other week. These mentors range from country doctors to multiphysician city practitioners and from
pediatrics to family practice to internal medicine.
Many students cite this yearlong relationship as their
most important learning experience of the basic science core.

Clinical Years

Halfway through the second year, students begin a
year of clinical core, which consists of required rotations through the major areas of medicine-surgery,
pediatrics, psychiatry, obstetrics and gynecology, family practice, and internal medicine. The rotations are
spread through three hospitals: Fletcher Allen in
Burlington, Vermont; Maine Medical Center in
Portland, Maine; and Champlain Valley in
Plattsburgh, New York. Most students say the experiences at all three are extremely positive, although the
quality of a given rotation varies with the attendings
and residents to whom students are assigned. The
population of Burlington is mostly white and middle
class, which makes for a fairly homogenous clinical
experience.

Most students—except those with children—are
required to spend at least two months (most spend
four or more) in Maine, which can be difficult for
those with spouses, pets, leases, or other obligations in
Burlington. The Plattsburgh rotations start and end
each day with a long commute and ferry ride. The
upside to this is that even on the first day of clinical
rotations, UVM students function at a reasonably high
level, thanks to their previous clinical training. This
clinical advantage seems to carries over into residen-

cies, with UVM students getting consistently high ratings from residency directors.

After one year of rotations, students return to the classroom for a month of advanced science, which consists of genetics, epidemiology, and a series of elective classes, including ACLS and embryology. Although these classes can help students prepare for the USMLE Step I (which UVM students tend to take a year or so after their colleagues around the country), many view them as a welcome break from the hectic pace of the hospital.

The last 1½ years are composed entirely of elective clinical rotations. The school requires that some rotations be completed in Vermont, and some of the rotations must be scheduled as acting internships (the actual requirements differ based on whether students choose the surgery major for this period or not), but most take this time to prepare for and take USMLE Step II, to travel to rotations around the country and the world, to interview for residencies, and to spend a little time with friends and family. Advising on postgraduate training is considered excellent, with between 85 and 90 percent of students matching at one of their top three program choices.

Social Life

Students are friendly. Most are laid-back people with some experience in fields other than medicine. The admissions process selects people with a history of community service, and the student body is active in the community and in supporting one another.

Students can enjoy hiking and skiing in the surrounding countryside, student-organized intramural athletics, movies, and the small-city club scene of Burlington. Crime is not a problem. Montreal is 1½ hours away, and Boston is 4 hours away. Although good housing can be hard to find, rent is reasonable: $600–$800 for a spacious two bedroom apartment, with higher prices for housing closer to the school.

The Bottom Line

Students who are looking for a nonclinical education, extensive experience with inner-city populations, or an ultramodern facility with a huge library should go somewhere other than UVM. Students looking to be treated like human beings in medical school and who desire some outstanding clinical training should consider UVM.

UNIVERSITY OF VIRGINIA SCHOOL OF MEDICINE

Charlottesville, Virginia

Tuition 1996–97: $23,952 per year
Applications: 4,474
Size of Entering Class: 139
Total Number of Women Students: 242 (44%)
Total Number of Men Students: 311 (56%)

World Wide Web: www.virginia.edu
Contact: Beth A. Bailey, Director, Admissions
Office
Charlottesville, VA 22903
804-924-5571

Nestled in the Blue Ridge Mountains, the University of Virginia (UVA) is the major tertiary-care center for southwest Virginia and has some of the country's top specialists (in areas such as infectious disease, neurosurgery, and endocrinology) on its faculty. While it is not a major metropolitan hospital with a bustling emergency department, the patient population is large and diverse. UVA has not adopted a systems-based teaching approach like many other schools, but the traditional curriculum has not been a disadvantage to the students, who average in the 80th percentile for Steps I and II.

The personality of the medical school is one of the most appealing factors for most of the students here. The program is traditional, and the curriculum has changed little. However, this is mostly a result of student input rather than reluctance from the faculty. Students work hard at UVA.

Preclinical Years

During the first year, faculty members try to coordinate the topics in the different classes in order to facilitate integrative learning, but at times students must incorporate topics on their own at the end of the semester in preparation for the exam. This is actually effective, as students are not spoon-fed the information; they must be proactive in their learning.

Consequently, many students work together in groups. Students at UVA are competitive, but cooperative study is common. Furthermore, faculty members are dedicated teachers who provide ready access for tutoring or mentoring. Most of the exams are Board-style exams, which gives students early exposure to the testing style. The two months after first year are a welcome time for students to travel, do research, and recuperate.

The second year is perhaps the most challenging because of the introduction of clinical reasoning and the exhaustive lecture schedule, small groups, and exam periods. The final exams are cumulative and are excellent review for Step I. Students are given a little more than two weeks to study for Step I and begin third-year clerkship within a week after taking the exam. There is no summer break after second year. That time is held over for the fourth year, when students can take up to three months of vacation time in addition to Christmas, Thanksgiving, and spring break.

Patient contact and exposure begins in the first year with Doctor, Patient, and the Interview (DPI), during which students practice interviewing patients.

The goal of these exercises is to acquaint students with the patients' personal histories and the effects of illness on their lives. This is an invaluable learning tool, as most students find that it is difficult to learn how to "relate" to patients. Learning how to elicit a good history and physical begins in the second year and continues throughout every doctor's career.

Clinical Years

The third year is the most rewarding year in medical school. Students often are the medical staff that patients interact with the most, and, consequently, they often become the primary caregivers. This level of responsibility is, however, dependent upon the student's interest and dedication. The attendings are all excellent role models who devote much of their time to teaching. Students are encouraged to develop their own medical personality and philosophy by being treated as contributing members of a team, managing their patients, and performing procedures. The residents at UVA are among the best in the country. There isn't a sense of a tight hierarchy between the house staff and the students, and interactions tend to be comfortable and informal. The residents at the VA and Roanoke aren't as uniformly qualified, and the students' experience at these two sites can be good or bad. However, the psych rotation at Roanoke is excellent, as students interact primarily with the attending and are given the same level of responsibility as interns.

Fourth year (the promised land) is the best year of medical school. The first three to four months are hectic, as students try to complete acting internships prior to residency application deadlines. The only mandatory elective is four weeks of neurology. Also, UVA requires that students pass Step II prior to graduation, and students typically take the test in the fall. After this, students are free to take whatever electives they want. Students are encouraged to do away electives and research. Humanities in medicine classes are offered throughout the year for those students who want a change of speed. However, most students take clinical electives in an effort to be better interns or to round out their medical experience. Graduation is in late May, and Charlottesville is beautiful in the spring.

Social Life

There is ample time in the first year to enjoy one's hobbies and to exercise. For those addicted to the rush of pumping iron or the thrill of competition, the University's fitness centers are world-class, and the intramural sports are challenging, as most of the undergrads tend to be in better shape than medical students. There are also weekly runs with Dean Pearson. The surrounding mountains provide for readily accessible hiking, camping, canoeing, fly fishing, and hunting.

Students who prefer nightlife find much to do. The "corner" has one of the best college bars in the country, the Biltmore, and the downtown mall has numerous watering holes for those with a more discriminating palate. Virginia's strong football tradition and even stronger tradition for tailgates are ideal for football fans. Furthermore, there are typically parties at the end of each exam period, which are funded by the classes' social budget.

The class raises funds throughout the first two years in order to throw the end of basic science party, which was held last year at Jefferson Vineyard.

UNIVERSITY OF WASHINGTON SCHOOL OF MEDICINE

Seattle, Washington

Tuition 1996–97: $22,251 per year
Applications: 4,464
Size of Entering Class: 174
World Wide Web: www.washington.edu/medical/som/

Contact: Pat Fero, Office of Admissions
Seattle, WA 98195
206-543-7212

The University of Washington (UW) School of Medicine is the only medical school in Washington, Wyoming, Alaska, Montana, and Idaho. This conglomeration of states is cleverly known as the "WWAMI" region and accounts for 28 percent of the U.S. landmass. One of the School's missions is training doctors for its rural population; therefore, it accepts a high number of primary-care students from small towns and sends clinical clerks to remote areas to learn community medicine. However, academic medicine plays a bigger role than advertised, and UW is home to world-class scientific inquiry and experimental therapy in fields as diverse as bone marrow transplant and injury prevention.

The School preferentially accepts students who reside in the five-state region. Underrepresented minorities and M.D./Ph.D. candidates are recruited from all fifty states, however, and these two groups comprise approximately 18 percent of each class. Women now comprise 50 percent of entering classes.

Tuition is $8,400 per year for in-state students, and students receive adequate financial aid.

Preclinical Years

Almost all students spend the first year in their home state learning the basic sciences. Washington residents, for example, start in Seattle with 100 fellow students and spend 25–35 hours per week in a 1970s-style lecture hall with brown plastic swivel chairs. Alternate first-year sites are Laramie, Wyoming; Anchorage, Alaska; Moscow, Idaho; Pullman, Washington; and Bozeman, Montana. During the second year, when the course work turns to organ pathology, all students come to Seattle, which produces a class of 176.

The first quarter is dominated by anatomy class. For the final, students must recite all relevant anatomic details on three of 153 different topics, chosen by the professor.

World-famous basic scientists teach courses in physiology, biochemistry, microbiology, immunology, and the various organs. The weakest classes are histology and pharmacology; both are poorly taught and currently under revision. With few exceptions, everything needed to pass exams is covered in course syllabi, which is distributed at the beginning of every quarter. In addition, many rely on the "Eugenia notes," the handwritten, near-verbatim lecture notes of a fastidious student who became a pediatrician (and medical student legend) long ago.

Grading at UW is honors/pass/fail; honors is usually given at the 85–90 percent level. There is no curve, and most students gravitate into study partnerships or groups. All but one or two students pass the USMLE Step I each year.

Exposure to clinical medicine begins in the first month of medical school, when students hit the wards to practice taking a social history. By spring quarter, students have learned the physical exam. Many elect to do preceptorships with an attending of choice, and during the first summer, they go to a rural site in the WWAMI region to learn to suture, deliver babies, and work up common medical problems. In Alaska, students might fly into the bush and immunize children in Eskimo villages; alternately, students might find themselvesthe surgeon's first assistant on trauma cases in a small Montana hospital.

Those interested in academic careers often spend the summer between first and second years doing research. UW sponsors the Medical Student Research Training Program (MSRTP), which offers stipends for projects undertaken with a research mentor. Doing summer research gets the much-bemoaned research requirement out of the way. The dean's office funds student presentations at scientific conferences, and many choose to attend a conference during the second year, an experience reputed to be one of the most enjoyable parts of the preclinical education.

Clinical Years

Clinical education takes place at six hospitals in Seattle and innumerable hospitals and clinics in the far-flung WWAMI region. This makes for an enormous and medically and culturally diverse patient base. The clinical experience is different at each hospital and often depends on the residents and attendings to which students are assigned. In general, teaching and patient-care experiences are top notch in core rotations.

Medical students are most excited about rotations in which they play a meaningful role in patient care. For this reason, Harborview, Seattle's 330-bed county hospital, is the most popular of the hospitals, where students both feel and act like real doctors, whether on surgery, medicine, or psychiatry. Harborview, the Pacific Northwest's only Level I trauma center, hosts another highly regarded rotation—ER. Masterminded by Dr. Michael Copass, the first to put defibrillators in ambulances, medical students work up and treat every patient who comes through the ER, under resident supervision. Students gain extensive exposure to myriad trauma situations.

University Hospital, a 331-bed tertiary referral center, is referred to as the Death Star and avoided if possible because of a weighty hierarchy that puts students at the very bottom of the food chain. Potentially troublesome rotations are surgery, famous for abrasive personalities and mind-crushing work hours—issues that turn out to be mostly hype—and rehabilitation medicine, which is roundly felt to offer little learning.

Rural WWAMI rotations are highly sought after for hands-on experience. Students on rural obstetrics/gynecology rotations report delivering twenty babies in a six-week period, for example. In pediatrics, motivated students simultaneously help manage patients in the neonatal intensive care unit, the pediatric intensive care unit, and the ward, in addition to clinic duties.

Two third-year rural tracks are offered for those who want a thorough primary-care experience. The Idaho track allows students to complete core rotations

in Idaho. And those interested in rural family medicine may elect six months with a rural family practice after basic training in relevant fields.

The fourth year provides ample time for electives and nearly six months of vacation. Ten to 20 percent of students stretch the last year into two to pursue further research or travel abroad, a move that the dean's office has supported in the past. Many UW students have done rotations in Central America, Asia, and Africa; it has become fairly routine to set up an international experience.

Although UW is reputed to be America's best primary-care school and top five in family practice and pediatrics, a number of students choose subspecialty and academic careers. Graduating classes match students into top residencies in ophthalmology, dermatology, ear-nose-throat, and neurosurgery every year. Ninety percent of students match in one of their top three programs.

Social Life

Lasting friendships most often form between students spending their first year together. During the second year, when all students come to Seattle, a retreat to Fort Warden on the Olympic Peninsula helps to mix up the tight groups that have formed.

Friday nights are active social nights at the School, since exams are usually on Monday mornings. Parties with themes are common. The medical school basketball team forms early on and is locked in a perennial rivalry with the law school. Students also organize Ultimate Frisbee, soccer, and crew teams to compete in city leagues.

Seattle has unique neighborhoods, excellent restaurants, arty bars, coffeehouses, and used bookstores. Students can go to the ballet, the theater, or a monster truck show at the Kingdome on a Friday night. Before bands such as the Presidents of the United States of America or Nirvana hit it big, they frequented bars around Seattle; live music remains a constant feature of nightlife.

Most students live near the University. Parking is a inadequate, so students rely on a bus line ($30 per quarter for unlimited riding) or bike in on the Burke-Gilman trail. Popular neighborhoods include trendy Freemont, Capitol Hill, Ravenna, and youthful Greenlake, where a two-bedroom apartment costs $800–$1,000.

One of Seattle's main attractions is its proximity to mountains and water. Although nearby trails are packed on weekends, beautiful, quiet terrain is close. Kayakers head for the San Juan Islands on sunny weekends, and climbers have no shortage of challenging faces and glacier climbs within a 2-hour drive.

The Bottom Line
For residents of a WWAMI state, the University of Washington offers a great education at a great price.

Students experience unique, hands-on clinical experiences, particularly in primary care. Students find highly respected academics at UW.

UNIVERSITY OF WISCONSIN–MADISON MEDICAL SCHOOL

Madison, Wisconsin

Tuition 1996–97: $22,826 per year
Size of Entering Class: 150
World Wide Web: medsch.wisc.edu/homepage. html

Contact: Dr. Phillip M. Farrell, Dean
500 Lincoln Drive
Madison, WI 53706-1380

The University of Wisconsin (UW) Medical School in Madison welcomes new students through a White Coat Investiture Ceremony that both solemnly signifies the entrance into the medical profession and exemplifies the faculty's pride in students. From that point on, the students become immersed in an institution recognized around the world for outstanding research, cutting-edge clinical techniques, and top-notch instruction. These qualities, combined with living in a beautiful and fun city, offer students an unbeatable experience.

The UW Medical School currently matriculates 143 students per class. Applicants selected to interview meet with one committee member who, in an easygoing manner, is interested in verifying that applicants match their identity on paper.

In 1998, 90 percent of accepted applicants were residents of Wisconsin, and 61 percent received their undergraduate degree from UW–Madison. Women constitute 55 percent of entering students, and members of minority groups comprise 14 percent. The student population is young, with an average age range of 20 to 23 years, but there are students age 30 or more. Yearly tuition is $15,512 for state residents and $22,826 for nonresidents. The Medical School provides ample help in securing any necessary financial aid.

Preclinical Years

The graduating class of 1998 was the first group of students to experience the new curriculum at the UW Medical School. The administration's goal was to reconfigure the science courses into a more integrated and interdisciplinary structure, minimizing rote fact memorization and introducing clinical, case-based learning. Curriculum design has been streamlined to provide less than 15 hours per week of lecture and several small, interactive group learning sessions with faculty members. Many of the courses, such as neuroscience, infection and immunity, and pathophysiology of organ systems, are headed by both basic scientists and clinicians. These changes in the style of education help foster skills in problem solving and offer better preparation for the clinical years. Best of all, the necessary accumulation of the gross facts and details needed for the National Boards exams has not been sacrificed.

Gross anatomy deserves to be mentioned as an outstanding first-year class with motivated faculty members who love to teach. Conversely, pharmacology lacks depth and attempts, but fails, to complement concurrent teaching in the pathophysiology series. Nevertheless, students can make up for this deficiency by taking a popular pharmacology elective during the fourth year. Progress throughout the first two years is measured by plentiful exams that follow a traditional letter grading system. Grades are typically downplayed by course instructors but, in reality, are important to final class standing.

A key goal of the UW Medical School is to place more than 50 percent of graduating students in primary care. The administration strives to meet this goal, beginning the first week of school, through the nationally funded Generalist Partners Program (GPP), in which students shadow a community-based primary-care physician in the outpatient setting. Many students enjoy the chance to see patients this early in their training, although the constant push toward generalist medicine can discourage students who are considering a subspecialty field of medicine. Additional early clinical exposure comes in the four-semester patient, doctor and society course, in which communication skills, the physical exam, and medical ethics are taught.

Between the first and second years of medical school, many students elect to do an externship with a community physician or apply for readily available NIH grant money to fund a summer research project. Others volunteer in the student-run medical clinics that provide free medical care for Madison's poor, homeless, or uninsured patient population.

Clinical Years

The University of Wisconsin Hospital and Clinics in Madison is the home base for medical students. This tertiary-care and referral center for Wisconsin and surrounding states has 479 inpatient beds and provides comprehensive clinical training. Faculty members are highly regarded by their peers and as top recipients of NIH funding for basic and clinical science research. Several programs, including the organ transplant program, have become world renowned. Students also rotate through the 122-bed VA hospital located on the same campus.

All students are required to spend a significant amount of time—usually five or more months—completing rotations in hospital or clinic sites around the state and train in cities such as Marshfield, La Crosse, or Milwaukee. Housing is provided; a car is a necessity.

Outstanding clinical rotations at UW Hospital include general surgery, transplant surgery, infectious disease, and the trauma and life support center. Teaching of medical students occurs in an earnest and friendly manner on both internal medicine and surgery rotations. At the outlying training sites, the friendliness of attendings, staff, and patients seems even more pronounced, although the overall quality of up-to-date clinical teaching is not as good.

A unique requirement for graduation is a two-month preceptorship during the fourth year. Students are sent to small communities around the state to work one-on-one with a family practitioner, general internist, pediatrician, or general surgeon. At this point in their training, students are typically offered a great deal of autonomy in providing medical care in the community-based practice.

When it comes time to send out residency applications, the faculty offers strong support. Many students choose to stay in Wisconsin or the Midwest

for residency; however, UW always has a solid contingency that moves on to train in top East and West Coast programs.

Social Life

Simply stated, Madison is a fantastic place to live. Recently voted the best city to live in the U.S. by *Money* magazine, Madison thrives as the state capital and as a university town of more than 200,000 inhabitants. The city is located on an isthmus between two beautiful lakes and exists as a progressive, cosmopolitan oasis surrounded by the rolling green hills of southern Wisconsin farmland and prairies.

The Student Union Terrace is the most memorable social spot for University of Wisconsin graduates. Located on the shores of Lake Mendota, the Terrace is the ideal place to hang out, meet friends, study for exams, rent a sailboat, drink a microbrew, and listen to free live music on the weekends. Every couple of months, the UW Medical School Alumni group funds a TGIF party at the Union that features free beer, food, and music for current medical students.

Overall, Madison offers the varied cultural experiences of larger cities, such as nearby Chicago, but is much safer and has a more affordable cost of living. Madison is not a nightclub city, but hip music venues, great ethnic restaurants, a ritzy lounge scene, and a variety of personality-laden coffee shops are available for entertainment. The city has been nicknamed "Mad Town" because of the rowdy college bar scene in the campus area.

For those who enjoy outdoor activities, opportunities abound to sail, hike, fish, camp, and rock climb during the spring, summer, and fall. Although the winter can be challenging, people willing to brave the elements can experience spectacular cross-country ski trails, snowshoeing, and ice-skating.

The Bottom Line

The University of Wisconsin Medical School provides fantastic training with a helpful and supportive faculty. Its program is geared toward primary-care education, but the final choice about residency training is limited only by one's drive. The downside to UW is that the winters are cold and people always ask students if they like cheese.

VANDERBILT UNIVERSITY SCHOOL OF MEDICINE

Nashville, Tennessee

Students Receiving Financial Aid: 81%
Applications: 5,838
Size of Entering Class: 104
Total Number of Women Students: 136 (33%)
Total Number of Men Students: 277 (67%)
World Wide Web: www.mc.vanderbilt.edu/
  medschool/

Contact: Dr. John N. Lukens, Chairman,
  Committee on Admissions
  Nashville, TN 37240-1001
  615-322-2145

Vanderbilt University School of Medicine is well-known in the South and has enjoyed a long tradition of producing some of the most influential doctors in the country. For those students who originally come from the Northeast or West, Vanderbilt turns out to be one of the best-kept secrets in medical education: students graduate with excellent training and a sense of pride and tradition.

Preclinical Years

Like most traditional medical schools, the first two years are classroom didactics. The curriculum continues to evolve, but in general, gross anatomy, biochemistry, microbiology, and physiology are taught during the first year. Pathology, histology, pharmacology, laboratory, and physical diagnosis are taught during the second year. Biochemistry and physiology are usually taught by basic scientists without any clinical training; microbiology tends to be more of a mixed bag.

The most time-consuming but rewarding class during the first year is gross anatomy. After an inauguration ceremony on the first day of medical school, students find themselves nervously meeting their cadavers for the first time. Needless to say, students spend much of their first semester reeking of formalin. Pathology is generally considered the best class during the second year.

The worst class in many students' opinion is pharmacology, which is taken during the second year. The Department of Pharmacology at Vanderbilt is a highly ranked department that produced the most recent edition of Goodman and Gilman's *The Pharmacological Basis of Medical Therapeutics*. The fact

that pharmacology has such bad reputation probably has more to do with the nature of the subject matter rather than the lack of depth or talent in the department.

The School still goes by the traditional letter grading system. However, a C is considered marginal rather than passing, and if a student receives two Cs in one year, he or she has to repeat the year. From most student experiences, the grading system, though harsh, has not created a competitive atmosphere. Students enjoy high morale and spirit of camaraderie.

Clinical Years

Students rotate through two main hospitals and two ancillary facilities. Vanderbilt University Hospital and the Nashville VA are physically adjacent to each other and are connected by walkways. The University Hospital is a nine-story building with very modern facilities. Vanderbilt is the only regional tertiary hospital with a Level 1 trauma center in the area, so the census can run high, and there are plenty of interesting cases for students to see. Like most places, the quality of experience is highly team dependent. Good attending/resident/intern equals good experience. The University Hospital has an advanced computerized patient information/ordering system. The drawback to student rotation is that many patients are private, and students may not get much hands-on experience.

The Nashville VA is similar to other VAs: a great place for "bread and butter" medicine. Most students like VA rotations, since they get to do more and are more involved in the decision-making process of patient care. St. Thomas and Baptist Hospitals are local institutions that compete with Vanderbilt for patients. They are private, nonteaching hospitals and are more efficient and have better fringe benefits (such as better food).

Social Life

Nashville is a thriving midsize (population 533,000) Southern metropolis known as the Music City. Country music writers, performers, and producers are prominent, but other forms of music are appreciated in the city. For example, Indigo Girls used to perform at the legendary Blue Bird Café, and the Police at the Exit Inn. Station Inn has excellent bluegrass music almost all year round. One of the advantages of Nashville is that major cultural events, though limited in number, are cheap and easy to attend. For example, classical music concerts do not tend to sell out, so $5 student rush tickets are fairly easy to acquire. Students can see Midori, Yo-Yo Ma, and Joseph Bell for that price. The same goes for operas and plays. In addition, Vanderbilt University itself invites its own fair share of cultural events to campus.

Professional sports are becoming a major part of city life. Two new professional sports teams are now in Nashville. The Houston Oilers are now the Tennessee Oilers. Before their new stadium is built, they will play at the Vanderbilt Stadium, which is within walking distance of the medical school. A new NHL expansion team, the Predators, has made Nashville its home. The franchise spared no expense in constructing a downtown hockey rink and in advertising its new presence. Outdoor activities include kayaking and white-water rafting in Ocoee River (an Olympics venue), and many beautiful state parks are within driving distance. Vanderbilt's recreation center organizes many outings throughout the academic year.

There are a number of good restaurants in Nashville. Most are continental, Italian, or Southern. Ethnic cuisine abounds. Cafés and microbreweries are beginning to thrive in Nashville. Atlanta is 4 hours away.

The Bottom Line

Vanderbilt is a special place. Students sense that their education is excellent. Tuition is expensive, but alumni attest to Vanderbilt's value.

VIRGINIA COMMONWEALTH UNIVERSITY MEDICAL COLLEGE OF VIRGINIA SCHOOL OF MEDICINE

Richmond, Virginia

Size of Entering Class: 170
Total Number of Women Students: 268 (40%)
Total Number of Men Students: 400 (60%)
World Wide Web: views.vcu.edu/html/schofmed. html

Contact: Cynthia Heldberg, Associate Dean for Admissions
901 West Franklin Street
Richmond, VA 23284-9005
804-828-9629

The Medical College of Virginia (MCV) offers a solid preclinical curriculum combined with high-caliber clinical training. MCV is a busy urban medical center with enormous opportunities for clinical experience. Most graduates feel that the breadth and rigor of patient exposure provides the cornerstone of their education. They emerge with strong feelings of confidence in their training and satisfaction with their experience. MCV also has a mission to train primary-care physicians, with approximately 40–50 percent of graduates choosing primary-care residencies.

Preclinical Years

The goal of the preclinical years is to provide students with enough exposure to the basic medical sciences to pass the boards and function on the wards. This is a considerable task, and despite a sympathetic faculty, most students find the first two years to be at least moderately painful. MCV provides a reasonably well-structured approach to the preclinical years, with an extremely intensive anatomy course, a nicely organized physiology course, and an entire second year based upon organ system pathophysiology that most students find to be intellectually practical.

The school has a number of outstanding professors. The Foundation for Clinical Medicine (FCM) course is probably the academic highlight of the first two years. This course teaches first- and second-year students the basics of history taking and physical examination and meets weekly in small groups or with primary-care physicians. This program has received excellent reviews from most students, who feel that it teaches excellent clinical fundamentals.

Mercifully, MCV provides a grading system that is based on a straight scale rather than a curve. This

permits students to work with, rather than against, each other. The biggest sources of stress come from the sheer volume of the workload and from students' expectations about their own performances. Students tend to score above average on Step I of the boards, thanks to an extensive review course and three weeks of designated study time at the end of second year. The administration is reasonably attentive to student concerns, with such recent improvements as a new lecture hall for first-year students, computer-based learning models, and a decreased amount of lecture time with more focused content.

Electives are offered six afternoons during the first two years, with a limited number of funded research opportunities and clinical electives during the summers. Students are provided six to eight weeks of vacation between the first two years. Most people make the decision to use this as leisure time.

Clinical Years

Most students are satisfied with their clinical training at MCV. The FCM course provides a solid basis of clinical skills in the first two years, and most students feel well prepared for the patient contact of third year. There is no secret recipe for the strength of MCV's third-year curriculum. Students are given significant patient-care responsibility, are exposed to a wide variety of pathology, and have faculty members who take their teaching responsibilities seriously.

Most of the training is done at the main MCV hospital in downtown Richmond, which features a largely urban, indigent population but also serves as a referral center for central Virginia. The McGuire Veterans Hospital also provides a significant amount of clinical exposure and functions as a referral center within the VA system. The training at these two main hospitals is supplemented to a lesser extent by private hospitals, such as St. Mary's in suburban Richmond and Riverside Hospital in Newport News. Students also spend one month of the third year in the setting of a primary-care practice. There is little managed-care exposure.

The internal medicine and surgery rotations are the strongest, most rigorous, and best organized. The majority of the others are quite good as well, but all vary with individual experience. The weakest links are the outpatient settings in rotations such as pediatrics and neurology, where students attend different settings on a daily basis in an effort to gain a variety of experiences, but in doing so, sacrifice continuity and consistency. Most of the grumbling about third year concerns the subjective grading system, "brown nosing" from fellow students, and personality conflicts with attendings and residents. These problems are not unique to MCV and will probably remain as long as the current medical education system is in place.

The fourth year at MCV is mentioned with reverence among its graduates and longing by members of the first three years. Students are given six to seven months of elective time and a month to travel and interview, with the one strict caveat that they complete a month's rotation as an acting intern in a selected field. As one might imagine, this year provides an experience of considerably less intensity than the previous three. However, most people feel that it has a distinctly salutary effect on their humanity.

MCV students have been performing extremely well on Part II of the boards in recent years. Last year, they featured a 99 percent pass rate, with nearly one third of the class scoring above the 90th percentile, a testimony to both excellent clinical training and a good review course. MCV (as well as the other two Virginia schools) has a grant from the state to encourage half of its graduates to choose residencies in primary care. MCV is very active in promoting the primary-care fields, especially during the first two years of school, but students who choose specialties (approximately half of the class) feel that they have excellent faculty and administrative support. MCV's career counseling service is a true asset to its students. It features a number of beloved figures at all levels who provide the aspiring resident with efficient and personable service. In 1998, 90 percent of students got one of their top three choices in the match.

Social Life

Life in Richmond is affordable, enjoyable, and, depending on location, usually safe. Apartments rent from $300 to $600, depending on size, location, and number of roommates. Single family homes are available beginning in the $70,000–$80,000 range. The MCV campus is located in downtown Richmond but has little residential area surrounding the campus. Many people choose to live in an area known as the Fan, which features older, charming apartments and beautiful, tree-lined streets; others prefer the suburban comforts of the West End or South Side of Richmond.

Richmond is the capital of the old South, and both the city and school are steeped in Southern tradition. At its best, this represents fine architecture, museums, and historical sites and monuments; at its worst, a preponderance of fried foods, cars with gun racks, and frequent NASCAR events. Richmond has some areas of violent crime, but they are isolated to certain areas in the inner city and South Side and, outside of trauma surgery, have little bearing on the life of the average MCV student. Campus security is good, and campus crime is usually limited to petty theft. Richmond offers a good selection of places for food and entertainment. Cary Street and various downtown locations have excellent restaurants, while Shockoe Bottom provides plenty of places to hear good music or drown one's sorrows.

MCV is a part of Virginia Commonwealth University (VCU), and students frequently participate in various activities such as intramural sports or elective classes. For students who find themselves in personal or academic difficulty, both MCV and VCU provide a substantial range of both academic and personal counseling support.

The Bottom Line

Like most traditional U.S. medical schools, MCV is an intense place. But contrary to its portrayal in the recent movie about MCV graduate Patch Adams, it is a place with heart and tradition that cares about its students and patients. Students who are ready to spend four years working hard to become a good physician won't go wrong with MCV.

WAKE FOREST UNIVERSITY BOWMAN GRAY SCHOOL OF MEDICINE

Winston-Salem, North Carolina

Tuition 1996–97: $26,500 per year
Applications: 6,855
Size of Entering Class: 108
Total Number of Women Students: 258 (42%)
Total Number of Men Students: 350 (58%)
World Wide Web: www.bgsm.edu

Contact: Dr. Lewis Nelson, Associate Dean for Student Services and Admissions
Reynolda Station
Winston-Salem, NC 27109
336-716-2883

Wake Forest University Bowman Gray School of Medicine in Winston-Salem, North Carolina, is a popular school for applicants. In 1998, one out of every seven applicants to a U.S. medical school applied to Wake Forest. Wake Forest is a friendly school that offers a top-rated education with an innovative, highly computerized curriculum.

Each incoming student receives a laptop computer on which to read e-mail from faculty members and fellow students, receive lecture notes, and view radiological and pathological slides. Most rooms and the library have computer connectivity. During the second year, students receive IBM WorkPads. In addition to e-mail, the hand-held devices are used to download patient data. Some internal medicine teams make rounds with portable computers that display patient data and perform literature searches, the results of which can be radiowaved to a nearby laser printer. Fast, up-to-date computers abound, giving students access to the Internet and a multitude of learning resources, such as a radiographic anatomy tutorial developed by Wake's own radiology residents.

Wake Forest attracts applicants from all over the country, but half come from North Carolina. Most students are in their early 20s, although several are in their late 20s, 30s, and 40s. In 1998, only 9 percent of applicants were interviewed and 3 percent were accepted. Eighty percent of students receive financial aid. The average student spends $15,425 for room, board, and miscellaneous expenses and graduates with an $83,870 debt.

Preclinical Years

The curriculum at Wake Forest has recently undergone major restructuring. The basic sciences and clinical medicine are now integrated throughout the four years, so students start seeing patients in the beginning of the first year and are studying basic science issues in the fourth. Integrated courses have taken the place of departmental ones. Now students enroll in human structure and development instead of separate anatomy, embryology, and physiology courses.

Much of the curriculum is case based: students are presented with a patient (described on paper or portrayed by an actor) who has a problem that needs to be explored. Students, in small-group discussions, come to a diagnosis. Along the way, students study topics that relate to the case.

Ten exam rooms provide a training ground for learning how to interact with nonintimidating actors posing as patients. Students start learning history taking and physical examination skills in the first weeks and practice these techniques in community practices fourteen weeks after beginning school. Lectures are usually well delivered. Students may subscribe to the student-run note service for typewritten transcripts.

Three months of vacation are available between the first and second years, but many students do research with receptive faculty members and/or participate in the funded summer research program.

Clinical Years

The clinical rotations of the third year are a test of endurance. Call can be as frequent as every fourth night during surgery and internal medicine. On less demanding rotations, call may be approximately once every week. Students have to spend the night, except for during obstetrics, when students await the opportunity to assist with deliveries every fourth night.

Attendings typically ask questions to challenge instead of to torment. An occasional surgeon will probe a student's memory of anatomy during a procedure and invariably find it lacking, even though anatomy instruction at Wake Forest has traditionally been extensive and excellent.

The morale of the house staff is high, with good resident-student interaction. Opportunities for meaningful patient involvement abound, but opportunities for placing IVs and suturing lacerations can be lacking, a fact that is mostly rectified by a required fourth-year emergency room rotation.

The affiliated 806-bed hospital is pleasant. The support staff is superb. In the 1998 *U.S. News & World Report* "America's Best Hospitals," Wake Forest University Baptist Medical Center ranked high in cardiology and cardiac surgery, neurology and neurosurgery, geriatrics, gynecology, orthopedics, oncology, rheumatology, urology, and otolaryngology.

Students get exposure to indigent care at a local public health center. To deliver babies, students travel three miles to the other hospital in town. In surgery, students hold retractors, cut sutures, and occasionally stitch while participating in everything from laparoscopic appendectomy to kidney transplantation.

Students learn office medicine in the eight-week required Community Practice Experience. Some choose to live away from Winston-Salem.

Most patients are private. Many come to the tertiary referral center from the outlying towns in rural North Carolina and as far away as the neighboring states. Students care for the Winston-Salem businessman as well as the small-town tobacco farmer. Spanish fluency comes in handy with the region's rising Hispanic population.

Social Life

Winston-Salem is ideally located in the middle of North Carolina, with the richly forested Blue Ridge Mountains 2 hours by car to the west and the relaxing beaches of the Atlantic 4 hours to the east. Washington, D.C., is 6 hours to the north, and Atlanta is the same distance to the south. The bigger city scene may be found in Charlotte, less than 90 minutes away.

For the culturally inclined, Winston-Salem boasts an impressive array of opportunities for a city its size (170,000), from the symphony to the Southeastern Center for Contemporary Art. The city also has a unique cultural and religious heritage in its Moravian founding. In December, students can enjoy Moravian coffee and love feast buns at a Moravian love feast.

The restaurant and bar scene may not be as rich as in larger cities, but students can find a limited selection of bars as well as Mexican, Indian, Thai, Chinese, Italian, and Japanese food, not to mention North Carolina barbecue. As for shopping, Winston-Salem has the largest mall in the Carolinas. The cost of living is below the national average, and the affordable housing in Winston-Salem—the quiet residential area surrounding the School—is safe. To learn more about the city, students can visit http://www.ci. winston-salem.nc.us.

Schoolwide activities, such as the Halloween Party, the formal Charity Holiday Ball, and the Spring Fling, are memorable. Free tickets to University sporting events are provided, including ACC basketball.

Recreational activities abound. A fitness center, complete with sauna, free weights, and Nautilus, is right across from the student study room. For those who want to get away from the medical center, the University's undergraduate campus is a 10-minute drive. The business and law schools are there, as well as cheap films and good libraries in which to study. City parks are plentiful. The well-equipped YMCA and YWCA are nearby. Medical students also participate in intramural sports on the beautiful undergraduate campus.

The Bottom Line

Wake Forest is a top-rated private school with a friendly feel in a medium-sized southeastern city.

WASHINGTON UNIVERSITY IN ST. LOUIS SCHOOL OF MEDICINE

St. Louis, Missouri

Tuition 1996–97: $29,670 per year
World Wide Web: medschool.wustl.edu/
Contact: Dr. W. Edwin Dodson, Associate Dean

1 Brookings Drive
St. Louis, MO 63130-4899
314-362-6848

Large portraits of the School's fifteen distinguished Nobel laureates hang in the main hall of the Washington University in St. Louis School of Medicine (WUMS). Since its founding in 1891, the School has contributed to groundbreaking discoveries in many areas of medical research. This dedication to being on the forefront of medicine permeates the School and defines its students. WUMS is the fourth-largest recipient of NIH money among the 124 U.S. medical schools, receiving more than $170 million per year. The School is generous with these funds in its provision of opportunity and facilities to its students but demands hard work and motivation in return.

Admissions/Financial Aid

The average WUMS class is 120 students, up to twenty of whom are enrolled in the M.D./Ph.D. program. Admission is competitive, with an emphasis placed on prior academic achievement and the MCAT. The student body is talented and diverse. For instance, the entering class of 1996 was 49 percent women and 11 percent members of minority groups, majored in twenty-five different subjects, represented fifty-four undergraduate institutions, and came from thirty states and seven countries. Scholarships for women and sixteen merit-based, full tuition scholarships are awarded annually, which helps to encourage the application of top candidates to the School. Tuition is comprehensive and is fixed for four years of study. Tuition is currently approximately $30,000 per year. Financial aid is awarded on the basis of need. The School often provides small scholarships and loans to students in need when low-interest government loans have been exhausted.

Preclinical Years

The first-year curriculum provides a solid foundation in the basic sciences, such as anatomy, biochemistry, molecular genetics, and histology. To account for the diversity of academic backgrounds among its students as well as the inevitable adjustments to the first year of medical school, all first-year courses are graded on a pass/fail basis. The second-year curriculum consists of studying pathophysiology by organ systems, including hematology, cardiology, and gastroenterology. The second year is graded more traditionally, with honors, high pass, pass, and fail. The passing grades are often figured on a curve, and competition for the highest grades can be extreme. Still, most students prefer to study in small groups. Students run an organized note-taking service funded by the administration, and there is widespread class participation. The professors and the administration remain very supportive of any student who falls behind and provides them with extra tutorials and occasionally a retest or a modified academic schedule. The opportunity to accelerate the timing of course work in the first two years is limited.

A three-month summer between the first and second years provides students with a well-earned rest. To encourage students to use their summer to pursue a research initiative, the School funds all students who present a research proposal and get a faculty project mentor. Faculty members, most of whom are involved in research themselves, are very receptive to the addition of students to their labs. The School helps to ensure the proper funding for students who wish to extend projects into master's degrees or doctorates.

The most popular classes during the preclinical years include practical labs, with such activities as culturing microbes in microbiology, identifying diseases from bone marrow specimens in hematology, and testing the live effects of cardiac drugs in cardiology. In the early 1990s, there was a movement to bring more clinical experience into the first and second years. A program in ambulatory care was designed to bring first- and second-year students into the clinics and get them talking with patients. Clinical scenarios appeared in lectures. X-rays and MRIs came into use as teaching adjuncts in anatomy lab. More importance was placed on the courses in history taking and physical examination. Students seemed to welcome these changes.

Clinical Years

The clinical years (three and four) are largely spent at Washington University's on-site hospital affiliates, Barnes-Jewish Hospital and St. Louis Children's Hospital. These hospitals house nearly 2,000 patient beds. *U.S. News & World Report* consistently recognizes Barnes-Jewish Hospital among America's best hospitals. Other teaching hospital affiliates provide a range of experience for the students and include the St. Louis Regional Hospital, the Veterans Administration Medical Center, the St. Louis Psychiatric Center, and the Christian Hospitals Northeast and Northwest.

The third year consists of the core clerkships of medicine, surgery, pediatrics, obstetrics/gynecology, neurology, and psychiatry. Emphasis is placed on formulating treatment plans and understanding underlying pathophysiology. Some students get more theoretical than hands-on training. Given its stature in the surrounding area, the Barnes-Jewish Hospital receives referrals from all over the Midwest, significantly enhancing the experience for its medical students. Residents and attendings are an integral part of each student's medical education and often take time to individually instruct students. Given the importance of the first clinical year for residency selection, the third year is the most competitive year.

The fourth year consists solely of electives. A lottery system is held at the end of third year for students to pick their fourth-year electives. The year can be as challenging or as relaxing as the student desires. There tends to be great demand for challenging subinternships in the critical first months of the fourth year. Research electives and anatomy teaching assistant electives become more popular during the final months of medical school.

After four years, WUMS students are remarkably well prepared. The passing rates for Parts I and II of the National Board Exams are approximately 99 percent, with WUMS students scoring an average of

20 points higher than their national counterparts. This translates into success in the long-anticipated match. The most popular career choices for students are internal medicine and surgery. In 1997, 80 percent of the class obtained residencies in one of their top three choices.

Social Life

Many first-year students live in Olin Hall, which also houses physical therapy and occupational therapy students. Olin Hall is a typical 1970s-fashion state school–type dormitory. It is a good way to get to know classmates and is convenient (attached) to the medical school and hospitals. It also has a number of drawbacks, including small rooms and no kitchen facilities. Most upperclass students move to apartments in the surrounding Central West End or the western suburbs. The medical center and hospitals are located at the western edge of the city in the Central West End.

The Central West End is an eclectic neighborhood of shops, restaurants, and apartments. It is bordered by Forest Park, one of the largest city parks in the nation. Owning a car is recommended. A recent addition to St. Louis is the Metro Link, which stops at the Barnes-Jewish–WUMS campus and connects to downtown St. Louis, the airport, and East St. Louis.

St. Louis's 2.5 million people are usually friendly and unpretentious. The city is home to several professional sports teams (the Cardinals, Rams, and Blues), many sports personalities (Mark McGwuire, Brett Hull, and Bob Costas), a variety of nationally acclaimed cultural events (the St. Louis Symphony and the annual VP July 4th Fair), and fabulous ethnic restaurants that are accessible and affordable. St. Louis is a family-oriented city. For those who want to travel on weekends, St. Louis is a 5-hour drive from Chicago and 6 hours away from Cincinnati. The climate is hot and humid in the summer, fair in the fall, and moderate in the winter.

The Bottom Line

WUMS provides its students with a state-of-the-art medical education and a tremendous opportunity for research. The work is demanding, but students are rewarded for their hard work. The prototypical WUMS student is smart and motivated.

WAYNE STATE UNIVERSITY SCHOOL OF MEDICINE

Detroit, Michigan

Tuition 1996–97: $21,812 per year
Applications: 4,174
Size of Entering Class: 276
Total Number of Women Students: 551 (40%)
Total Number of Men Students: 816 (60%)

World Wide Web: www.wayne.edu/med.htm/
Contact: Dr. James Collins, Assistant Dean
656 West Kirby Street
Detroit, MI 48202
313-577-1466

The Wayne State University School of Medicine is the largest medical school in the country, with 280 students per class, and is set in the Detroit Medical Center, one of the country's largest multihospital complexes. The School's focus is to educate students in areas other than basic science, which is reflected in the recent creation of an alternative medicine component of the curriculum.

Preclinical Years

The first year consists of gross anatomy, histology, biochemistry, clinical nutrition, physiology, neuroanatomy, Introduction to the Patient, evidence-based medicine, and genetics. Students are also required to shadow physicians in their offices six times. The second year consists of immunology, microbiology, pathobiology, pathophysiology, psychiatry, preventive medicine, pharmacology, physical diagnosis, and medical ethics. Pathophysiology is particularly strong, while pharmacology, because of scheduling concerns, tends to be a weaker course.

Wayne students are minimally competitive in a healthy way that does not seem to interfere with friendships and camaraderie. Everyone seems to fill their own niche and, for the most part, welcomes interaction with others. Faculty members are extremely helpful, hosting extra sessions and providing old exams and extra slides. Individual tutors and group review sessions run by second-year students are available free of charge.

Beginning in the second half of the second year, free noontime review sessions are offered by faculty members in preparation for the USMLE. Students can also obtain CD-ROM Boards study assistance in preparation for the institution of computerized Boards.

Clinical Years

The Detroit Medical Center consists of Harper Hospital, Hutzel Hospital, Children's Hospital, the Rehabilitation Institute, Detroit Receiving, Gershenson Radiation Oncology Center, Kresge Eye Institute, and Huron Valley Hospital. The medical school also maintains affiliations with Providence Hospital, Oakwood Hospital, Beaumont, Veterans Administration Hospital, and other major urban and suburban hospitals in the Detroit metropolitan area.

In particular, Hutzel is a recognized leader in obstetrics and gynecology. Children's Hospital is one of the country's largest hospitals of its kind. Detroit Receiving is a Level 1 trauma center. In general, residents and attendings take care of their students. Hours are long, but the experience and knowledge gained are outstanding.

The third year consists of rotations in neurology, psychiatry, surgery, obstetrics and gynecology, internal medicine, pediatrics, and one elective. Although students must complete these rotations on-site, performing rotations at off-site locations may soon be a possibility. A minimum of eight electives comprise the fourth year. One of the electives may be a month off for credit earned through the cocurricular program. The administration rewards participation in community service through this program, which requires that students attend monthly seminars and perform 150 hours of community service.

Social Life

Wayne State is culturally diverse, a fact that is celebrated each fall during Ethnic Week, which brings noontime guest speakers, food, and a weekend party. Intraclass and interclass socializing is common. More than fifty student organizations offer the opportunity to perform community service, which is very popular. Students recently ventured to a local senior citizen center, where they took blood pressures and medical histories, administered medications, and created a keychain for each patient.

The School is situated in the heart of the cultural center, which includes the Fox Theater, the Detroit Institute of Arts, the Science Center, and the Museum of African American History. Within walking distance of the campus are the Attic Theater; the New

Center Area, which is a shopping area; and restaurants, such as Mexican Town. Apartments cost $250 or more per month.

The Bottom Line

At Wayne State, students get hands-on experience, beginning on the first day, fostered by a helpful administration. Training at the Detroit Medical Center is outstanding.

WESTERN UNIVERSITY OF HEALTH SCIENCES COLLEGE OF OSTEOPATHIC MEDICINE OF THE PACIFIC

Pomona, California

Applications: 4,007
Size of Entering Class: 181
World Wide Web: www.westernu.edu/comp.html
Contact: Susan M. Hanson, Director of
Admissions

309 E Second Street College Plaza
Pomona, CA 91766-1854
909-469-5335

Western University of Health Sciences (WUHS) is located in Pomona, California, a suburb of Los Angeles, and occupies the site of a restored downtown mall. Following the tradition of osteopathic medicine, education is geared toward producing primary-care physicians.

Admissions/Financial Aid

In general, WUHS attracts a wide spectrum of students and many races, religions, and philosophies. Students tend to be older (average age 29), and many are pursuing a second career, having developed a personal interest in osteopathy. Most are from the West, with 72 percent from California. Admission is weighted heavily on candidate interviews, and the school actively pursues a diverse student mix. It is essential that each applicant be knowledgeable about the differences between osteopathic and allopathic medicine. Because WUHS is a private school, the majority of students use financial aid, and many have military scholarships or help from their home states. Interviews are comfortable, with committees consisting of one or two professors, an admissions counselor, and a clinician. The atmosphere tends to be friendly and open, and interviews usually involve one ethical dilemma question.

Preclinical Years

The first semester is spent taking classes in the basic sciences as well as Osteopathic Principles and Practice (OP&P). The average amount of time spent in class per week is 36 hours, including labs. Exams are held every Monday. The second semester is dedicated to finishing gross anatomy and beginning organ system–

based instruction, which continues into the second year. In theory, the systems approach is meant to integrate all aspects of science involved in an organ system. Unfortunately, teaching styles vary and some systems are taught better than others.

During the first two years, the clinical medicine experience varies. OP&P is taught throughout both years and includes one week of cranial manipulation during the second year and timed practical exams one or two times a semester. There are a one-week class in clinical medicine during the end of the first year and an elective family medicine track that pairs students with preceptors. Most students, however, gain experience through clubs on campus dedicated to emergency medicine, surgery, sports medicine, and community health. Students can work in several free clinics, including one that volunteers in Tijuana.

The grading system is A–F, but the class tends not to be competitive. There is no note service, but professors bring their notes to class, and study books of old exams are handed down from class to class. Opportunities for research and clinical work between the first and second years are limited and usually occur through clubs or personal initiative.

Clinical Years

WUHS is not based out of a main hospital, and it has a system of clinical education that seems to change a little from year to year. Each student is assigned a block of five 4-week rotations at one of several hospitals in either southern California or Phoenix, Arizona. For the other seven months, there is one vacation rotation, and the other six are set up individually by each student from a list of thousands of approved rotation sites around the U.S. This allows a lot of freedom to travel and to see various facilities, but it can also be frustrating because there is little guidance from the school as to how to shape the educational experience. Each student has a different clinical experience.

The best hospitals at which to perform rotations tend to be the larger county hospitals, specifically San Bernardino County. There are also good rotations at Long Beach Community Hospital, Western Medical Center, Downey Hospital, Mesa General Hospital, and Tempe St. Lukes. Private preceptors are usually picked based on advice from previous students and written evaluations kept on file. For students on military scholarships, there is a lot of freedom to pursue rotations at military hospitals, and these rotations are generally very good.

During the third and fourth years, there are three weekends when students are required to be in Pomona. Essentials of Family Medicine consists of three days of classes, exams, and clinical work. Students are required to travel from their current clinical site (possibly anywhere in the U.S.) to Pomona for these weekends.

Social Life

Extracurricular life revolves primarily around an amazing array of student clubs, which are dedicated to ethnic and religious affiliations or hobbies. A thespian club produces one or two plays per year. The exam schedule during the first semester makes it difficult to do much on the weekends, but after Christmas, exams are held every three or four weeks, so students get more free time. The weather is beautiful in the winter and extremely hot in the summer; smog is particularly troublesome. The beach is approximately 45 minutes away, and many students invest their free time in surfing. Los Angeles is nearby and offers a bounty of urban activities.

Most students live near school, though not in the city of Pomona. Pomona can be quite unsafe, and there are guards on campus to reinforce that point. Safer communities are approximately 10–15 minutes away, and there is a decent social scene around the Claremont Colleges. Students often study at Claremont libraries in the evenings. There is no on-campus housing. Affordable single and family housing is available but may require some looking. Many single students room with each other, and the school facilitates the roommate search.

The Bottom Line

Students at WUHS leave with fond memories of their diverse classmates and club activities but often lament administrative problems and sometimes erratic teaching practices. Overall, WUHS offers reasonable didactic instruction with a chance to customize each student's clinical experience.

WEST VIRGINIA UNIVERSITY SCHOOL OF MEDICINE

Morgantown, West Virginia

Tuition 1996–97: $22,704 per year
Size of Entering Class: 88
Total Number of Women Students: 404 (56%)
Total Number of Men Students: 322 (44%)
World Wide Web: www.hsc.wvu.edu/som/

Contact: Dr. John W. Traubert, Associate Dean
University Avenue
Morgantown, WV 26506
304-293-2408

The West Virginia University (WVU) School of Medicine offers a small, laid-back, student-oriented program located in Morgantown, West Virginia. The School prides itself on turning out excellent clinicians and places an emphasis on primary care.

Preclinical Years

The basic sciences at WVU are currently in flux, as the more traditional schedule has been replaced by a curriculum that seeks to integrate similar subjects and give a greater clinical exposure in the first two years. For example, physiology has been condensed into one semester and is combined with biochemistry and genetics into a class entitled Human Function. Ultimately, the system involves the same subjects, lectures, and professors but a different schedule. More self-study is required compared to the old curriculum, which many students dislike and think is a bad idea. Fortunately, one of the best aspects of WVU is how responsive the administration is to student concerns. The new curriculum began in 1998–99, so students should be prepared for many modifications to the grand experiment.

It is hard to say how much the new curriculum affects the first two years. In general, medical students at West Virginia, as much as their counterparts elsewhere, disdain the first two years and look forward eagerly to their clinical years. To address this concern, WVU has been quite proactive. First years learn how to interview patients and get their first taste of the real world by shadowing a private physician. In the second year, students practice taking histories and physicals in the hospital. In the summer between first and second year, several departments in the hospital offer paid externships, where students are often treated as third years for a few weeks.

Clinical Years

This is where WVU shines. The School teaches by having students actually work (and work hard) in the hospital, not just look over their attending's shoulder. Working hard means no electives during the third year, and the vacation time is limited to two 2-week breaks. In the fourth year, students get four months for electives, as well as two weeks guaranteed off for residency interviews. This tends to pay off, as students usually do quite well in the match.

For the clerkships, there are two campuses: Morgantown and Charleston. One third of the class must spend its third year in Charleston, but it is possible to return to Morgantown for the fourth year. In Morgantown, the hospital complex is connected, but in Charleston, students work at three different hospitals, which are far enough apart to require transportation. In addition, some of the fourth year can be spent in Wheeling, West Virginia, or at an approved out-of-state hospital.

The hospital in Morgantown is a tertiary-care university facility in a rural setting. The size of the hospital means that patient exposure is more varied than would be expected for the area. The Charleston hospitals are more heterogeneous, as the capital city is as urban as West Virginia gets. Both campuses require the same rotations, but the individual requirements for each clinical clerkship can vary. A primary-care rotation at a rural site is necessary in both years.

Social Life

WVU students are as laid back as students find in medical school. The relaxed atmosphere is helped by an accommodating and sympathetic administration and an approachable faculty. As for a social life, students need to bring their own fun to Morgantown because it is hard to find. West Virginia is known for its many outdoor activities, but beyond that, choices are limited. WVU sports are popular, and the football stadium and basketball arena are close to the hospital. In general, if the University does not provide an activity, students are not going to find it in Morgantown. The last resort is the bars downtown, but medical students tend to feel out of place here unless they attend WVU for college. If you really miss city life, Pittsburgh is only 80 miles to the north. Morgantown does have enough appeal that most of the class wants to stay in town for their clerkships.

Although Charleston is much more urban, it is still close to wilderness for the outdoor enthusiast. It is also more bike friendly than Morgantown. Charleston has more of what a city can offer: a vibrant downtown, large shopping centers, and several good restaurants. With a population of just more than 100,000 in the greater area, it retains a small-town feel and is free of many urban problems.

West Virginia has one of the lowest crime rates in the country, and both campuses are safe. The cost of living is low compared with the rest of the nation, but housing is better in Charleston, as landlords in Morgantown enjoy raising the rent because of the great student demand. The School offers housing at both campuses at a very reasonable price. Few students live in University housing in Morgantown, as the apartments are small and rather old. The Charleston campus offers a variety of housing that ranges from old, small efficiencies to newer apartments on the Kanawha River to houses close to the hospital.

The Bottom Line

WVU turns out great clinicians in a user-friendly environment. While the preclinical years are not particularly enjoyable, the School offers a relaxed atmosphere, caring faculty, an administration that is student oriented, and numerous opportunities for other clinical sites in the state. Unless students need to live in a big city, WVU is the school for them.

WRIGHT STATE UNIVERSITY SCHOOL OF MEDICINE

Dayton, Ohio

Tuition 1996–97: $19,488 per year
Size of Entering Class: 90
Total Number of Women Students: 206 (54%)
Total Number of Men Students: 175 (46%)
World Wide Web: www.med.wright.edu

Contact: Dr. Paul Carlson, Associate Dean for
Student Affairs and Admissions
Colonel Glenn Highway
Dayton, OH 45435
937-775-2934

Wright State University School of Medicine, named for the brothers who pioneered flight, was established in 1973 in Dayton, Ohio. The School strives to serve Dayton's surrounding communities, with a strong emphasis on primary care. Wright State is among the top three schools producing primary-care physicians. The benefits of a young medical school include state-of-the-art basic science facilities, from the gross anatomy lab to the new computer labs, as well as an enthusiastic, progressive, and young faculty dedicated to teaching.

Typically, more than 50 percent of Wright State's class are women, and approximately 30 percent are members of minority groups. All facilities are wheelchair accessible.

Preclinical Years

Orientation begins in mid-August, when the class of approximately ninety-five students spends a week getting to know one another in events such as ropes courses and fun runs. The first-year curriculum starts with gross anatomy, an intensive course that lasts a little more than two months. During anatomy, students begin to appreciate the strong link between the medical school and the community. Cadaveric donors' death certificates are displayed in the anatomy lab, and the end of the year is marked by a Unitarian interment ceremony attended by the donors' relatives and the students.

Once anatomy is over, students rest and prepare for the remainder of the curriculum, which is entirely systems based and relies heavily on computers. Computer testing is being phased into the curriculum in preparation for the USMLE's move to computer-based testing. The grading is numerical, with no letter grades. Students who score between 60 and 70 percent are allowed to repeat exams to bring their average to

70. Students with lower averages must retake the course. Fortunately, the administration believes their commitment to admitting students lasts through graduation. The school offers 4+1, 4+2, and (in extreme cases) 4+3 programs. Tutors are provided free of charge.

During breaks between blocks of courses, students choose two-week electives, which range from experiences in urban or rural private practice offices to plastic surgery. A student can also create his or her own elective. Students say these experiences serve to remind them of why they are in medical school and forestall the disillusionment many face during two years of tedious basic sciences courses. The curriculum also exposes students to clinical medicine every Friday starting the first week of school, when groups of two to four students spend time with preceptors at Franciscan Hospital learning the art of the history and physical.

Students can opt for a variety of options during the summer between the first and second years. Some choose to take more electives, which gives them more free time during second year. Others take advantage of eight-week research opportunities funded by the American Heart Association or four-week funded opportunities in urban or rural medicine.

Clinical Years

Because Wright State does not have its own teaching hospital, it makes use of the resources of the Dayton community, which include five hospitals (Miami Valley, Franciscan, Good Samaritan, Kettering, and Wright Patterson Air Force Base Hospitals) and numerous private practices. These hospitals provide an incredible array of patient experiences. Students are exposed to patients in urban and rural settings as well as suburban settings.

Students enjoy their experiences at the East Dayton Health Center, an urban practice dedicated to community health and patient education in an economically depressed area of Dayton. Obstetrics and gynecology at Wright Patterson offers the benefit of a hospital where the nuclear family still exists, with complete family planning and prenatal care. On the other end of the spectrum is the high-risk and teenage clinic at Miami Valley, the largest hospital in Dayton.

Fourth-year students are required to complete rotations in neurology, orthopedics, emergency medicine, and primary care. The rest of the year is filled with electives. Students have two months off to interview and for vacation.

Social Life

There are many extracurricular activities available to students. Sports leagues are popular (soccer, volleyball, basketball, etc.), and the nightlife is about 15 minutes from the School in downtown Dayton's Oregon district. Downtown Cincinnati and Columbus are within an hour's drive as well. For the past few years, students have joined law students at the University of Dayton for M.D./J.D. parties.

One of the benefits of Dayton is the cost of living. Most students find apartments off campus, with many quiet communities within a 10- or 20-minute drive. Students willing to live with a roommate can easily find a nice apartment for $250 to $350 per person per month. A single spacious apartment runs from $350 to $500 per month. Dayton is a great place to raise a family, given the low cost of living and the quality of the schools. These two factors have been important aspects for professors at Wright State as well.

The Bottom Line

Wright State's primary-care emphasis, reinforced by community projects, provides graduates of this young school with an excellent foundation for residency training.

YALE UNIVERSITY SCHOOL OF MEDICINE

New Haven, Connecticut

Size of Entering Class: 102
World Wide Web: info.med.yale.edu/medical/

Contact: Applicable degree Program
New Haven, CT 06520

The Yale University School of Medicine offers an excellent medical education and ample time for outside pursuits. Initiative and independence are essential qualities for students who wish to make the most of a Yale medical education. Those who take advantage of the Yale System can become first-rate physicians and physician-scientists while enjoying their years in medical school.

Preclinical Years

Yale offers lectures and problem-based tutorials. Instead of one professor teaching an entire course, each class is taught by multiple physicians and basic science experts on a given topic. The first-year curriculum reflects Yale's excellence in basic science as well as its high expectations for students. For example, first-year cell biology offers a parade of international luminaries, with the result that some complain that the material is not all clinically relevant.

Physiology, biochemistry, and neuroscience do a better job of satisfying the students' desire for clinical relevance, with basic science lectures balanced by weekly patient-based cases. Anatomy lab is fairly standard: groups of four dissect two mornings per week until spring break. The course also uses X rays and computer software to emphasize important structures. The first year is rounded out by classes in professional responsibility, health policy, and child and adult development.

Students are not required to attend class or to sit for midterm exams. Everyone must take a qualifier at the end of each course, but these are graded anonymously and are pass/fail. Those who fail can usually see the professor, and most end up resitting for the exam and passing. The system fosters a noncompetitive environment in which students are given the responsibility for their own education. Despite the lack of grades, students are well prepared for the wards and the Boards; the average score on the USMLE Part I is usually in the 220s.

The second year is broken down into blocks of one to four weeks that focus on the major body systems: e.g., cardiovascular, gastrointestinal, and endocrine. Within each module, the relevant pathophysiology, pharmacology, radiology, physical exam, and public health issues are neatly addressed in a series of well-integrated lectures, labs, and problem-based seminars.

Yale is the last medical school in the country to require an independent research project for graduation, and, like so much of the School, the thesis is what each student makes of it. It can be as simple as a chart review or so involved that students choose to take a fifth year to complete it. Many begin their project during the summer after the first year, and there is plenty of funding available for research. The stellar facilities at the Cushing Medical Library include comfortable study space (both social and secluded), abundant computers, and hundreds of journals.

Clinical Years

The quality of clinical rotations is generally high but variable. Students rotate through a number of hospitals, including Yale–New Haven Hospital, the West Haven Veterans Administration Hospital, St. Raphael's, and many community hospitals throughout Connecticut. Students generally receive their top choices for sites.

Internal medicine is a strong clerkship at Yale. The department, one of the finest in the country, is filled with attendings and residents who are eager to teach. Didactic sessions are well organized and comprehensive. Similarly, the psychiatry department is outstanding, and students emerge from that rotation better able to think about their patients and themselves, regardless of their chosen specialties. Psychiatry can be done at an outside institution.

Other rotations are team dependent because they offer fewer didactics. Pediatrics is friendly and flexible; the rotation offers the option of many subspecialties, primary care, or a month away. The twelve weeks of surgery are broken into one month of general surgery and eight weeks of subspecialties. The philosophy of the department is that all physicians should understand surgery and perioperative management.

Obstetrics and gynecology is the one of the weakest clerkships at Yale; still, many students choose this as their specialty. Neurology and primary care, both of which can be completed at other institutions, are required. In the fourth year, students must take Integrated Clinical Medicine. Fourth-year students devote time to one or more subinternships, electives, applications, and the thesis.

A noticeable gap is family medicine. Although students protest the absence of such a department at Yale, no change seems imminent. The bias of the School remains specialization and research. Students are nonetheless encouraged to perform rotations elsewhere to gain other perspectives.

Clerkships are graded, unlike the first two years. There are no written exams at the end of each rotation, which makes grading subjective and unpredictable. The dean's letter highlights student accomplishments, and every year, students match at the top hospitals in the country.

Social Life

New Haven is a great place to live as a student, and most students are happy because of the curriculum and the high quality of life. Housing options include lovely old houses with inexpensive rents and big yards, as well as high-rise apartment buildings two blocks from the School. Rents start at approximately $500 per month for large one-bedroom apartments; two-bedroom apartments can be had for $800 to $1,000 per month.

Because of Yale's presence, New Haven offers the cultural diversity of a larger city. It does help to have a car for travel to outlying hospitals as well as for taking advantage of the area around New Haven, which offers beaches, hiking, and restaurants. New York and Boston are nearby and easily accessible by train. Thanks to the Yale System, students actually have time to go.

Perhaps because New Haven is more of a small town than Boston or New York, the Yale community is quite tight-knit. Students form close friendships. Club Med, a Thursday night bar at the dormitory, is hosted by a different professor each week. Every year, the second-year class puts on a musical comedy show spoofing medical school life (recent titles include *The Rx Files* and *Live and Let Diagnose*). Professors often invite students to their homes for dinner, and the dean hosts students at events ranging from backyard barbecues to picnics at the world-class Pilot Pen tennis tournament.

Like many older cities, New Haven has its share of urban problems, making it a fitting site for medical training. Most students become involved in the life of the city through community service programs that provide health care to the homeless, teach children about AIDS and substance abuse, and tutor high school students in science.

In terms of safety, the medical school offers numerous security escorts, shuttles, and patrols. Unfortunately, the city remains unsafe mostly for its economically disadvantaged citizens.

The Bottom Line

Yale offers a first-rate medical education, and most say they chose Yale because when they came to visit, they found unusually happy and relaxed students.

YESHIVA UNIVERSITY ALBERT EINSTEIN COLLEGE OF MEDICINE

New York, New York

Tuition 1996–97: $27,650 per year
Applications: 9,136
Size of Entering Class: 180
Total Number of Women Students: 399 (0.44%)
Total Number of Men Students: 507 (0.56%)
World Wide Web: www.aecom.yu.edu

Contact: Noreen Kerrigan, Assistant Dean for Admissions
500 West 185th Street
New York, NY 10033-3201
718-430-2106

Albert Einstein College of Medicine (AECOM) is the medical epicenter of the Bronx, one of the five boroughs of New York City. While some parts of the Bronx are notorious for their levels of social dysfunction, Einstein is surrounded by a stable and amicable community.

Einstein students pride themselves on being friendly, cohesive, and noncompetitive. The administration, the faculty, and most of the attendings in the affiliated hospitals create a comfortable environment for students, are easily accessible, and facilitate exchanges on improving medical education. In fact, the administration is open to suggestions and encourages student input in revising the curriculum. Because Einstein is the medical school for Yeshiva University, the school shuts down before sundown on Fridays.

Preclinical Years

The preclinical curriculum at Einstein is undergoing major transformations and has adopted an interdisciplinary approach to medical education; cell biology, genetics, biochemistry, and immunology have been interwoven into one course entitled Molecular and Cellular Foundations of Medicine (MCFM), and system-based courses combine physiology, pathophysiology, pathology, and pharmacology. Case-based learning is pervasive, and the administration hopes that it will become the primary teaching device as lecture hours are reduced.

Students have mixed reviews about the new curriculum. Many enjoy learning by juxtaposing the normal and abnormal, but others protest that this approach does not devote enough emphasis to the fundamentals of physiology and pharmacology. In

general, however, the system-based courses are taught well by experienced faculty members who care about teaching. The inclusion of a ten-week parasitology course is called excessive by many students.

The main exposure to clinical medicine comes from participation in case-based learning. Einstein also offers a required Introduction to Clinical Medicine (ICM) course, which helps students develop the skills to establish meaningful doctor-patient relationships. In the first year, ICM sponsors weekly visits to a primary-care facility, substance abuse clinic, or prenatal-care clinic. A voluntary Generalist Mentorship program provides early exposure to primary care under the supervision of an internist. The second year of ICM is the traditional physical diagnosis course.

In order to reduce competition and allow students to adjust to the rigors of medical school, grades for the first year are pass/fail, but in the second year, an honors category is added. The school provides free tutoring, counseling, and tracking of exam performance. Students who fail exams are encouraged to stay in school and spread out their preclinical courses over three years.

Between the first and second years, students have the option of taking the summer off, engaging in scientific or clinical research, or acquiring early exposure to the clinical world by working in Einstein's affiliated hospitals or elsewhere. A few students rotate through the Jacobi ER, a level-one trauma center that is one of New York City's busiest.

Einstein, known for its high-quality basic and clinical research, encourages students to work in labs, and the school provides multiple opportunities to get involved. For example, students are required to write a paper that is suitable for publication before graduation. During the summer months, the school offers a stipend of roughly $2,000 for eight to ten weeks of research. Many students are fortunate enough to publish during this experience, while others continue with their research over the next three years. For those students who want more intense laboratory experiences, Einstein has ranked in the top 10 percent for obtaining prestigious Howard Hughes medical student fellowships.

Clinical Years

AECOM has six affiliated hospitals located in the Bronx, Manhattan, and Long Island, with a variety of environments and patient populations. In general, there is more hands-on experience at the public hospitals (Jacobi and Bronx Lebanon) than in the private hospitals (Long Island Jewish, Beth Israel, and Weiler Hospitals).

Montefiore Medical Center (MMC), Einstein's largest and strongest teaching hospital, includes neighborhood maintenance health satellites throughout the Bronx and Westchester County. Jacobi Hospital is distinguished for its ER training. Beth Israel is Einstein's Manhattan campus, where students are provided with free housing during their rotations and the call schedule is generally lighter.

Einstein emphasizes primary-care training in eleven weeks of internal medicine, seven weeks of pediatrics, six weeks of family medicine, two weeks of geriatrics, eight weeks of ambulatory medicine, and eight weeks of a subinternship in medicine or pediatrics. Internal medicine is one of the strongest rotations. At MMC, the attendings and the house staff provide excellent training, and the subinternship is essentially equivalent to a two-month internship experience. In pediatrics, MMC also offers one of the stronger experiences in outpatient care, while at Long Island Jewish Children's Hospital (Schneider), inpatient training is excellent.

Surgery is the one of the weakest experiences at Einstein because of the high ratio of scut work to learning. At MMC and Long Island Jewish, however, interested students relish the number of procedures they can observe. Bronx Lebanon stands out because of the high proportion of residents who, as graduates of international medical schools, were formerly

attendings in other countries and are more comfortable with teaching.

The obstetrics/gynecology clerkship also needs improvement. With some exceptions, students must be very aggressive to acquire any training in deliveries and procedures. This is particularly true at Beth Israel.

Psychiatry offers a good variety of strong sites. Four Winds Hospital, an open facility in suburban Westchester County, is notable for providing drama therapy and managing adolescent patients who are battling drug abuse. Students who prefer a locked facility that houses mostly psychotic patients find Bronx State Psychiatric Center ideal. Jacobi's psychiatric ER offers an invaluable opportunity to gain hands-on experience with patients who have made suicide and drug overdose attempts.

Einstein's most popular electives, which are not available until the fourth year, are emergency medicine at Jacobi, cardiology at Weiler Hospital, and nephrology at Montefiore. Popular externships can be performed in Israel at Hadassa and Soroka hospitals, in Costa Rica, or on a Native American reservation in the Dakotas. One month is allotted for official vacation time, but most people consider the entire fourth year (other than ambulatory medicine and the sub-I) less stressful.

Social Life

Students have mixed feelings about living in the Bronx. Housing and parking are inexpensive and convenient. Apartments at Einstein come in three varieties: studio apartments ($380 per month), one-bedroom apartments ($528 per month for two people), and two-bedroom apartments ($700 per month for three people). During the preclinical years, students have ample time to explore other interests. Community-based projects include homeless shelters, vaccination programs, violence prevention, and public school health education. On the other hand, Einstein has no bookstore or gift shop. Instead, a book service sells the recommended or required books for each class at cost, and a monthly, nomadic kiosk sells Einstein paraphernalia.

The area immediately surrounding Einstein is barren—there are a food truck, one bar, one pizza restaurant, and two other fast-food restaurants that constantly change ownership. Within a 10-minute walk are banks, grocery stores, a video store, and a neighborhood popular for its Italian cuisine. For more expensive restaurants, Arthur Avenue is a 10-minute car ride away, as are two movie theaters. On campus, there are two cafeterias, both kosher.

With express buses leaving hourly, travel to and from Manhattan is easy and convenient. The Botanical Gardens, Bronx Zoo, and Orchard Beach provide pleasant entertainment. Nearby golf courses and horseback riding are other advantages to living on the outskirts of Manhattan.

The Bottom Line

Einstein is a top-twenty-five medical school that is ideal for the outdoor-oriented, noncompetitive student interested in primary-care medicine, research, or both.

AUTHORS OF
Medical School Profiles

Steve Anisman, University of Vermont College of
Medicine

Christopher Blewett, University of Texas Southwestern
Medical Center at Dallas Southwestern Medical
School

James L. Bockhorst, Saint Louis University School of
Medicine

James E. Bradner, University of Chicago Pritzker
School of Medicine

Michael J. Brenner, Northwestern University Medical
School

Derrick Brooks, Louisiana State University School of
Medicine in New Orleans

Christopher Brown, University of Kentucky College of
Medicine

Melissa E. Brunsvold, University of North Dakota
School of Medicine

Krisczar Bungay, State University of New York Health
Science Center at Brooklyn College of Medicine

Atul Butte, Brown University School of Medicine

Monique Carroll, Western University of Health
Science College of Osteopathic Medicine of the
Pacific

Kristen A. Carter, University of California, Los
Angeles, UCLA School of Medicine

Daniel H. Chang, Duke University School of Medicine

Joseph R. Check, New York Medical College

Tae Chong, University of Virginia School of Medicine

Alice W. Chuang, University of Tennessee, Memphis,
College of Medicine

Siren Chudgar, State University of New York Health
Science Center at Syracuse College of Medicine

D. Chris Chung, MCP-Hahnemann University School
of Medicine

Al Cohn, Medical University of South Carolina
College of Medicine

Michael DeMarco, University of Medicine and
Dentistry of New Jersey School of Osteopathic
Medicine

Kimberly DeVore, University of New England College
of Osteopathic Medicine

Armen Dikranian, University of Southern California
School of Medicine

Adam Dorfman, University of Michigan Medical
School

Marguerite Duane, State University of New York at
Stony Brook School of Medicine, Health Sciences
Center

Nick Dutcheson, Michigan State University College of
Human Medicine

Kristine Dziurzynski, University of South Alabama
College Of Medicine

Melissa Ehlert, Loyola University Chicago Stritch
School of Medicine

Larry K. Fan, University of California, San Francisco,
School of Medicine

Anne Forrest, Wayne State University School of
Medicine

Robert Galamaga, Lake Erie College of Osteopathic
Medicine

Dan Godbee, Mercer University School of Medicine

Mita Sanghavi Goel, University of Medicine and
Dentistry of New Jersey New Jersey Medical School

Ravi D. Goel, University of Medicine and Dentistry of
New Jersey Robert Wood Johnson Medical School

Robert Goodwin, Georgetown University School of
Medicine

Scott Gottlieb, Mount Sinai School of Medicine of the
City University of New York

Brian A. Greenlee, Marshall University School of
Medicine

John Hamilton, Kirksville College of Osteopathic
Medicine

Vikram Hatti, Meharry Medical College School of
Medicine

Joseph Herman, University of Maryland School of
Medicine

Mark Hiatt, Wake Forest University Bowman Gray
School of Medicine

Dan Higgins, Medical College of Wisconsin

Christopher J. Hoimes, New York Institute of
Technology New York College of Osteopathic
Medicine

Li-Yu Huang, Texas A&M University Health Science Center College of Medicine

Melissa Hurwitz, Tufts University School of Medicine

Faith Jackson, Harvard University Harvard Medical School

Wenny Jean, University of Missouri–Kansas City School of Medicine

Tinisha Jordan, Ohio University College of Osteopathic Medicine

Aparna Kambhampati, Baylor College of Medicine

Tory Katz, University of Colorado Health Sciences Center School of Medicine

Paymon Kayhani, University of New Mexico School of Medicine

Richard Kettelkamp, University of Osteopathic Medicine and Health Sciences College Of Osteopathic Medicine and Surgery

Mohammed Khan, University of Texas Health Sciences Center Medical School

Michael Kia, Touro University College of Osteopathic Medicine

Brian Kim, University of Kansas School of Medicine

James Kirkpatrick, Loma Linda University School of Medicine

Daniel Kovnat, Case Western Reserve University School of Medicine

Suzanne L'Ecuyer, University of Louisville School of Medicine

Elizabeth Leman, Wright State University School of Medicine

Daniel Lerer, Yeshiva University Albert Einstein College of Medicine

Eloisa Llata, Eastern Virginia Medical School

Jonathan Lu, Vanderbilt University School of Medicine

M. Albert Malvehy, University of Miami School of Medicine

James McCallum, University of South Carolina School of Medicine

Kristina M. McLean, University of South Florida College Of Medicine

Karen McNiece, University of Arkansas for Medical Sciences Medical School

Nicholas Mehta, Pennsylvania State University College of Medicine Milton S. Hershey Medical Center College of Medicine

Sejal Mehta, Thomas Jefferson University Jefferson Medical College

Anna Mendenhall, Ohio State University College of Medicine and Public Health

Eleanor R. Menzin, University of Pennsylvania School of Medicine

Jim Michelson, University of Utah School of Medicine

Sarah Minor, Oklahoma State University College of Osteopathic Medicine

Courtenay Moore, Albany Medical College

Sarah Nehls, University of Wisconsin–Madison Medical School

Ryan Nielsen, Creighton University School of Medicine

Jorge Nieva, University of California, Irvine, College of Medicine

Benjamin R. Nordstrom, Dartmouth College Dartmouth Medical School

Ivan Oransky, New York University School of Medicine

Osaguona Osa, Howard University College of Medicine

Sharvari Parghi, University of Missouri–Columbia School of Medicine

Rose Pham, University of Texas Health Science Center at San Antonio Medical School

Ernest Poortinga, Rush University Rush Medical College

Eric J. Poulsen and Gregory J. Poulsen, University of California, Davis, School of Medicine

David Priebe, University of Nebraska Medical Center College of Medicine

Melissa Reinhardt, University of Minnesota-Twin Cities Campus Medical School-Minneapolis

Suzanne Reuter, University of South Dakota School of Medicine

Francisco Rhein, Louisiana State University School of Medicine in Shreveport

Tim Rogers, University of Connecticut Health Center School of Medicine

Andrew Russman, Michigan State University College of Osteopathic Medicine

David Peter and Eric Russo, University of North Texas Health Science Center Texas College of Osteopathic Medicine

Barrett Ryan and Daphne Ryan, Midwestern University Chicago College of Osteopathic Medicine

David Ryan, Virginia Commonwealth Uiversity Medical College of Virginia School of Medicine

Darshak Sanghavi, Johns Hopkins University School of Medicine

Ankur Saraiya, Columbia University College of Physicians and Surgeons

Laura Sass, George Washington University School of Medicine and Health Sciences

Sean I. Savitz, Yeshiva University Albert Einstein College of Medicine

Kathy Schaeffer, Philadelphia College of Osteopathic Medicine

Susannah Schlichter, East Carolina University School of Medicine

Matt Schwartz, University of Nevada School of Medicine

J. Jewel Shim, Loma Linda University School of Medicine

Ryan Simovitch, Finch University of Health Sciences/ The Chicago Medical School

Justin Smith, Mayo Medical School

Cara Smith, University of Minnesota-Duluth School of Medicine

Eugene Soh, Uniformed Services University of the Health Science F. Edward Hébert School of Medicine

Merrill Sparago, University of Maryland School of Medicine

Judi Stanton, University of Florida College of Medicine

Elizabeth Steele, University of North Carolina at Chapel Hill School of Medicine

Scot Stewart, Medical College of Georgia School of Medicine

Asha Subramanian, Oregon Health Sciences University School of Medicine

Chris Suhar, Medical College of Ohio School of Medicine

Harsh Sulé, University of Illinois at Chicago College of Medicine

Antoinette Sweet, Morehouse School of Medicine

Erik Thingvoll, University of Rochester School of Medicine and Dentistry

Bertha Tsai, University of Arizona College of Medicine

Krista Burris, Tulane University School of Medicine

Ellen Turner, Texas Tech University health Sciences Center School of Medicine

Jay K. Varma, University of California, San Diego, School of Medicine

Deep K. Varma, University of Pittsburgh School of Medicine

Chris Vashi, Northeastern Ohio Universities College of Medicine

Kristofer Wagner, University of Oklahoma Health Sciences Center College of Medicine

Seth Walker, West Virginia University School of Medicine

John Watring, Pikeville College School of Osteopathic Medicine

Brook Watts, University of Alabama at Birmingham School of Medicine

Kathleen Weigle, Washington University in St. Louis School of Medicine

Deborah J. Wexler, Yale University School of Medicine

Audrey Young, University of Washington School of Medicine

INDEX OF
Schools by State